Twenty-Six Portland Place

The early years of the Royal Society of Tropical Medicine and Hygiene

Gordon C Cook

MD, DSc, FRCP, FRCPE, FRACP, FLS

Visiting Professor, University College London
President, Royal Society of Tropical Medicine & Hygiene, 1993–5

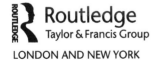

Routledge
Taylor & Francis Group

LONDON AND NEW YORK

First published 2011 by Radcliffe Publishing Ltd

Published 2018 by Routledge
2 Park Square, Milton Park, Abingdon, Oxon OX14 4RN
52 Vanderbilt Avenue, New York, NY 10017

First issued in paperback 2018

Routledge is an imprint of the Taylor & Francis Group, an informa business

British Library Cataloguing in Publication Data

A catalogue record for this book is available from the British Library.

Typeset by Phoenix Photosetting, Chatham, Kent
Cover designed by Meaden Creative

ISBN 13: 978-1-138-11764-8 (pbk)
ISBN 13: 978-1-84619-485-6 (hbk)

'Zonae Torridae Tutamen'*

*Guardian of the Torrid Zone

Contents

Preface

This book records the first fifty years of the *Society of Tropical Medicine and Hygiene* (STMH), founded in 1907 (over a century ago), which was to add *Royal* to its title in 1920. As a former president (1993–5), I have for long felt that a history of these years was much overdue, largely because this Society had such an enormous impact on the fledgling medical specialty in the early days of the twentieth century.[1]

The STMH was formed in order to provide a forum at the 'heart of Empire' for discussion and development of ideas and current research by physicians and *clinical* parasitologists into the 'exotic' diseases of warm climates, about which the average medical practitioner in London's 'medical quarter', and also a wider audience in Britain, knew little or in many cases nothing.[2]

Although its venue in the initial years of its existence was far from stable and to a large degree unsatisfactory, for some seventy years, from 1931, it operated from its own premises – 26 Portland Place – a *permanent* memorial to its first president, Sir Patrick Manson FRS (1844–1922), the 'father of modern tropical medicine'.

Twenty-six Portland Place in many ways became in the minds of countless Fellows of the Society, throughout the world, synonymous with the organisation itself, and following the unfortunate sale of this property in 2004, the focal point of the Society's various activities over these years was lost forever.

It is perhaps worthy of note that George Bernard Shaw's (1856–1950) well-known polemic on the contemporary medical establishment – *The Doctor's Dilemma* – was written in 1903, *ie* a mere four years prior to the foundation of the STMH; furthermore, the action of the play is set in nearby Queen Anne Street, the location of Manson's London residence.[3]

I have quoted liberally from the Society's minute books (most written in longhand) – both those of *Council* and *Ordinary* meetings. My editing has been minimal, alterations being aimed solely at easier reading. Although I have referred at times to the Annual Reports, these have had a far lesser part to play in the genesis of this story. The presidential addresses (which I have both edited and shortened – the originals being reproduced in entirety in *Transactions*) over these fifty years form a close reflection of the formative years of the *new* discipline. Where I have used the abbreviation *CM*, reference to *Council* minutes is indicated.

I am extremely grateful to Caryl Guest, for some twenty years the Society's Administrator, for much invaluable assistance with the archival material, and to Maureen Moran for typing the entire book from my longhand manuscript.

G C Cook
St Albans, June 2010

References and notes

1. F M Sandwith, W C Brown. *The Society of Tropical Medicine and Hygiene: first annual report of the Council*. 1908.
2. G C Low. The history of the foundation of the Society of Tropical Medicine and Hygiene. *Trans R Soc trop Med Hyg* 1928; 22: 197–202; G C Cook. Presidential address – Evolution: the art of survival. *Trans R Soc trop Med Hyg* 1994; 88: 4–18; G C Cook. *Tropical Medicine: an illustrated history of the pioneers*. London: Academic Press 2007: 118–25, 136–41.
3. S Weintraub. Shaw, George Bernard (1856–1950). In: H C G Matthew, B Harrison (eds). *Oxford Dictionary of National Biography*. Oxford: Oxford University Press 2004; 50: 83–97; B Shaw. *The Doctor's Dilemma*. London: Penguin Books 1957: 188.

Prologue

Tropical medicine contains two separate but closely related components; although linked, for practical purposes they can be considered separately.[1]

The first is 'medicine in the tropics'. This has been practised in some form or other since the origin of *Homo sapiens*, and will continue until that species ceases to inhabit the earth; in its early days, the practice of medicine in tropical countries was of course primitive in the extreme. This entity is not primarily dependent on ambient temperature *per se* but on the prevailing absence of health infra-structure and, more importantly, poverty; in fact the disease spectrum is very similar to that which existed in England (and indeed the whole of northern Europe) in the nineteenth century. And that includes *malaria*, 'ague' being a major cause of morbidity in mid-nineteenth century England.[2] Of course the spectrum of disease is constantly changing – one significant development relatively recently being the emergence of HIV/AIDS, which is currently affecting both tropical and non-tropical populations alike.[3]

The second component is the formal discipline of *tropical* (or *colonial*) *medicine*, which according to G C Low (president from 1929 to 1933) grew up in a twenty-year period – 1894–1914 – for political reasons in those countries which possessed colonies or territories in warm climates.[4] There are a number of reasons for its development at this time – and these have been reviewed.[5] Joseph Chamberlain (1836–1914)[6], British Secretary of State for the Colonies from 1895 until 1903, considered this to be an essential component of 'constructive imperialism', the *raison d'être* of which was to prevent or cure disease in those servants of Empire and Raj living in a country situated in the tropics – the most notorious location of severe morbidity and mortality being West Africa. Chamberlain exploited the newly developing discipline, headed by Patrick Manson (1844–1922)[7] primarily for *political* purposes. In order to establish a focal point for the *new* discipline, a group of individuals (almost all, *clinically* qualified) established in the capital city of the British Empire, London, a Society where the pioneers of this new pursuit could meet to discuss recent developments.

Some writers have dated the *origin* of *tropical* (or *colonial*) medicine to Manson's demonstration that a vector (the mosquito) played a significant role in transmission of a human disease, *ie* demonstration of the man-mosquito transmission of lymphatic filariasis, in 1877.[8] The early decades of the twentieth century were therefore extremely exciting ones for proponents of this newly founded discipline.

It was upon this broad canvas therefore that the *Society of Tropical Medicine and Hygiene* emerged a little more than a century ago.

References and Notes

1   G C Cook. *Tropical Medicine: an illustrated history of the Pioneers*. London: Academic Press 2007: 278; G C Cook, A I Zumla (eds). *Manson's tropical diseases* 22nd ed. London: Saunders 2009: 1830.

2   G C Cook. *From the Greenwich Hulks to Old St Pancras: a history of tropical disease in London*. London: Athlone Press 1992: 338; G C Cook. *Health-care for all: history of a 'third-world' dilemma*. St Albans: Tropzam 2009: 226.

3   *Op cit*. See note 1 above.

4   G C Low. A retrospect of tropical medicine from 1894 to 1914. *Trans R Soc trop Med Hyg* 1929; 23: 213–32.

5   *Op cit. See* note 1 above (Cook: 33–50).

6   P T Marsh. Chamberlain, Joseph (Joe) (1836–1914). In H C G Matthew, B Harrison (eds). *Oxford Dictionary of National Biography*. Oxford: Oxford University Press 2004; 10: 923–34. [*See also: Op cit.* Note 1 above (Cook, 2007: 251–4)].

7   P H Manson-Bahr, A Alcock. *The life and work of Sir Patrick Manson*. London: Cassell and Co Ltd 1927: 273; J W W Stephens, M P Sutphen. Manson, Sir Patrick (1844–1922). In: H C G Matthew, B Harrison (eds). *Oxford Dictionary of National Biography*. Oxford: Oxford University Press 2004: 36: 553–5.

8   P Manson. Further observations on *Filaria sanguinis hominis*. *Med Rep Imperial Maritime Customs China* Special Series no 2 (14th issue) 1877: 1–26. [*See also*: P Manson. *Tropical Diseases: a manual of the diseases of warm climates*. London: Cassell and Co Ltd 1898: 607].

Chapter 1

Foundation of the Society

The Society was conceived in December 1906, when James Cantlie FRCS (1851–1926)[1] remarked to Dr George Carmichael Low MRCP (1872–1952)[2] (*see* Chapter 8), after they had met for a joint consultation on a patient, 'What do you think of a *Society of Tropical Medicine and Hygiene*?'. Low replied that he considered the idea excellent, and they agreed to take soundings from others with an interest in *tropical medicine*. Both Cantlie and Low were subsequently to become presidents. Low approached: Sir Patrick Manson (1844–1922)[3], Dr F M Sandwith (1853–1918)[4], Dr C W Daniels (1862–1927)[5] and others. Cantlie subsequently wrote, or spoke to, the Director-General of the Army and the Navy – Lt Gen Sir Alfred Keogh (1857–1936)[6] (*see* below), Professor W J R Simpson (1855–1931)[7], Dr W Carnegie Brown (1859–1913)[8], Dr C F Harford (1865–1905)[9], Dr William Hartigan (?–1936)[10] and 'one or two more'. Reactions were mixed: Manson himself was apparently 'at first a little doubtful about the idea, thinking that the time was not yet ripe'; he had also heard that the Royal Army Medical Corps (RAMC) were considering starting a comparable organisation; Fleming Sandwith was, however, keen on the project, while Charles Daniels was somewhat guarded.

Cantlie and Low, however, decided upon a meeting, which was arranged for **4 January 1907** at the Conference Hall of the Colonial Office (*see* Figure 1.1); the Society's first Minute Book records (*see* Figure 1.2):

> … Sir Patrick Manson was voted to the chair [at that meeting].
>
> Mr Cantlie explained the steps he had taken, [as early as] 1899, to form a Society of Tropical Medicine, and the correspondence he had with the Royal Medico Chirurgical Society upon the subject, as well as more recently with the Colonial Institute, the Epidemiological Society, the Polyclinic, the Royal Institute of Public Health, the Director-General of the Army Medical Department and with those interested in the amalgamation of the Medical Societies of London.

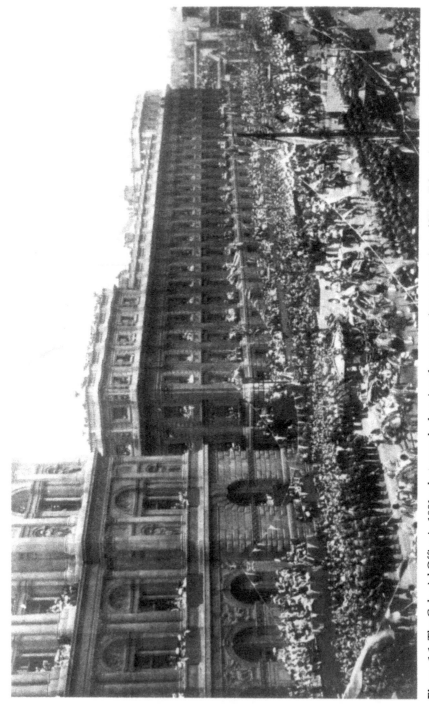

Figure 1.1: The Colonial Office in 1901: photograph showing the coronation procession of King Edward VII (courtesy: The National Archives, Kew – reproduced with permission).

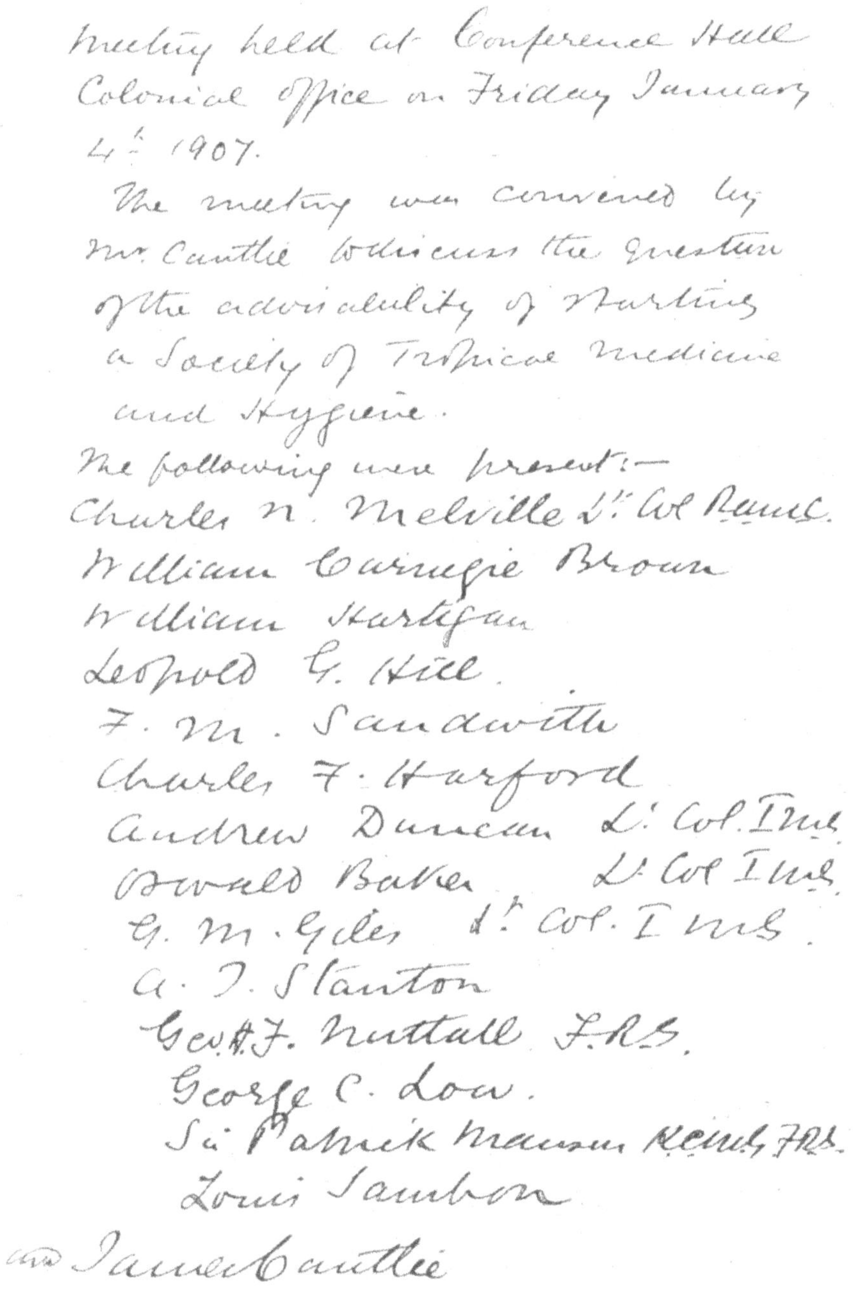

Meeting held at Conference Hall
Colonial Office on Friday January
4th 1907.
The meeting was convened by
Mr. Cantlie to discuss the question
of the advisability of starting
a Society of Tropical Medicine
and Hygiene.
The following were present:—
Charles H. Melville Lt. Col R.A.M.C.
William Carnegie Brown
William Hartigan
Leopold G. Hill.
F. M. Sandwith
Charles F. Harford
Andrew Duncan Lt. Col. I.M.S.
Donald Baker Lt Col I.M.S.
G. M. Giles Lt. Col. I.M.S.
A. T. Stanton
Geo. H. F. Nuttall F.R.S.
George C. Low.
Sir Patrick Manson K.C.M.G. F.R.S.
Louis Sambon
and James Cantlie

Figure 1.2: Beginning of the meeting at the Colonial Office held on **4 January 1907** (extract from the first minute book of the Society).

After most of those present had expressed their opinions on the subject, Professor Nuttall [1862–1937][11] proposed and Dr. Fleming M Sandwith [*see above*] seconded, and it was unanimously decided to form a Society of Tropical Medicine and Hygiene [STMH]. A Sub-Committee [was appointed] consisting of:

Sir Patrick Manson, Colonel [C H] Melville[12], Dr Sandwith, Dr [W] Carnegie Brown, Representative from Liverpool, Mr James Cantlie [with] Dr Geo. C Low as Secretary to the Sub-Committee.

The meeting then adjourned.

Patrick Manson
10th May 1907

Thus plans to form the Society were well underway and the sub-committee was destined to meet at Cantlie's house – 140 Harley Street (*see* Figure 1.3) – on four occasions during January. At the first meeting, *'The Society of Tropical Medicine and Hygiene'* was suggested as a suitable title; the constitution and laws were framed and discussed, and referred to the next meeting:

11 January
... The following [were] present: Sir Patrick Manson, Col Melville, Dr Sandwith, Dr Carnegie Brown, Mr Cantlie, and Dr Low. Sir Patrick Manson read two letters from Director-General Keogh [*see above*], the general content of which was that the RAMC [Royal Army Medical Corps] was starting an Institute which would embrace *Tropical Medicine* amongst its subjects. After discussion it was agreed that Col Melville should [discuss] the subject ... with Director-General Keogh to see if the proposed *new* Society could amalgamate with his in some way or other. Mr Cantlie then brought forward a series of suggested rules he had drawn up [*see* Appendix I], and after [discussion] they were finally adopted.

16 January
The following members [were] present: Mr Cantlie, Dr [W] Carnegie Brown, Dr Sandwith and Dr Low.

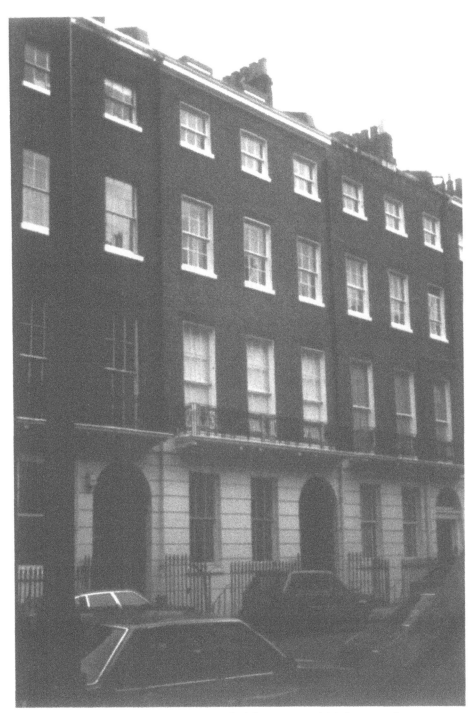

Figure 1.3: 140 Harley Street – James Cantlie's house – in which four meetings were held in January, 1907.

23 January
Present [were]: Col Melville, Dr Sandwith, Dr Brown, Mr Cantlie, Sir Patrick Manson, [and] Dr Low.

30 January
Present [were]: Sir Patrick Manson, Mr Cantlie, Dr Brown, Col Melville, Dr Sandwith and Dr Low.

The first General meeting

Minutes of [a General] meeting held at the Royal College of Physicians London [*see* Figure 1.4] on **15 March 1907**:

Present [were]: Dr William Hartigan, Dr Henry D McCulloch, Fleet Surgeon P W Bassett Smith RN[13], Dr J M H Macleod, Dr W Carnegie Brown, Professor W M Haffkine[14], Dr John Anderson CIE, Dr R N Moffat, Dr Andrew Duncan, Dr F P Beddoes[15], Dr Francis Fremantle, Dr Charles F Harford, Dr Leopold George Hill, Dr A T Stanton, Professor R Smith, Dr F M Sandwith, Mr James Cantlie, Jhn A Moore Lt Col, IMS.

Dr F M Sandwith was voted to the chair.

... The subcommittee appointed to draw up [the] constitution & rules of the Society submitted their proposals. Some alterations were suggested & the subcommittee were instructed to draft the rules in accordance with the generally expressed opinion & to have the alterations suggested printed and submitted to the next meeting.

Proposed by Dr Hartigan & seconded by Fleet Surgeon [PW] Bassett Smith [1861–1927] that the laws as prepared by the subcommittee be approved with the exception of several [which were] referred back. The rules referred for further consideration related to the methods of election of the President & Vice-President, & to the number of members of Council.

Patrick Manson
14th May 1907

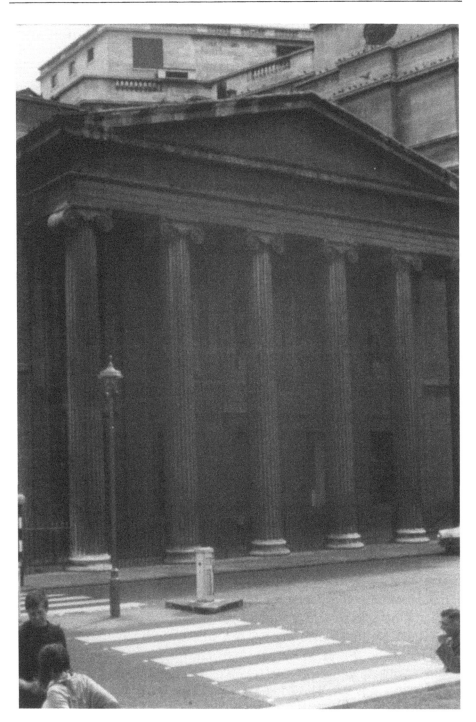

Figure 1.4: The Royal College of Physicians (RCP), Pall Mall: venue for the *general* meeting on **15 March 1907**.

The Society's first full meeting

In its issues for 27 April and 4 May, *The Lancet* carried the following notice:

> *Society of Tropical Medicine and Hygiene* – A meeting of the Society will be held at 5.30 pm on Friday **May 10th 1907**, at the rooms of the Royal Medico-Chirurgical Society [RMCS], 20 Hanover Square, London W [*see* Figure 1.5] to receive the report of the Sub-Committee appointed to draw up the rules and constitution [*see* above], to elect members of *Council*, and to appoint the officers of the Society.

At this meeting the following were present:

> Sir Patrick Manson, Mr Cantlie, Dr Sandwith, Dr Hartigan, Fleet-Surgeon Bassett-Smith, Dr T S Kerr[16], Dr G C Low, Dr Harford, Mr W M Haffkine, Mr T P Beddoes and Dr Carnegie Brown.
>
> It was proposed by Mr Cantlie and seconded by Dr Sandwith that Sir Patrick Manson take the Chair.
>
> Sir Patrick Manson having taken the Chair, Dr Sandwith read the notice, published in the medical papers, calling the meeting [*see above*] …
>
> Laws IV, V, and VI were passed as amended.
>
> Law VII was amended by adding after 'Representatives' the words 'of the Biological Sciences', after 'Services' the word 'and', and by striking out the last two words 'Biological Science', the Law being thereafter passed as amended.
>
> Law VIII was passed as amended.
>
> Law XXXVII was amended by leaving out all the words after 'September' and substituting 'at 8.30 pm, or on such other day, and at such hour as the *Council* may direct', the Law being thereafter passed as amended.
>
> Law XIII was passed as amended.
>
> [The amended Laws are set out in Appendix I; they were published by the STMH in late 1907 and printed by John Bale, Sons & Danielsson of 83–91 Great Titchfield Street, Oxford Street, London W]. The Chairman said that these Laws having been amended in accordance with the recommendations of the previous meeting and of the *Council*, and duly passed, the

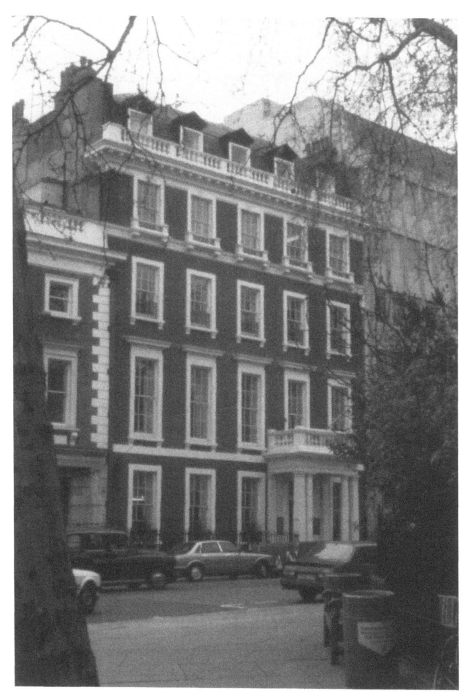

Figure 1.5: 20 Hanover Square: the 'home' of the Royal Medico-Chirurgical Society (RMCS), which became the Royal Society of Medicine in 1907, and moved to 1 Wimpole Street in 1912. This was the venue for the first *ordinary* meeting.

Constitution of the Society was now complete, and he declared the Society duly constituted.

The meeting proceeded to the Election of Officers. On the motion of Fleet-Surgeon P W Bassett-Smith RN, seconded by Dr Carnegie Brown, Sir Patrick Manson was unanimously elected first President of the Society. On the motion of Sir Patrick Manson, seconded by Dr Sandwith, Professor Ronald Ross [1857–1932][17] was elected first Vice-President.

The following members of *Council* were then elected:

> Ernest E Austen FZS, Fleet-Surgeon Bassett Smith RN, W Carnegie Brown MD, James Cantlie FRCS, C W Daniels MB, Lt-Col G M Giles IMS FRCS, W M Haffkine CIE, C F Harford MD, W Hartigan MD, T S Kerr MB, G C Low MB, Professor E A Minchin FZS, Lt-Col C H Melville RAMC, Professor G H F Nuttall MD FRS, L W Sambon MD, F M Sandwith MD FRCP, Arthur Everett Shipley MA FRS[18], J W W Stephens MD [and] Fredk. V Theobald MA.
>
> Dr W Hartigan MD (of 5 Bond Court, Walbrook, London EC) was elected Treasurer and Drs F M Sandwith FRCP (of 31 Cavendish Square, London W) and W Carnegie Brown MRCP (of 32 Harley Street, London W) Secretaries of the Society until the first meeting of *Council*. It was resolved that the first [*ordinary*] meeting of the Society be held at 20 Hanover Square (*see above*) on a date to be fixed by *Council*.

The Society had thus been established and the first Minute Book continues with the:

> Minutes of [the first] meeting of *Council* held at 31 Cavendish Square London W [*see* Figure 1.6] on Wednesday **22 May 1907** at 5.30 pm.
>
> Present [were] Sir Patrick Manson, Lt Col Melville, Drs Sandwith, Hartigan, Kerr, Carnegie Brown, and Mr Austen.
>
> Dr Hartigan, who had been temporarily elected treasurer at the [10 May] meeting, was unanimously elected Treasurer of the Society.
>
> Drs Sandwith and Carnegie Brown who had been temporarily elected Secretaries at the same meeting were unanimously elected Secretaries of the Society.

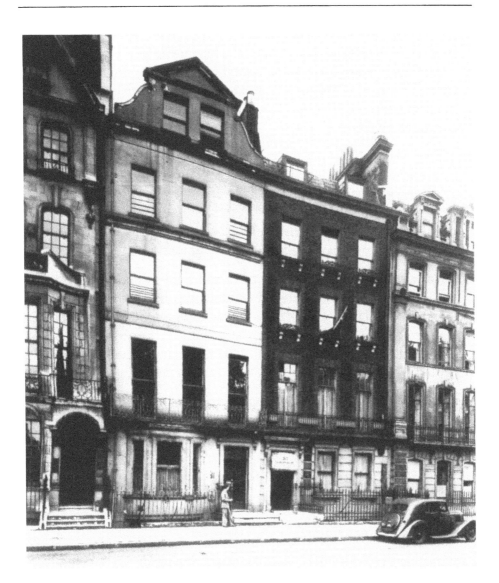

Figure 1.6: 31 Cavendish Square – the house belonging to Dr F M Sandwith, and venue for the first meeting of the newly elected *Council* on **22 May 1907**. This house (second from left) was demolished in a redevelopment plan in the late 1950s (courtesy: London Metropolitan Archives – reproduced with permission).

Dr Carnegie Brown reported that he had been in communication with the [RMCS regarding] permanent quarters for the Society at 20 Hanover Square; he 'brought up' a letter from the Secretary of that Society, dated May 18th 1907, in which accommodation was offered at an inclusive rental of forty guineas per annum.

Dr Carnegie Brown was instructed to reply that the Society agreed to accept the terms of the [RMCS], the tenancy to be a yearly one.

Dr Carnegie Brown was instructed to draft an announcement of the formation of the Society, and to forward it, with a list of the members of *Council*, to the following papers, for publication (if approved by them)

> *The Lancet*
> *The British Medical Journal*
> *The Journal of Tropical Medicine*
> *The RAMC Journal*
> *The Indian Medical Gazette* [and]
> *The Annals of Tropical Medicine*

It was resolved, on the proposal of Dr Sandwith, seconded by Sir Patrick Manson, that a letter of condolence on the death of Sir Joseph Fayrer [1824–1907][19] [*see* Figure 1.7] be sent on behalf of the Society to Lady Fayrer.

The following [21] applicants [all medical graduates] were elected Fellows under Law IV:- [They included:

> 34   J H Christopherson MD Khartoum
> 37   Aldo Castellani MD, Colombo, Ceylon
> 39   Col W B Leishman RAMC Junior United Services Club SW].

Patrick Manson
26th June 1907

The Society's Minutes continued with those of:

> a meeting of *Council* held at 20 Hanover Square on Wednesday **26 June 1907** at 6pm.
>
> Present [were] Sir Patrick Manson, Professor R Ross, Drs Sandwith, Carnegie Brown, Hartigan, Kerr, Low, Fleet Surgeon Bassett Smith, Professor Minchin, and Messrs Austen, Haffkine and Shipley. …
>
> Dr Sandwith stated that as instructed by the *Council* he had written a letter of condolence to Lady Fayrer [*see above*], and read the reply which he had received from the family of the late Sir Joseph Fayrer.
>
> The following candidates were elected Fellows of the Society under Rule IV [the names of 42 candidates are recorded, including:

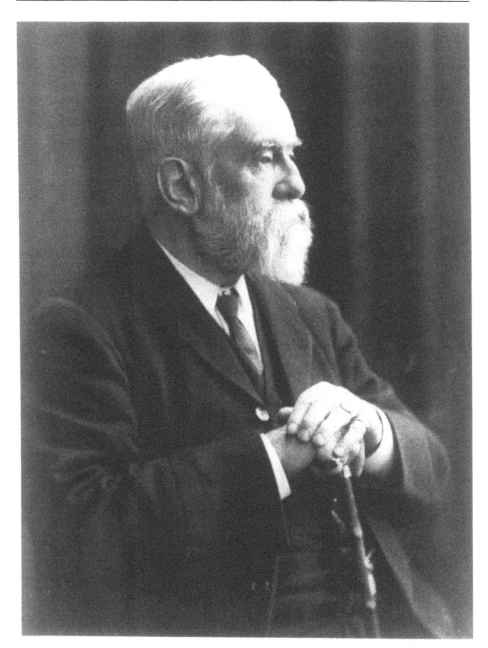

Figure 1.7: Sir Joseph Fayrer (1824–1907) (reproduced courtesy the Wellcome Library, London).

48   W J Prout MB CMG, 17 Canning St. Liverpool
50   Charles Begg MD Ed, 62 Pulteney St Bath
53   Miss Grace Mackinnon LRCP, 51 Bukenhall Mansions

> 60   Hugh Basil G Newham
> 62   St George Gray MB, Sierra Leone
> 66   John Anderson CIE MD FRCP, 9 Harley Street, W
> 73   Andrew Balfour MD MRCP (Ed) Court Lodge, Deal, Kent
> 75   Professor Osler MD FRS, 13 Norham Gardens, Oxford
> 76   Andrew Davidson MD, 19 Erith Road, Belvedere, Kent.

The following [distinguished gentlemen] were elected [original] *Honorary* Fellows:

> Professor Robert Koch MD Kurfurstendamm [sic] 25, Berlin
> Professor Dr Paul Ehrlich, Direktor Konigl. Instit. Exp.
> Therapie Frankfurt a/m
> Professor A Laveran, Membre de l'Académie de Medicine, Paris
> Professor Raphael Blanchard, Membre de l'Académie de Medicine, Paris
> Lt Col W C Gorgas, USA Chief Sanitary Officer, Panama
> Dr Theobald Smith, Prof of Comp. Pathology, Harvard Univ.
> Prof Camillo Golgi, University of Pavia
> Professor Ettore Marchiafava, University of Rome
> Prof. Vasili F Danilewski, University of Kharkov
> Catherdratico Carlos Findlay, Universidad de la Habana, Cuba
> Jonathan Hutchinson, MD FRCS FRS, 15 Cavendish Sq.
> Prof Shilamiro Kitasato, University of Tokio, Japan, [and]
> Dr K Shiga, Tokio (Director of the Institute of Infectious Diseases).

Professor Ross suggested that the days of the *Ordinary* meetings should be changed to Fridays, as being most convenient to provincial Fellows. The Secretaries were instructed to inquire what arrangements could be made to carry this proposal into effect.

Patrick Manson
Chairman
14th July 1907[20]

Following this, the first *ordinary* meeting was held at 8.30pm (*see* Chapter 2).

References and Notes

1   Anonymous. The late Sir James Cantlie (obituary). *Times, Lond* 1926, 31 May; Anonymous. Sir James Cantlie (obituary). *Lancet* 1926 i: 1121–2; Anonymous. Sir James Cantlie (obituary). *Br Med J* 1926 i: 1971–2; Anonymous. Cantlie, Sir James (1861–1926). *Plarr's Lives: London: Royal College of Surgeons of England* 1930 l: 192–3; N Cantlie, G Seaver. *Sir James Cantlie: a romance in medicine.* London: John Murray 1939; 279; P Manson-Bahr. Sir James Cantlie KBE, FRCS (1851–1926). In: *History of the School of Tropical Medicine in London (1899–1949).* London; H K Lewis 1956: 129–32; J C Stewart. *The Quality of Mercy: the lives of Sir James and Lady Cantlie.* London; George Allen and Unwin 1983: 277; M Harrison. Cantlie, Sir James (1851–1926). In: H C G Matthew, B Harrison (eds). *Oxford Dictionary of National Biography.* Oxford: Oxford University Press 2004; 9: 962–4.

2   Anonymous. G Carmichael Low (obituary). *Times, Lond* 1952, 1 August: 8; Anonymous. George Carmichael Low (obituary). *Lancet* 1952 ii: 296–7; Anonymous. George Carmichael Low (obituary). *Br Med J* 1952 ii: 341–2; N H Fairley (obituary). George Carmichael Low. *Trans R Soc trop Med Hyg* 1952; 46: 571–3; Anonymous. Low, George Carmichael. *Munk's Roll.* London: Royal College of Physicians 4: 594–5; G C Cook. George Carmichael Low FRCP: twelfth president of the Society and underrated pioneer of tropical medicine. *Trans R Soc trop Med Hyg* 1993 87: 355–60; G C Cook. George Carmichael Low FRCP: an underrated figure in British tropical medicine. *J R Coll Phys Lond* 1993 27: 81–2; M Worboys. Low, George Carmichael (1872–1952). In: *Oxford Dictionary of National Biography.* Oxford: Oxford University Press 2004; 34: 550–1. G C Cook. *Caribbean Diseases: Dr George Low's expedition in 1901–02.* Oxford: Radcliffe Publishing 2009: 229.

3   Anonymous. Sir Patrick Manson (obituary). *Br Med J* 1922 i: 623–6, 702–3; A Alcock. Patrick Manson, 1844–1922 (obituary). *Trans R Soc trop Med Hyg* 1922 16: 1–15; H B Guppy. A reminiscence of Sir Patrick Manson at Amoy. *Trans R Soc trop Med Hyg* 1925 18: 285–6; P H Manson-Bahr, A Alcock. *The Life and Work of Sir Patrick Manson.* London: Cassell and Co Ltd 1927: 273; R Ross. *Memories of Sir Patrick Manson.* London 1930: 26; P H Manson-Bahr. British Masters of Medicine: Patrick Manson (1844–1922). *Med Press Circ* 1935, 6 February: 120–4; Anonymous. Manson centenary: 'Father of Tropical Medicine'. *Times, Lond* 1944 15 December; H H Scott. *A History of Tropical Medicine* London; Edward Arnold 1939: 1068–76; P Manson-Bahr. The Manson saga, 3 October 1844 – 9 April 1922. *Trans R Soc trop Med Hyg* 1945 38: 401–17; Anonymous. Manson of Tropical Medicine. *Lancet* 1945, 6 January; *Ibid. Indian Med Gazz* 1945, August; P Manson-Bahr. *History of the School of Tropical Medicine in London (1899–1949).* London: H K Lewis 1956: 113–25; P Manson-Bahr. *Patrick Manson: The Father of Tropical Medicine.* London 1962: Thomas Nelson and Sons Ltd: 192; G C Cook. Emergence of Dr Patrick Manson on the London medical scene. In: *From the Greenwich Hulks to Old St Pancras: a history of tropical disease in London.* London: Athlone Press 1992:

68–79; J W W Stephens, M P Sutphen. Manson, Sir Patrick (1844–1922). In: H C G Matthew, B Harrison (eds). *Oxford Dictionary of National Biography*. Oxford: Oxford University Press 2004; 36: 553–5.

4   P Manson-Bahr. Dr Fleming Mant Sandwith. In: *History of the School of Tropical Medicine in London (1899–1949)*. London: H K Lewis 1956: 145–6; Anonymous. Sandwith, Fleming Mant. *Who Was Who, 1916–1928* 5th ed. London: A & C Black 1992: 722.

5   P Manson-Bahr. Dr Charles Wilberforce Daniels, In: *History of the School of Tropical Medicine in London (1899–1949):* London: H K Lewis 1956: 162–5; Anonymous. Daniels, Charles Wilberforce. *Who Was Who, 1916–1928* 5th ed. London: A & C Black 1992: 202; G C Cook. Charles Wilberforce Daniels (1862–1927): underrated pioneer of tropical medicine. *Acta Trop* 2002; 81: 237–50.

6   Anonymous. Keogh, Lieut-Gen Sir Alfred. *Who Was Who, 1929–1940* 2nd ed. London: A & C Black 1967: 747–8.

7   Anonymous. Simpson, Sir William John Ritchie. *Who Was Who, 1929–1940*. 2nd ed. London: A & C Black 1967: 1240.

8   **William Carnegie Brown** (1859–1913) received his education at Aberdeen, King's College London and St Thomas's Hospital, and qualified in 1880. After service as a ship's surgeon, he served in the Middle and Far-East. Returning to England in 1904, he entered private practice. He wrote books on sprue and amoebiasis. Anonymous. W Carnegie Brown. *Br med J* 1913; ii: 969. [*See also:* Anonymous. William Carnegie Brown. *Trans Soc trop Med Hyg* 1913–14; 7: 57–8].

9   **Charles Harford** was the Principal of Livingstone College at Leyton (where Manson gave some of his early lectures in London). He was the youngest son of Canon Harford-Battersby but by the time he became a Secretary of the STMH he had dropped the 'Battersby'! He had been a medical missionary in Nigeria, serving with the Church Missionary Society. G B Price. Charles Forbes Harford. *Trans R Soc trop Med Hyg* 1925; 19: 98–9;. Anonymous. Charles Forbes Harford. *Lancet* 1925; ii: 93; *Who Was Who, 1916–1928* 5th ed London: A & C Black 1992: 358. [*See also*: M Davies. *It's only me: Mary Kingsley and health in the tropics*. Hawkshurst, Kent: Wealden Advertiser Ltd 2005: 80].

10 **William Hartigan** (? – 1936). Qualifying in Dublin in 1876, he later served in Hong Kong where he was undoubtedly known to Manson. Hartigan was subsequently Treasurer (1907–9), Councillor (1907–21) and Trustee (1921–36) of the Society. *See*: Anonymous. *Trans R Soc trop Med Hyg* 1936–7; 30: 274; *Medical Directory*. J & A Churchill 1908: 171; 1937: 138.

11 Anonymous. Nuttall, George Henry Falkiner. *Who Was Who, 1929–1940* 2nd ed. London: A & C Black 1967: 1013; G S Graham-Smith, M E Gibson. Nuttall, George Henry Falkiner (1862–1937). In: H C G Matthew, B Harrison (eds). *Oxford Dictionary of National Biography*. Oxford: Oxford University Press 2004: 41: 294–5.

12 Anonymous. Melville, Chas Henderson. *Medical Directory 1915.* J & A Churchill 1915: 1628.

13   Anonymous. Bassett-Smith, Surgeon-Rear-Admiral Sir Percy William. *Who Was Who, 1916–1928* 5th ed. London: A & C Black 1992: 49–50.

14   Anonymous. Waldemar Haffkine, CIE (obituary). *Lancet* 1930: ii: 995–6.

15   Anonymous. Beddoes, Thomas Pugh. *Medical Directory 1910.* London: J & A Churchill 1910: 78. [*See also*: Anonymous. Beddoes, Thomas Pugh (1861–1930) *Plarr's Lives 1930–1951*: 67–8].

16   Anonymous. Kerr, Thomas S. *Medical Directory 1910.* London: J & A Churchill 1910: 214.

17   R Ross. *Memoirs, with a Full Account of the Great Malaria Problem and its Solution.* London: John Murray 1923: 547; R L Mégroz. *Ronald Ross: discoverer and creator.* London; George Allen & Unwin Ltd 1931: 282; Anonymous. Sir Ronald Ross: the conquest of malaria (obituary). *Times, Lond* 1932, 17 September; Anonymous. Ronald Ross 1857–1932. His life and work. *Lancet* 1932, ii: 695–7; Anonymous. Sir Ronald Ross KCB, KCMG, MD, LID, DSc, FRS (obituary). *Br Med J* 1932 ii: 609–11; G H F Nuttall. Sir Ronald Ross (1857–1932). In: *Obituary Notices of Fellows of the Royal Society.* London; Harrison and Sons 1933: 108–15; C M Wenyon. Colonel Sir Ronald Ross, KCB, KCMG, MD DSc, LID, FRCS, FRS, IMS (retd) 1857–1932 (obituary). *Trans R Soc trop Med* 1933; 26: 473–8; J O Dobson. *Ronald Ross Dragon Slayer: a short account of a great discovery and of the man who made it.* London; Student Christian Movement Press 1934: 162; H H Scott. Ronald Ross (1857–1932). In: *A History of Tropical Medicine.* London; Edward Arnold 1939: 1086–90; E F Dodd. *The Story of Sir Ronald Ross and his Fight against Malaria.* London; MacMillan & Co Ltd 1956: 81. J Rowland. *The Mosquito Man: the story of Ronald Ross.* London; Lutterworth Press 1958: 150; J Kamm. *Malaria Ross.* London; Methuen & Co Ltd 1963: 181; R Ross. *The Great Malaria Problem and its Solution: from the memoirs of Ronald Ross.* London; Keynes Press 1988: 236; G C Cook. Ronald Ross (1857–1932): 100 years since the demonstration of mosquito transmission of *Plasmodium spp.* – on 20 August 1897. Trans R Soc trop Med Hyg 1997, 92: 487–8; E R Nye, M E Gibson. *Ronald Ross, Malariologist and Polymath: a biography.* London; MacMillan Press Ltd 1997: 316; W F Bynum, C Overy (eds). *The Beast in the Mosquito: the correspondence of Ronald Ross and Patrick Manson.* Amsterdam; Rodopi B 1998: 528; W F Bynum. Ross, Sir Ronald (1857–1932). In: H C G Matthew, B Harrison (eds). *Oxford Dictionary of National Biography.* Oxford: Oxford University Press 2004; 47: 842–6. [*See also*: N Hawkes. DNA scientists join war against malaria. *Times, Lond* 1997 13 August: 7].

18   [S F H]. Sir Arthur Everett Shipley, 1861–1927. *Proc Roy Soc B* 1928; 103: i–viii.

19   **Joseph Fayrer** was the doyen of the Indian Medical Service (IMS). Fayrer, Sir Joseph, 1st Bt. *Who Was Who, 1897–1916* 5th ed. London: A & C Black 1966: 239–40.

20   Minute Book 1 [*see*: Appendix III]: Society of Tropical Medicine and Hygiene 1907–1920; The Society of Tropical Medicine and Hygiene: first report of … Council 1908; G C Low. The history of the foundation of the Society of Tropical Medicine and Hygiene. *Trans R Soc trop Med Hyg* 1928; 22: 197–202.

Chapter 2

The Society established and Manson's presidency – 1907–9

The first *Ordinary* meeting of the Society was held at 20 Hanover Square (the venue for all meetings until October 1908 – *see* Chapter 1), at 8.30pm on Wednesday **26 June 1907**.

> Present [were]: Sir Patrick Manson [*see* Figure 2.1] President, Professor R Ross Vice-president, the Treasurer, Secretaries, 32 Fellows and 33 Visitors …
>
> The President, Sir Patrick Manson, delivered his inaugural address [see below] to the [newly formed] Society.
>
> Dr C W Daniels [*see* Chapter 1], Superintendent [of the] London School of Tropical Medicine, gave an Epidiascope Demonstration of objects of interest in *Tropical Medicine*.
>
> The President [then] proposed a vote of thanks to Dr Daniels for his demonstration, which was carried unanimously.
>
> Mr [A E] Shipley [*see* Chapter 1] proposed, and Professor Ross seconded a vote of thanks to the President, which was carried unanimously.
>
> The meeting closed at 10.10pm.
>
> Patrick Manson
President
10th July 1907.

Figure 2.2 indicates the attendance at that meeting.

Manson's inaugural Address to the newly formed Society

Manson was the first of 23 presidents during the first fifty years of the Society (*see* Appendix II). He seems to have been far too busy to prepare

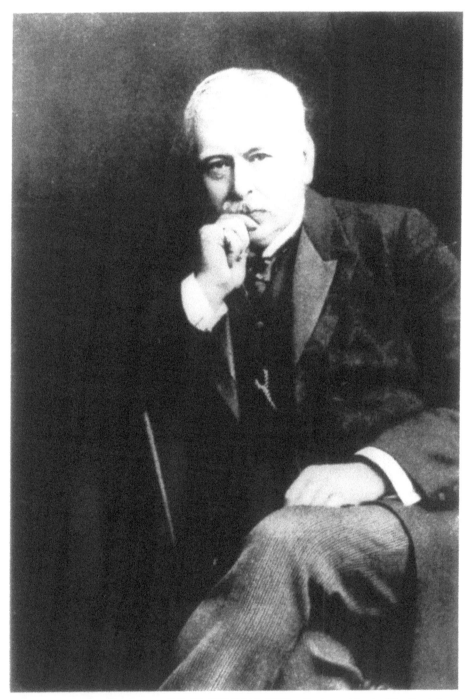

Figure 2.1: Sir Patrick Manson GCMG, FRS (1844–1922) – first president of the Society (RSTMH archive).

his Address properly, and concentrated on summarising modifications which rapid emergence of the *new* discipline[1] had exerted to the standard medical texts of the day:

> I trust that it does not augur badly for the success of the [STMH] that its first President has to commence his Inaugural Address with an apology. Such, unfortunately, is the case. I intended to devote some time to preparation, but have been called on unexpectedly to take part in the recent International Conference on *Sleeping Sickness* [author's italics], I have been so occupied that I have not been able to find adequate time or to give that care to preparation that the importance of this occasion demands. I apologise in advance, and trust you will be indulgent to my shortcomings.
>
> [He continued] I wish to express my appreciation of the compliment the Council has paid me in electing me the first President of the Society, a Society which, although the youngest, has some reason to expect that it will be one of the most useful and fruitful of the medical institutions of the country. During nearly the whole of my professional life tropical disease has interested me, and as opportunity offered I have endeavoured to follow up the subject, and, if I may be allowed the expression, to forward the interests of the cause. Now that I am fast approaching the end of my career [Manson was then aged 63], to find that these efforts, however humble, are appreciated by my colleagues is to me most gratifying. I need hardly say that I thank you sincerely for the compliment, and that I shall do my best to discharge the duties of the office with which I am entrusted, and to forward the interests of our Society.

Manson next outlined certain objectives of the Society:

> ... An important [object] is to bring together the men who are interesting themselves in *tropical medicine*, with the idea that by so doing the subject itself will be advanced and we ourselves benefited. With a view to securing these objects, the Society has been placed on a basis as broad as possible. Although domiciled in the Metropolis, it is open to any member of the profession, whether domiciled in London, Great Britain and Ireland, or abroad, and also to those followers of any science or profession capable of forwarding, directly or indirectly, the interests of *tropical medicine*.

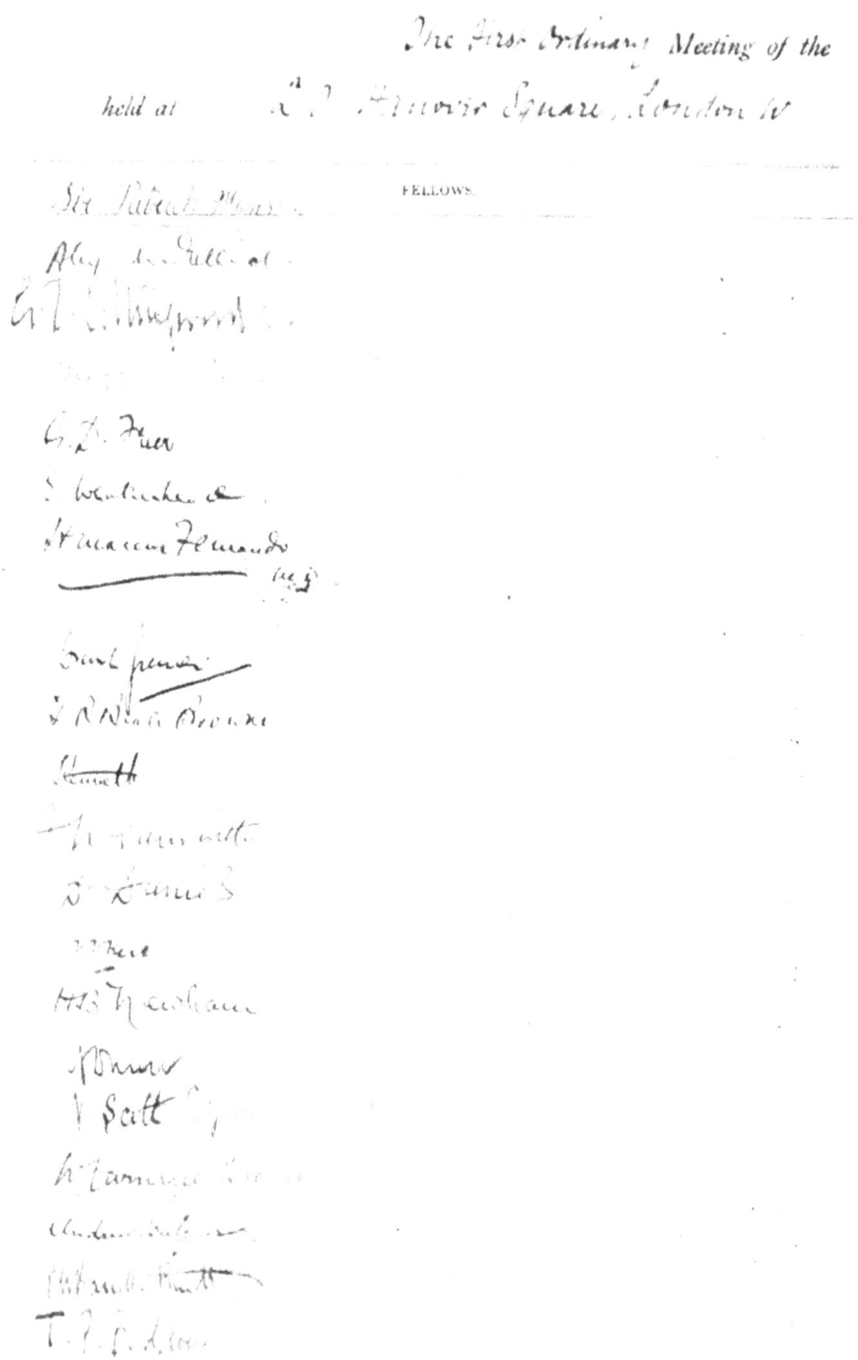
Meeting of the
held at
Square, London
FELLOWS.

Figure 2.2: Extract from the first attendance book showing signatories of Fellows and visitors present at the first *Ordinary* meeting on Wednesday 26 June 1907.

Society of Tropical Medicine and Hygiene,

on *Wednesday June 26th, 1907.*

FELLOWS.

VISITORS.

NAME OF VISITOR.	NAME OF INTRODUCER.
Samuel Evans	*Dr. Evans*
Cristino Wilson	Dr Daniels
Catherine P. Anderson	Dr Newman
James Anderson	Dr Newman
John Stoddart	Dr Basset Smith R.N.
Francis Lovell	Sir Patrick Manson
C.F.A. Moss	Dr Elliot
Michelli	Dr A. M. Wandsworth
Sir Wm. Thresher	Dr Carmine Brown.
Kenneth A. Crawford	

The First Ordinary Meeting of the

held at 20 Hanover Square London.

FELLOWS

[handwritten signatures of Fellows, mostly illegible]

31 Fellows

Figure 2.2 continued: Extract from the first attendance book showing signatories of Fellows and visitors present at the first *Ordinary* meeting on Wednesday 26 June 1907.

Society of Tropical Medicine and Hygiene,

on *Wednesday June 20*

FELLOWS.

VISITORS.

NAME OF VISITOR.	NAME OF INTRODUCER.
Russell H.S. Marshall	Dr Daniels
J. Colin C. Ford	do.
J.C. Hepburn	
L.G. Barbour	"
E. Mackintosh	
Gertrude McKinnon	
	Brandwork
W.J. Wellman	Dr. Daniels
Austin Forster	"
C. Hurt	

It is apparent to anyone who has followed the discoveries of recent years that *tropical medicine*, more than any other branch of medicine, is dependent on several of the collateral sciences, more especially on the various branches of natural history. Our basis therefore has to be a broad one, and in drawing up the constitution of the Society this point has been kept steadily in view.

At one time the specialising of *tropical medicine* was looked on somewhat askance, and still more so the establishment of special schools for [its] teaching ... Doubtless the formation of this Society will be regarded by some in a similar way, but as time goes on and the general body of the profession becomes acquainted with our objects and our work, I have no doubt, as has been the case with the special teaching of *tropical medicine*, that we shall soon be tolerated and ultimately approved.

How important it is for the subject itself, as well as for those who are engaged in its study, that the latter should have opportunities, such as this Society is calculated to afford, of placing themselves abreast of the times will be readily understood when we think of the rapid progress that *tropical medicine* has made within the last few years. This progress has been as remarkable as it has been great; indeed, it is hard to keep pace with it. *No sooner have we settled down to digest some new and important discovery than a fresh and perhaps more startling one is offered us* [author's italics]; and this, too, we must digest and assimilate if we are to practise, or to teach, or to work to the best advantage.

The rapidity of advance(s) in the new discipline over the previous twenty years[2] now became the subject of his attention, and he gave an illuminating account of the 'state of the art' in 1907:

... if we come from abroad after an absence of years, or if we compare the state of knowledge, say, of twenty years ago with that of to-day, we shall find that the stripling has not only altered in feature, but has grown into a veritable giant.[3]

I sometimes take from their shelves the text-books of my student days and compare their contents with those of the text-books of to-day – Watson's[4] with, say Osler's *Principles and Practice of Medicine*.[5] The contrast is remarkable. A perusal of Osler's shows how nearly all the old theories have been upset; how new diseases have been brought to light, old drugs and methods of treatment abandoned, pathology and etiology in most instances completely changed. If the contrast be great between the general medicine of to-day and that of forty or fifty years ago, it is even still greater in the case of *tropical medicine*. As regards the latter, it is unnecessary to go back to the days of Watson to recognise a striking contrast. It suffices to compare the *tropical medicine* of the early 'nineties as represented, say, by Dr Davidson's *Hygiene and Diseases of Warm Climates*, published in 1893[6], with one of the recent text-books, say, the section on *Tropical Medicine* in the new edition of Allbutt's *System of Medicine* edited by Rolleston.[7] Of the 1000 pages in Allbutt's book, the first 200 are exclusively devoted to protozoa, mosquitoes, blood-sucking flies, and ticks. In Davidson's work there is hardly a sentence on these subjects.

Practically, this is a new and a big and rapidly growing branch of *tropical medicine*. In Davidson's work the first chapter in the section on General Diseases relates to malaria. It is a very complete, carefully-written article, embracing all the most important knowledge and views of the time; yet in that article there is not a single word on the mosquito as a carrier of malaria. In those days, although Laveran's great discovery[8] had already been before the world for twelve years, we had got no further than the conviction that the air was the common medium of infection, and there was still a lingering belief in the Hippocratic idea that the drinking of marshy water produced enlargement of the spleen. Now a large part of the tropical section of Allbutt's system is occupied with the part played by the mosquito in the malarial drama. Everyone knows that the mosquito is the sole vector of malaria, and an enormous literature has grown up around a discovery which has changed radically our views, not only as regards the etiology and prophylaxis of malaria, but has given a powerful stimulus to the study of the protozoa in general, and also the *rôle* of insects in the transmission of disease germs. Taking the chapters in Davidson's book in their order, we come next to Tropical Typhoid Fever. Since this chapter was written, [Almroth] Wright's[9] bold and apparently successful prophylaxis has been introduced, and is being extensively practised. This, although not relating to a specially tropical disease, may in time be shown to be a great advance in the prophylaxis of one of the most serious diseases occurring in the Tropics.

When he wrote the chapter on Malta Fever, [Sir David] Bruce[10] had already discovered the *Micrococcus* [renamed *Brucella*] *melitensis*; but, just as was the case with Laveran's discovery, we had to wait a long time before the discovery bore practical fruit. Now, however, we know that the micrococcus is acquired in what, when Davidson's book was written, was an entirely unsuspected medium and manner. Both from a scientific and practical standpoint, Zammit's discovery that the germ of Malta Fever is eliminated in the milk of apparently healthy goats is a discovery of a little more than a year's standing.[11] It carried with it important practical results, as has already been proved.

Yet more important are the recent discoveries in regard to the still undiscerned germ of yellow fever, especially its dependence for propagation on the offices of the *stegomyia* mosquito [renamed *Aëdes aegypti*] and the efficiency of the prophylactic measures founded on that circumstance.[12]

We cannot claim any definite or important advance in our knowledge of dengue; but in plague, the subject of the next chapter in Davidson's book, the *rôle* of the rat in its diffusion[13] – so familiar to the ancients – has once more been rediscovered and more soundly established than ever, this time not by observation only but also by experiment. This is a discovery that promises to be of great practical value in the struggle against a terrible disease; its establishment on carefully observed facts is quite a recent occurrence.

We cannot claim that there has been much material advance in any of the subjects treated in the next three chapters of Davidson's work, namely, those on Cholera, Leprosy, and Beri-beri; but, as regards the subject of the succeeding chapter, Negro lethargy, or the Sleeping Sickness, it may be claimed truly that the whole subject, both as regards etiology, symptoms, diagnosis, and treatment, has been completely revolutionised and placed on a sound, and, it may be, hopeful, basis. We now know that the sleeping sickness is a terminal phase of a trypanosome infection[14] – a type of disease hitherto unrecognised in human pathology – that the immediate cause of the sleeping symptom is an infiltration of the lymphatic spaces of the brain with certain small mononuclear cells, that the disease is conveyed by the tsetse fly, and that it is amenable to some extent to arsenic, mercury, and certain dyes – all absolutely recent discovery.

Turning to the next chapter in Davidson, we are obliged to remark that the battle is still in progress as to whether yaws is syphilis or an entirely independent disease. [Sir Aldo] Castellani's[15] recent discovery of a spirochete in yaws, though interesting, has by no means solved the question.

In connection with the subjects of the next four chapters of Davidson, much work has been done and is going on; but it is to be regretted that these strenuous efforts have not proved more fruitful. The tropical fluxes – diarrhoeas and dysenteries – in the aggregate constitute, I believe, the most important department of *tropical medicine*. Unfortunately they are still, both as regards etiology and treatment, in an unsatisfactory state. It is true that the amoeba is creeping into favour, and that we have got the length of recognising a bacillary dysentery; but the amoeba and bacillus dysentariae [*Shigella* spp] do not, I feel sure, cover the entire field, and unfortunately, the knowledge of their existence, although it may have done a little for diagnosis, has not materially strengthened our powers of treatment. Sprue remains a mystery. [16] It is a specific disease undoubtedly, but the specific element has not been detected. On the other hand, the specific relation of the amoeba to a certain type of dysentery and to liver abscess may now be regarded as thoroughly established. This at least is a gain. Its complete recognition is of recent years. There are still spurs to be won in this field of the tropical fluxes.

Almost equally important in their own line are the numerous additions to tropical helminthology. They are far too numerous to mention on the present occasion. I might allude to one or two of them, as they are of special interest. Chief among these is Looss's discovery[17] that the larval ankylostome obtains access to the intestinal canal by penetrating the skin on the surface of the body – a discovery suggesting possibilities which have to be reckoned with in regard to other nematodes, or even parasites in general, when we study the route by which they obtain access to the human host. The intact epidermis can no longer be regarded as the impenetrable coat of mail it was supposed to be. Leiper's experimental demonstration[18] that the guinea-worm may be acquired through swallowing its cyclops intermediary, and also the discovery of two new and probably important parasites, *Schistosomum japonicum* and *Amphistomum watsoni*, are important additions to this department of *tropical medicine*. The linking up of the larval *Filaria diurna* with its parental form *F. loa*, as well as the recognition of this parasite as the cause of Calabar swellings, is a modern event. As regards the chapter on Skin Diseases, similar advances could be credited to recent years.

The text-book of to-day has therefore to be in many respects a very different work from that of Davidson's. Besides amplification and alteration there have to be many absolutely new additions. Kala-azar[19], for instance, is an entirely new chapter, dealing with a subject absolutely unknown when Davidson wrote, and it is one which will soon be found to be of far-reaching importance, both practically and theoretically. The modern text-book must have chapters on spirillosis, seeing that the term 'relapsing fever' which Murchison and others used, and which Carter also used in his studies in India, covers not one but a number of infections, spread probably by a corresponding number of previously unsuspected ticks or other blood-suckers.[20]

... the tropical pathologist must take cognisance of a number of diseases of the lower animals, important in themselves, but more important in their bearing as illustrating principles applicable to human pathology, especially tropical pathology. The study of the arthropod blood-suckers and the correlated diseases has grown to be so vast a subject that for its proper appreciation special studies have to be made and its teaching relegated to special men. In Davidson's day a single *culex* was all that we had to bother ourselves about; but nowadays we have to know something about some 600 species of mosquitoes; and so in a less degree with ticks, tsetse flies, and several other though less important blood-suckers. Truly the burden of the student of *tropical medicine* has become a heavy one.

Manson then proceeded to focus his attention on the *future* of the new discipline:

... Not only has recent discovery widened our horizon, but many additional works are now in the field, and hitherto untrodden departments of natural science having a bearing on tropical pathology have been opened by the tropical pathologist. The multiplication of workers is extraordinary, and doubtless is accounted for by the establishment of the several tropical schools in

Great Britain and elsewhere; not least by the sympathy and active encouragement that research in tropical pathology has received at the hands of the British Government. Time was when with justice we could reproach our rulers for indifference in this matter. Nowadays quite a different feeling obtains in official circles, and instead of being repressed and cold-shouldered the investigator in tropical pathology is encouraged in every possible way by the British Government and its officers.[21] Other Governments, too, have ceased to be indifferent; some are actively sympathetic.

The interest which the British Government has shown in sleeping sickness promises well for our object. The fact that His Majesty's [King Edward VII] Government has called a Conference of the Foreign Powers to discuss this subject from an international point of view shows that we are entering on a new era as regards the Governmental element in the study of tropical disease. It may be that this Sleeping Sickness Conference is but the prelude to similar discussions and international agreements on other important tropical diseases, a matter of more importance than at the first glance it might appear to be.

All over our own tropical possessions laboratories are being established for the special investigation of tropical disease, and for the assistance of the tropical practitioner. These laboratories have just begun to bear fruit, and I have not the slightest doubt that ten years hence we will have important discoveries as well as an enormous accumulation of important data as a result of this enlightened policy.

And regarding the future role of the STMH he considered the first priority was:

> ... to try and bring ourselves and our fellow-practitioners abreast of what is being done by this army of workers; so that those of us who have to teach in this country, and those of us who go abroad to practise or to investigate, shall be thoroughly abreast of what has been done and of what is being done, and be in the best position to do full justice to tropical patients and to tropical communities, and to lend a hand at advancing our subject.

But the Society also had other functions to fulfil and Manson proceeded to highlight one of these, with examples from his own career:

... Thirty odd years ago [in the 1870s] and after eight years of experience of medical work in the Tropics, during which I succeeded in learning this much, namely, that I knew nothing about tropical disease, I came home on furlough. After a month or two with my people, I came to London principally with the view to rub myself up in recent medicine and surgery, more especially in their bearing on tropical subjects. But it was like fishing in a big lake for the two or three fish the big lake might or might not hold. I did not know where the particular fish I wanted lay, and I found no one to tell me where they lay or how to set about hooking them. I finally landed at the Reading Room of the British Museum. Dreary enough and profitless enough was the fishing, there, as you may imagine. Nowadays things have improved vastly in this respect. There are post-graduate classes of all sorts; but I am not quite sure that a visitor from abroad with only a few months – it may be only a few days – to spare could put his hand at once on the special information he might be in search of, or on the person or persons who could or would guide him to that information. Nor – and that is an important consideration from the standpoint of a bashful man – would he feel quite certain that he was heartily welcomed by those who might be able to supply his wants.

Had such a Society as ours existed thirty-three years ago, I would not have had to go to the British Museum for my tropical pathology; I would have been put in touch at once with those who could have taught me, or been put in the way of being taught. Notwithstanding the greatly-increased facilities of recent times, there is still, in my opinion room in London in the way I indicate, and especially in our particular branch of practise. The stranger might still have to search, perhaps in vain, for the hand that would welcome and assist him. I trust that our Society will supply this welcome and this assistance.

... I once more came to London on furlough in the year 1882–3 with the same object in view – to learn the latest in medicine and surgery, especially in their application to *tropical medicine*. I heard plenty about the tubercle bacillus [*Mycobacterium tuberculosis*], but although I visited the Societies and became acquainted with many medical men of standing, I did not once hear of Laveran's important discovery of the malaria parasite [*see above*]. Indeed, it was not until I returned to [Amoy] China that I heard about it. I read Laveran's first book with great interest, and as I had abundant material at my command, I set to work to find the organism he described. Although repeated and prolonged attempts were made, I completely failed in my search, and almost became a sceptic about the existence of the plasmodium, and it was not until I returned to England in 1889, and not until I had renewed opportunities of working on the subject at the Seamen's Hospital [the Albert Dock Hospital],[22] that I saw for the first time the malaria parasite. But by that time my chances of fruitful work had gone. I had no longer abundance of material at my command. My failure to find the parasite when in China was entirely attributable to faulty technique, not from want of opportunity. Had there been a Tropical Society in 1883, doubtless Laveran's discovery would have been a prominent subject for discussion, the technique for its demonstration would have been familiar to the Fellows, and I should have gone back to China in a satisfactory position to pursue its study under favourable circumstances. I lost ten years by this.

Manson was not alone, however, in suffering the effects of these deficiencies, and he knew of others interested in *tropical medicine* who had suffered similar disadvantages:

... They have had no opportunity of seeing these things, in their flying visits to this country, or of learning how to recognise them. They go abroad, and, although anxious to work, they are not in a position to work in a fruitful way. The tropical schools do much, but they do not adequately supply the wants of the flying visitor. I take it that our Society has a distinct *role* in this direction. It will be powerfully educative, and no one wishing to get abreast of the actual position of *tropical medicine* at the time of his visit to London need go away ignorant on any particular point, no matter how recently it may have cropped up.[23]

Although the main thrust of Manson's Address now assumes *historical* interest, the potentially important role(s) of the Society which he outlined so vividly, remain very much the same today; present Fellows would do well to take note of words uttered by its first president as long ago as 1907!

The Society during Manson's Presidency

Appendix III shows the dates of the first ten Minute Books of the Society. The following passages (most of which were signed by the president) are taken from the first Minute Book (which includes both *Council* and *Ordinary* meetings) during Manson's two-year presidency. I have included a great deal of detail so as to provide a complete picture of the Society in its earliest days:

> Minutes of a Meeting of *Council* ... on Wednesday **10 July 1907** at 8pm.
>
> Present [were]: Sir Patrick Manson, Drs Hartigan, Sandwith, Carnegie Brown, Kerr, Low, Sambon, Stephens & Messrs Austen [and] Haffkine ...
>
> [18] candidates were put forward for election as Fellows under Law IV. [these included]:
>
> > 91 Andrew Duncan MD FRCS MRCP, 24 Chester St. Grosvenor Pl. SW
> >
> > 92 J L Todd MD Liverpool School of Tropical Medicine, Liverpool
> >
> > 93 Sir Francis Henry Lovell CMG London School of Tropical Medicine E
> >
> > 99 Signor A Terzi, 23 Russell Road, Addison Road W.
>
> On the motion of Dr [F M] Sandwith, seconded by Dr [W] Carnegie Brown it was unanimously resolved that the usual day for the *ordinary* meetings of the Society be changed to the third Friday of every month except August and Sept; and the *annual general meeting* to the third Friday in June.

Following this, the second *Ordinary* meeting of the newly formed Society took place at 8.30pm. It should be noted that not all communications minuted were published in Transactions and *vice versa*.

> Forty-three Fellows and visitors were present.
>
> Sir Patrick Manson, having taken the Chair, stated that the number of Fellows who had been elected by *Council* under Rule IV up to the present time was 102, and that 10 Honorary Fellows [*see* Chapter 1] had also been elected. *Council* had, to meet the wishes of many of the Fellows, changed the day for the

ordinary meeting [*see above*]. The Secretaries were now preparing a Syllabus of the work for next session, and would [therefore] be glad to have notice of papers, communications, etc. ...

Dr J W W Stephens [a member of *Council*], [from the] Liverpool School of *Tropical Medicine*, gave a description of some ... researches recently carried out at the Runcorn Laboratories, and described the development of *Piroplasma Canis* in the dog-tick – *Rhipicephalus Sanguineus* – as traced by Capt. [SR] Christophers IMS in India.[24] He also touched on the morphology of *Spirochaeta Duttoni*, and *Histoplasma Capsulata* (Darling), and showed a specimen of *Dibothriocephalus* from Tasmania, which had been taken from a patient who had recently come from Syria, and two nematodes (*Echinorhynchus*) from British Honduras. He afterward demonstrated Capt Christopher's specimens illustrating the development of *Piroplasma*, in which the club shaped bodies in the intestine and the sporoblasts in the salivary glands of the tick were well seen [*see* Table 2.1].

Dr Breinl [also] of the Liverpool School of *Tropical Medicine* described the morphology of *Trypanosoma Gambiense* & the changes which it exhibited (1) during reproduction and (2) during treatment of its host by atoxyl [an arsenical preparation]. [25] He said that the effect of Atoxyl was to cause the parasite to secrete a capsule, and retire to the internal circulation. There was no evidence of sexual conjugation at any time in the circulation, reproduction being always by division after distinctive changes in the nucleus and blepharoplast. He demonstrated the changes by microscopic specimens.

Dr Nierenstein of the Liverpool School, spoke of the treatment of *trypanosomiasis* (1) by atoxyl (2) by atoxyl in combination with organic compounds and aniline derivatives (3) by atoxyl followed by a course of mercury.[26] He indicated the latter method as being that which in his opinion was most promising, and said he believed the mercury acted on the encysted conditions.

Dr J L Todd of the Liverpool School ... gave a description of parasitic protozoa of various sorts observed by him in the Congo, including a *Leucocytozoon*, described by Schaudinn of which male and female forms were seen. He further described the stages of development of *Trypanosoma Loricatum* in the frog.[27]

Sir Patrick Manson [from the chair] said the Society was greatly indebted to the Members of the Liverpool School who had at considerable inconvenience to themselves travelled to London to give their excellent demonstrations and observations which they had listened to that evening. The development of *Piroplasma* was of great interest and importance, and the researches of Capt Christophers would, he believed, throw much light on a problem in proto-zoology of which little had hitherto been known. At the request of Dr Todd, Sir Patrick Manson described the results he had experienced in the treatment of Europeans affected with *Trypanosomiasis*. He regarded the clinical question as being in many ways parallel to that of syphilis, and said that with care, abundant nourishment, and treatment in the earlier stages, there was a moderately hopeful prospect of ultimately controlling the disease, or, at least, materially reducing the mortality. He further described at length the cases of several Europeans, and said that he agreed that atoxyl followed by mercury was a rational, and, possibly, would be found to be a successful treatment.

The meeting terminated at 10pm.

The fourth *Council* meeting was held at The Royal Devon and Exeter Hospital (the Section of Tropical Diseases, B M Association) on Thursday **1 Aug 1907** at 3pm.

The following [18] candidates were elected Fellows ... under Law IV [they included]:

107 Major Leonard Rogers IMS, Professor of Pathology, Calcutta
108 Oswald Baker MD Durh, 2 Montagu Mansions, Baker St W
111 Sir Rubert Boyce FRS School of Tropical Medicine, Liverpool.

From then, *Ordinary* meetings were always held after *Council* meetings; subjects and speakers at the latter are summarised in Table 2.1.

Table 2.1: Communications at *Ordinary* Meetings during Manson's presidency

Date	Subject	Speaker
1907		
26 June	*Inaugural address* (*see above*)	Sir Patrick Manson
10 July	*Piroplasma Canis, Rhipicephalus Sanguineus, Spirochaeta Duttoni, Histoplasma capsulata, Dibothriocephalus, Echinorhynchus, and Piroplasma.*	J W W Stephens (Liverpool School of Tropical Medicine)
	Trypanosoma Gambiense	Dr A Breinl (Liverpool School of Tropical Medicine)
	Trypanosomiasis: treatment with atoxyl	Dr M Nierenstein (Liverpool School of Tropical Medicine)
	Leucocytozoon	J L Todd (Liverpool School of Tropical Medicine)
18 October	*Trypanosomiasis*	H Johnston (Uganda), A R Cook (Mengo, Uganda)
15 November	*Oriental Sore*	Sir Patrick Manson
	Morphology of Spirochaete duttoni	The late [JE] Dutton and J L Todd (Liverpool School of Tropical Medicine)
	Serology in *Spirochaeta duttoni* infection	R Strong (Manila)
	Hamburg School of Tropical Medicine	F M Sandwith
20 December	*Ankylostomiasis* in Australia	T F MacDonald (Geraldton, Queensland, Australia)
	Physaloptera Mordens	R T Leiper
	Recent advances in helminthology	L Sambon
1908		
17 January	Distribution of *filariasis* in tropics	G C Low
	Biography of Fritz Schaudinn	W Carnegie Brown
21 February	*Kala-azar* in the Royal Navy	P W Bassett-Smith
	Plasmodium falciparum infection	J Cropper
20 March	Intestinal Entozoa	A E Shipley FRS (Cambridge)
	Disease caused by filariae	W T Prout (Liverpool School of Tropical Medicine)
15 April	Dysenteric diarrhoea	W T Prout (Liverpool School of Tropical Medicine)
	White races in the tropics	T F MacDonald (Geraldton, Queensland)
15 May	Discussion on Prout's paper (*see above*)	
	Quinine in pregnancy and the puerperium	J Preston Maxwell (Amoy)

Date	Subject	Speaker
19 June (1st AGM)	Tick fevers of Africa	C F Harford
17 July	Tropical skin diseases	A Castellani
16 October	Spinal meningitis in the Gold Coast	A E Horn (Gold Coast)
20 November	Elephantiasis and its surgical treatment	W Sampson Handley
	Colorectum in diarrhoea and dysentery	J Cantlie
18 December	Rat-flea theory of *plague*	W C Hossack
1909		
15 January	Parasite of *Kala-azar*	W Scott Patton (King Inst. Of Preventive Medicine, Madras)
	'Jeddah' ulcer	Dr Creswell (Suez)
19 February	New pathogenic spirochaeta	H G Waters
	Tropical notes from Barbados	T F McDonald
	Yellow fever in Brazil	E Ribas (São Paulo, Brazil)
19 March	*Kala-azar* treated with atoxyl	Sir Patrick Manson
	Interesting questions in 'tropical medicine'	C F Craig (NSA)
16 April	Aetiology of *beri-beri*	L Braddon
21 May	Discussion of Braddon's paper.	
	History of *beri-beri*: a 1629 account	Dr Stanton (Kuala Lumpur)
	Epidemiology of pneumonic plague	C A Gill (IMS)
18 June (2nd AGM)	Ross's *presidential address* (*See* Chapter 3).	R Ross (Liverpool School of Tropical Medicine)

Significant contributions to Council and Ordinary meetings during Manson's presidency

At a *Council* meeting on Friday **18 October 1907**:

The following [21] candidates were elected Fellows of the Society under Law IV [these included]:

> *121* Capt J Percival Mackie FRCS IMS, Asst. Director, Bombay Bacteriological Laboratory, c/o Grindley Groom & Co, Bombay
>
> *123* Arthur G Bagshawe MA MB Camb. (Uganda) 7 Beauchamp Avenue, Leamington

> 126 Hugh Stannus Stannus MB Lond MRCS, Fort Johnston,
>   Brit Central Africa
> 129 Lt Col Leishman RAMC College, Millbank SW
> 134 Professor Looss, School of Medicine, Cairo, Egypt. …

A memorandum from Professor Nuttall as to the formation of an *International Society of Tropical Medicine* [ISTM], a letter from Professor Ronald Ross, and correspondence between one of the Honorary Secretaries and Professors Ross and Nuttall were read. [But] discussion of these papers was deferred until a future opportunity.

And at the following *Ordinary* meeting:

> Dr Sandwith read a letter from Sir Harry Johnston KCMG [1858–1927], [Britain's Special Commissioner in Uganda – 1899–1901] saying that he much regretted his inability to be present. He sent, however, a historical and geographical narrative of the progress and extension of *Sleeping Sickness* in Central Africa[28], which was read by Dr Sandwith.
>
> The president [Manson] said the Society was much indebted to Sir Harry Johnston for his interesting and lucid description of the spread of the mysterious malady which was to be their subject that evening, and he asked that the thanks of the Society should be recorded for the excellent paper which had just been read. This was unanimously agreed to.

[Dr Albert Cook's paper]

Dr [later Sir] Albert Cook of Mengo, Uganda read a paper entitled '*Sleeping Sickness as met with in Uganda, chiefly with regard to treatment*'. After sketching the researches in the *tropical medicine* of Central Africa that had been made during recent years, and dealing specially with the advances of knowledge as to African disease which had occurred from that work, Dr [A R] Cook enumerated the various steps that had led up to our present knowledge of Human *Trypanosomiasis*. He referred to the original observation of Col [D] Bruce that the area of endemicity coincided with the distribution of *Glossina Palpalis*, and the discovery by Capt [E D W] Greig of the early implications of the cervical lymphatic glands, and their importance in diagnosis, as discoveries of great and practical benefit, the one as being the foundation of our attempts at prophylaxis, the other offering a tolerable, rapid and reliable method of identifying the disease. He also called attention to premonitory mental symptoms, sometimes seen as mania, more often as morbid consciousness of infection, and said that these conditions had received insufficient notice. Our knowledge of the disease was as yet incomplete and unsatisfactory, and this was especially true of treatment.

Dr Cook traced the various methods that had been adopted in prophylaxis, such as segregation of persons who were infected, clearing areas of jungle, and instruction of chiefs as to sanitary measures, and said that these, so far as they went, had been successful, but that the amount of work that had to be done was so enormous, that progress was necessarily slow, and, in reality, it was only in very limited areas that the disease had been stayed. He further described the various methods by which he had attempted to combat the disease when established, the results which had been attained in the Mission Hospital at Mengo, in which there were 140 beds, and the cost of the various drugs which had been employed. Sodium arsenite was inexpensive, but the injections were painful and apt to be followed by arsenical intoxication. It diminished the symptoms but did not cure the disease. Atoxyl was expensive, but the results were more satisfactory. Alleged cures were, however, to be deprecated until we had more experience of the malady. With regard to combinations of mercury, an element of great moment was the exceptional susceptibility of natives of Africa to that drug. That idiosyncrasy was a most important consideration in treatment.[29]

Dr G C Low [who had led the first Sleeping Sickness expedition to Uganda in 1902–3] said [in discussion] that with regard to segregation, experiments were necessary to show how far the disease might be transmitted by infected animals. It was useless to remove infected natives, if monkeys and other fauna were equally efficient hosts. *Trypanosomiasis*, like many other grave epidemics, seemed to appear at intervals; waves of sickness were followed by periods of comparative health; nature, therefore, had a remedy, and much might be gained if our knowledge of this natural immunisation were more complete. Professor [E A] Minchin spoke as to the anatomical characteristics of glossina, and compared the fitness for the transmission of trypanosomes of various species of tsetse flies with that of *Stomoxys*, and other suctorial insects. Mr [E E] Austen said that further experiments were required to settle the question whether other species than *G. palpalis* conveyed the disease, and a point of importance was the possibility of extension to South Africa. In [northern] Rhodesia [now Zambia], the only tsetse flies known at present was *G morsitans* but on the extreme north western border of that territory, there was a district where three species *morsitans, palpalis* and another overlapped. A tsetse fly had been discovered in the Aden hinterland. Dr [L] Sambon referred at some length to the biological affinities and distribution of various species of *trypanosomes*. (As it was now ten o'clock it was moved by Dr [F M] Sandwith and seconded by Dr [C F] Harford, and agreed to that the discussion be continued).

Sir Patrick Manson referred to the effects of mercury in the treatment of *trypanosomiasis*, and to its action in combination with organic compounds of arsenic. He said that on the whole the therapeutic position was encouraging, though some of the later remedies had been unsuccessful. A supply of parafuchsin, a drug which had been under observation and experiment at the Frankfurt Institute for Therapeutic Research had been sent him by Prof [Paul] Ehrlich, but he was sorry to say his experience had not been favourable. He was satisfied that the human organism presented great natural resistance to the *trypanosomes* of sleeping sickness which tended ultimately to die out, if the patient could be kept going. Research was required to further elucidate the facts as to the life history of *Trypanosomes* and their hosts; insufficient knowledge was at our disposal to enable us to supply Governments with responsible and authoritative advice as to preventive measures.

Dr Cook replied to the arguments and criticisms of the various speakers, and said that the urgency of the matter was insufficiently appreciated. Research was no doubt imperative, but it would be useless unless it resulted in effective measures before there was no further need of them.

The meeting terminated at 10.25pm.

The sixth *Council* meeting was held on Friday **8 November** at 5.30pm.

… [17] candidates were elected …[These included]:

> 154 A J Stanton MD MRCS Inst for Medical Research, Kuala Lumpur
> 156 Lt-Col Alcock IMS FRS London School of Trop Medicine.

The [Hon] Secretary intimated that these were the last elections which according to the Laws of the Society could take place under Law IV.

Another meeting of *Council* took place on Friday **15 November** at 5.30pm:

> … Professor [G H F] Nuttall made a communication on the subject of the [ISTM], and laid a memorandum on the table as to the circumstances of the formation of the Society at a meeting of those interested in *Tropical Medicine* at Berlin. He further asked that this Society should appoint two representatives on the provisional Committee of the International Society, which was being formed to draft a Constitution and Rules. Letters from Professors [R] Ross and Nuttall were considered, and after some discussion it was proposed by Dr [C F] Harford, and seconded by Fleet Surgeon [P W] Bassett-Smith:
>
> > That this Society appoint two Representatives to the provisional Committee of the [ISTM], on the understanding that this Society is not committed to any special policy by this action, and that they report to this Society.
>
> On being put by the President this motion was unanimously carried.
>
> It was further proposed by Lieut Col [C H] Melville, and seconded by Dr Hartigan that this Society be represented on the provisional Committee by Professor Ross and Dr Sandwith. On being put by the President, this was unanimously agreed to.
>
> The [Hon] Secretaries stated that it was desirable to take into consideration the question of the appointment of *Local Secretaries*, and that a definite proposal on the subject would be brought forward at an early date. This was approved.

The penultimate *Ordinary* meeting for the foundation year took place at 8.30pm:

[ORIENTAL SORE]

... Dr [F M] Sandwith took the Chair while the President [Manson] gave a demonstration of *Oriental Sore*[30], and showed the patient, Dr Johnson to whom Sir Patrick Manson said the Society was much indebted for his complacency [sic] and courtesy in subjecting himself to examination. Several specimens in which the *Leishman-Donovan* parasites could be well seen were shown under the microscope, and the clinical history of the case, with the general characteristics of the disease were fully described. The points which were of special interest were the fact that *Oriental Sore* was protective against itself, that the incubation period was uncertain, and that it appeared on exposed parts of the body, that it was inoculable and that the parasite after being virulent and active for an indefinite time, passed through involution stages, during which time it was uninoculable or inoculable only with great difficulty, but more important than any of these was the connection between the disease and Kala-Azar, and the prospect that was opened of being able to combat that terrible fatal malady by the virus *of oriental sore.*

Dr Low [in discussion] called attention to the prevalence of *oriental sore* in dry countries in contra-distinction to Kala-Azar, essentially a disease of hot, moist climates. Spirochaetes, too, were an important feature of such infections; had any variety been found in oriental sore? Lt Col [A] Duncan spoke of the application of metallic lead compounds, a cure in vogue on the frontiers of India, as having, to his knowledge, been efficacious. Dr [L] Sambon said that though the disease, doubtless, produced immunity against itself, there was often recurrence, which was a different thing. It showed, too, the systemic nature of the disease, which like others of the *Leishman-Donovan* group of parasites, was thought to be conveyed by flies. After Drs Hartigan, Freemantle, MacDonald, Johnson and Newham had taken part in the discussion, the President replied in detail to the points made by the various speakers.

The President [then] resumed the Chair and Dr Sandwith read a paper by the late Dr [J E] Dutton [1874–1905] and Dr Todd on the morphology of *Spirochaeta Duttoni*.[31]

Dr Sandwith also read a letter from Dr R Strong [Manila] in which he said he had been able, by means of serum reactions, agglutinations, and bacteriolysis to confirm Mantengel's [sic] results in the differentiation of *Spirochaeta duttoni* and the Spirochaete of American relapsing fever; Dr Sambon also spoke on that subject.

Dr Sandwith [also] read a paper on the Hamburg School of Tropical Medicine and the work which had been done there[32], for which he received the thanks of the Society. The meeting terminated at 10.30pm.

The last of the Society's meetings for 1907 (the inaugural year) took place on **20 December**:

… At the *Council* meeting the Secretaries announced the names of six candidates [nominated] for the Fellowship of the Society. [They included]:

Sir Richard Havelock Charles KCVO MD [a future president], 9 Manchester Square
Robert Thomson Leiper MB, London School of Tropical Medicine.

The names were approved and a ballot was ordered to be taken at the next [Ordinary] meeting.

It was agreed that Fellows elected this month should be on the same terms as regarded subscription as those elected in January next.

The *Ordinary* meeting then took place at 8.30pm.

[ANKYLOSTOMIASIS IN AUSTRALIA]

… Dr T F MacDonald, Geraldton, N Queensland, Australia, read a paper entitled *'Experiences of Ankylostomiasis in Australia'*.[33] He said that the question had assumed very great importance on account of the decision of the Australian Government to replace Kanaka* labour on the sugar estates by white labour, and thus to substitute a population that did not possess the same

---

* An Australian term referring to 'a native of the South Sea Islands'.

resistance to *ankylostome* infections as did the Coloured races. He himself had advocated the ability of white men to till and mill sugar cane in Queensland, and believed that they were able to do so efficiently and healthily, but increased sanitary precautions would have to be taken and especially against *ankylostomiasis*. The infection had spread very rapidly, and it was now extremely prevalent. Dr MacDonald also called attention to the frequency of geophagia, and mental and moral deterioration. He classed these as definite symptoms. *Ankylostomiasis* was easily cured in individuals, the problem was to stamp it out in Communities. Possibly it was an aboriginal disease, but there was a definite history of its introduction by Italian labourers from Pisa in Italy. Dr MacDonald further emphasised the necessity for family surveillance and treatment, on account of its great frequency in children.

Dr Sambon [in discussion] reviewed briefly the present condition of Italy and Sicily with regard to *ankylostome* infections. Dr Sandwith said that Eucalyptol, which had been recommended by Dr MacDonald was now generally adopted in Egypt. Dr [R T] Leiper [1881–1969] and Dr Alex M Elliott also spoke. Sir Patrick Manson asked which species of *ankylostome* was prevalent in Queensland, also whether it was associated with Rhabdonsoma [sic], and if Beta-naphthol had been used as a remedy. He remarked that a study that was particularly germane to this Society was the epidemic relations of the disease, as Governments frequently wished to be advised as to its prevention in communities. Dr MacDonald replied to the various speakers and said that the one species he had seen was the Old World ankylostomum; the *Necator Americanus* had *not* been encountered. He stated that he had found ankylostomes in a child of eight months old.

Dr R Leiper, Helminthologist to the London School of Tropical Medicine described and demonstrated a new intestinal nematode parasite of man which he named *Physaloptera Mordens*[34], and which he had obtained at Entebbe in Uganda from Dr Gray. The patient had died of sleeping sickness and many of the worms were found in the stomach and oesophagus. Dr Leiper compared the parasite with *Physaloptera Caucasica* found only once before by Linston [sic] in South Russia, with which it had generic affinities.

Dr Sambon read a paper on the '*Rôle of Helminthology in Tropical Medicine*', in which he emphasised the importance of the subject, and discussed the recent additions to our knowledge, especially with reference to the method of infection in ankylostomiasis, bilharziasis and other conditions.

Drs Sandwith and Low [in discussion] criticised Dr Sambon's views as to the schistosome named by him *Schistosumum mansoni*, while Dr Leiper stated that Looss recognised that ankylostome infection could take place by the intestine as well as through the skin. The President spoke as to arguments in favour of a Schistosome with a lateral spined ovum, and said that the view of its specific nature was supported by pathology and geographical distribution. Dr Sambon briefly replied to the arguments of the various speakers and the meeting terminated at 10.30pm.

1908

The first *full* year in the Society's existence started on Friday **17 January 1908**:

> ... The [Hon] Secretaries announced [the names of three candidates for election]. The names were approved, and a ballot was ordered to be taken at the next meeting.
>
> The Treasurer presented a statement of the financial position of the Society, which was considered satisfactory, and approved. ...

The sixth *Ordinary* meeting followed at 8.30pm:

> [The following were amongst those approved by *Council* and duly elected by ballot]:
>
> 165 Sir Richard Havelock Charles KCVO, 9 Manchester Sq, W, [and]
> 166 Robert Thomson Leiper MB, London School of Tropical Medicine.

The President said that Dr Johnson, who had so kindly exhibited in his own person [*see* above], an example of *oriental sore*, was again present, and would show the effects of scraping in comparison with expectant treatment.

[FILARIASIS IN THE TROPICS]

Dr G C Low read a paper on the distribution of *Filariasis* in Tropical Countries, and adduced figures which he had compiled as the result of a very large number of observations made both in the Eastern and Western tropics. He showed that there were great and often surprising variation in the index of infection which were extremely difficult to explain, in different regions, and that it varied greatly in places that were quite adjacent. He urged that further research in this direction, systematically carried out and carefully recorded was urgently required.[35]

Dr Sambon [in discussion] said research was also requisite to settle the identity of observed helminths; *Filaria Bancrofti* for example might be found to comprise several varieties; reports of authorities such as Looss and Thorpe indicated that was probable. Hyperparasitism explained many facts, however, and that should not be left out of sight. Dr Leiper discussed the statements of Dr Low as to the infection of natives in Uganda by *filaria nocturna* and *filaria perstans*. Sharp tailed embryos did not occur in man in Central Africa, but they were found there in monkeys. He agreed with Dr Sambon that *F. Bancrofti* might include several species; definite statements should not be founded on blood examination only; and parental forms were necessary for identification. Dr Sandwith said filariasis was not very common in Egypt proper; as to the Sudan, he had no reliable information. At DamietIa[?] and Rosetta where water had formerly for some months in the year to be stored in cisterns, the disease was common, but when an improved water service was instituted, it became less prevalent. Hayward, now of Port Said had found 15 per cent of the patients in the Kasr El Assingo [?] Hospital infected by filariasis; that perhaps indicated it might be more common than the previous failures to find the parasite would lead them to believe.

The President [Manson] thanked Dr Low on behalf of the Society for a very admirable paper, which he said would stimulate much needed research. A point was that contrary to what might be expected in the poorer and less instructed classes, an extreme degree of infection in man was rare. He did not agree with Dr Sambon that hyperparasitism was a cause. The actual nature of elephantiasis had not been fully explained, and both points required further study.

Dr Low replied to the various points raised. He said that in very many feeding experiments which he had made, he had never seen hyperparasitism. He was convinced that elephantiasis was a filarial disease.

Dr [W] Carnegie Brown read a biographical sketch of the late Professor Fritz Schaudinn[36], for which the President thanked him on behalf of the Society.

The meeting terminated at 10.30pm. …

The second *Council* meeting for 1908 was held on **21 February** at 8.00pm. At the following *Ordinary* meeting (41 Fellows and Visitors were present):

[Kala-azar]

… Fleet-Surgeon [P W] Bassett-Smith [a member of Council] read a paper on a case of *Kala-azar* which had occurred in a [?]-of-war's-man who had had service on the East Indian Station. The diagnosis had been confirmed by the demonstration of *Leishman-Donovan* bodies in smears of liver blood, specimens of which were shown by the speaker. The treatment had been unsatisfactory and protracted, and the patient was still very ill.[37]

Sir R Havelock Charles on being asked by the President to open the discussion said that he would not criticise the very interesting paper to which they had listened further than to cite a case of successful treatment by no other means than abundant sea-air. A patient of his in an apparently hopeless condition had got well by voyaging for four months between Colombo and Australia. Personally, he was of opinion that no drug would cure *Kala-azar*; the only treatment was immediate removal from the place where the disease had been contracted and complete change of air. Major [W B] Leishman said that he had come to the meeting hoping to get a clue to a successful treatment. He had some experience of atoxyl, and he thought it the most promising drug yet put before them though in the last case he had it was carefully tried unfortunately without benefit. A method of inducing a collection of polynuclears by pustulation suggested by Major [S L] Cummins seemed to him worth a trial. With regard to development, he had, during the last few days, received cultivation forms made by M Nicolle from cases of *Kala azar* in Tunis showing segmented bodies which looked as if they had been split off the flagellated form which he thought were the same as he had previously described, and he would be glad of any opinions on the nature of those bodies. Dr Low stated that he was of opinion that no case could be pronounced *Kala azar* until the parasite had been demonstrated; and cited several instances which, clinically, closely simulated the signs and symptoms of that disease, but which had either been shown to be of an entirely different nature, or had remained doubtful. Dr Harford said that the points of most interest were the insidious way in which the disease had commenced in Sir Patrick Manson's case, and asked for information as to its connection with antecedent fever which had been of long standing. Dr Sambon said that similar bodies to which Major Leishman had referred were seen in trypanosome cultures; they were certainly not artefacts. Dr Sandwith asked the authors of the paper to state their views as to whether there was real danger in puncturing spleen or liver, and if so what precautions should be taken to avoid or mitigate it.

… Bassett-Smith admitted the great difficulties of diagnosis in some cases after a negative result obtained by spleen puncture. That proceeding was not without danger, but he thought liver puncture safe.

The President [Manson] replied to the various points raised by the speakers. He said that drugs had a decided effect on diseases analogous to *Kala azar*, and which clinically closely resembled it, and he should place his next patient on atoxyl with considerable hope. He did not think splenic puncture justifiable; but liver puncture had no dangers if carefully done. He thought Dr Harford's patient had [had] the disease for several years.

Dr [J] Cropper [also] described a case of severe malarial infection with phenomenal abundance of parasites in the peripheral circulation, and showed a large number of blood films, in which malignant tertian parasites were present in all stages of development.[38] After remarks by Drs Low, Col Leishman and Fleet Surgeon Bassett-Smith, the President asked what interpretation Dr Cropper put on the marked clumping of parasites in corpuscles which was shown in one preparation. Clumping might be an explanation of the thrombosis which so frequently occurred in malarial infections. He said the Society was much indebted to Dr Cropper for the demonstration of the finest collection of malarial preparations that he … had ever seen.

Dr Cropper said that in such cases immature crescents were often seen, which had probably been forced into the blood vessels by contraction. In ordinary infections crescents were never seen unless fully formed.

The meeting terminated at 10pm. …

At the meetings on **20 March**, *Council* approved the following amendments to the laws:

All papers, contributions, reports and other literary matter accepted by the Council shall be the property of the Society, and every such paper shall be delivered to one of the Secretaries not later than seven days after it has been read in order that it may be published in the *Transactions* or dealt with in such manner as the Council may direct.

Notwithstanding any provision to the contrary however accepted papers may be published by the authors in any scientific periodical approved by the Council provided that due acknowledgement is made of their having been read before the Society. …

At the subsequent *Ordinary* meeting at 8.30pm (43 being present), two papers were presented, only the first of which was published in *Transactions*:

[AN HELMINTHIC CAUSE OF APPENDICITIS?]

… Mr A E Shipley [*see* Chapter 1] of Cambridge read a paper on *'The Relation of Entozoa to the Mucous Lining of the Alimentary Canal'*. In his communication which was illustrated by a large number of excellent epidiascope slides, Mr Shipley traced the various entozoal infections of the lower animals and man, and demonstrated the injuries and septic consequences which might result from the presence of parasites in the alimentary canal. After describing various intestinal parasites of the grouse, the common fowl, and the horse, he reviewed the state of our knowledge as to the influence of entozoa in originating disease in man, and suggested that appendicitis might be caused by *Trichocephalus trichiurus*.

Sir Patrick Manson [who was again in the Chair] said the Society was much indebted to Mr Shipley for his excellent and most interesting paper, and invited criticism. Dr Daniels stated that he did not agree to the connection of *Trichocephalus* and appendicitis; he thought he was supported in this by the fact that though natives of the tropics were deeply infected by the parasite, appendicitis was very rare. Sir Havelock Charles said that his experience was that appendicitis was not uncommon in natives of Lower Bengal. After remarks by Drs Sambon and Leiper both of whom agreed that *Trichocephalus* had no influence in originating appendicitis Sir Patrick Manson said that it was generally believed by medical men, and statistics fully supported the belief, that *Trichocephalus* and appendicitis had no definite connection.

Dr [W T] Prout of Liverpool [also] read a paper on '*The Rôle of Filariasis in the production of Disease*'[39] and exhibited the sword of a sword-fish which he had removed from a man who had been transfixed by it.

As it was now 10.30 the President said that discussion on Dr Prout's very valuable paper, with the reading of his other communication would have to be deferred until next meeting. ...

At a meeting of *Council* on **15 April**:

The Treasurer presented his Report for the year ending March 31 1908 [and] a Subcommittee of the *Council* to consider the question of publications and of the best method of meeting requirements of the Society was appointed as follows: Drs Sandwith, Low, Brown and Messrs Cantlie and Austen. ...

The following papers were read at the subsequent *Ordinary* meeting (only ten Fellows being present) under the Chairmanship of Dr Sandwith.

... In the absence of Dr Prout, the Chairman [Sandwith] read a paper which he [and Prout] had contributed on the subject of an outbreak of Dysenteric Diarrhoea at Bathurst, W Africa, which has been caused by locusts' faeces having been washed into the tanks of drinking water.[40] Mr Cantlie, and Drs Hartigan and Carnegie Brown briefly criticised the paper.

Dr [T F] MacDonald, Geraldton, Queensland read a paper on *'Tropical lands and White Races'* in which he expressed the view that Climate *per se* did not materially prejudice the tropics as a place of permanent residence for the White Races and that if endemic disease could be eradicated, Europeans could live and propagate families without any ill effect.[41] After a discussion in which Mr Cantlie, Mr Austen, Col [O] Baker and Drs Sandwith and Hartigan took part, Dr MacDonald replied.

The meeting terminated at 10.15pm [instead of the customary 10.30pm]. ...

On **15 May**, *Council* approved a draft (consisting of a summary of proceedings so far) of the first *Annual Report of Council* – see below:

The *Ordinary* meetings continued however to be only moderately well attended, 41 being present that day to hear:

... An adjourned discussion ... on Prout's paper [of 20 March] on the *'Rôle of Filariae in the production of Disease'*, in which Dr Low, Mr Cantlie, Dr Carnegie Brown, Sir Havelock Charles and the President took part.

Dr Hartigan [also] read a paper for Dr [J] Preston Maxwell of Amoy, on *'The use of Quinine during Pregnancy, Labour and the Puerperium'*[42] and a discussion followed in which Drs Hartigan, Sandwith, Harford and the President took part. ...

First AGM

The first *Annual General meeting* was held, following a short *Council* meeting, on **19 June 1908** at 8.30pm. The main business was to approve various amendments to the Society's Laws:

... Law II [which had been alluded to at the last Council meeting] was brought up for consideration:

A limited number of members of the medical profession and others engaged in scientific pursuits bearing on *tropical medicine* shall while resident abroad be eligible for election by the Council as *Corresponding* Fellows. A Corresponding Fellow so elected, who afterwards takes up his residence in the

United Kingdom, may on making application and on paying the subscription due for the current year become an *Ordinary* Fellow of the Society without ballot or further election, but should such application not be made he shall cease to be a Corresponding Fellow and any privileges he has enjoyed as such shall determine.

Law 28 was deleted.
Law 29 was amended:

Honorary and Corresponding Fellows shall pay no entrance fee or subscription.

The following *New* Laws were adopted:

(1) All papers, contributions, reports and other literary matter accepted by the *Council* shall be the property of the Society and every such paper shall be delivered to one of the Secretaries immediately after it has been read, in order that it may be published in the *Transactions* or dealt with as regards the *Transactions* in such manner as the *Council* may direct.

(2) Authors of papers accepted by the Society shall not thereby acquire a right to have such papers or abstracts of them inserted in the *Transactions*, but should the Council decide to publish papers in an abridged or altered form the authors shall be entitled to prepare the abstracts for publication, and any question that may arise as to the form or matter of such abstracts, or the method of their publication shall be finally decided by *Council*.

(3) Notwithstanding any provision to the contrary, accepted papers may be published by the authors in any scientific periodical approved by the *Council* provided that due acknowledgement is made of their having been read before the Society.

(4) Except by permission of the President the time to be occupied in reading any paper or moving any resolution before the Society shall not exceed 30 minutes and the time occupied by a Fellow in speaking to a resolution or discussion shall not exceed 10 minutes. ...

At the *Ordinary* meeting following the AGM:

> Dr Harford read a paper on *'The Tick Fever of Africa with Special reference to its clinical manifestations, and its relation to the Relapsing Fever of India and other parts of the world'*.[43] Drs Sambon, Sandwith, Bagshawe, Castellani, Low, C J Baker, L Hill and Sir Patrick Manson spoke on the subject and Dr Harford replied. …

At a *Council* meeting held on **17 July** (to complete the first full year of the Society's existence):

> … Dr Carnegie Brown informed … Council that the work of publishing the *Transactions* would be completed within the next month, only the proceedings of that night [*see* below] remaining to be included – and said that it would be necessary to appoint an Editor for next year. Dr Carnegie Brown stated that it would not be possible for him to continue after the first volume had been published, but after some conversation it was agreed to defer making another appointment until October. …

And at the following *Ordinary* meeting, when 22 Fellows and visitors were present:

> … Dr Aldo Castellani read a paper on *'Some tropical skin diseases'*. [44] Dr Pernet, Fleet Surg Collingwood, Mr Cantlie, Dr [W] Carnegie Brown, Dr Sandwith, Dr Sambon, Dr Graham Little and Sir Patrick Manson spoke on the subject, and Dr Castellani replied.
>
> Before the meeting terminated, the President [Manson] thanked Dr Castellani on behalf of the Society for a complete and extremely interesting paper, and said that the Society was also much indebted to the Dermatologists for their presence and for the remarks which they had contributed to the discussion. …

The Society's (and Manson's) second twelve months; accommodation problems begin

The first meeting of *Council* for the second year was held at 6pm on Monday **28 September** at *32 Harley Street* with Lt Col [C H] Melville in the Chair – problems with accommodation at the RSM were first aired at this meeting:

... Dr Carnegie-Brown read letters from the Secretary of the [RSM] dated Sept. 23 and Sept. 25, in which it was stated that in consequence of a misunderstanding the Room hitherto occupied by the Society, had been let to the Quekett Society for next session, and suggesting that the date of meetings should be altered. After consideration ... it was moved by Dr Hartigan and seconded by Dr Daniels:

> That the Society accept an offer of the Medical Society of London [MSL – *see* reference 8 page 121] to place suitable accommodation at their disposal for the ensuing year at a rate of twenty guineas per annum, and that the Secretaries be instructed to make arrangements to carry that arrangement into effect.

It was further moved by Dr Hartigan and seconded by Dr Harford that the Secretaries be instructed to make a claim for Twenty guineas from the [RSM], being six months rent in lieu of notice.

Both resolutions were carried unanimously. ...

And at the next *Council* meeting on Friday **16 October** (at 11 Chandos Street):

> ... Correspondence between the Honorary Secretaries and the Secretary of the [RSM] relative to the Society's occupancy of quarters at [20] Hanover Sq was read and approved.
>
> Correspondence with Mr G Bethell [Registrar of the MSL] relative to the occupancy of 11 Chandos St was [also] read and approved.
>
> A letter from the Secretary of the [RSM] was read in which it was stated that he would be glad to receive suggestions as to the addition to the Library of books on *Tropical Medicine*. The Secretaries were instructed to thank Mr [John] MacAlister [sic] [the RSM's librarian and Secretary] for his offer, and to say that a list with suggestions would be forwarded. They were also instructed to suggest that consideration might be given to a proposal that the Members of the [RSM] interested in *Tropical Medicine* should be represented on the Library Committee. ...
>
> The a/c of the Bedford Press amounting to £79.8.6 for printing and publishing last years *Transactions* was approved and ordered to be paid. ...

Only 24 Fellows and visitors were present at the following *Ordinary* meeting, to hear:

> ... Dr A E Horn ... on *An investigation of Cerebro-Spinal Meningitis in the Northern Territories of the Gold Coast* [now Ghana] in which he described the epidemiology, bacteriology, clinical manifestations and treatment of the disease, with special reference to prophylaxis.[45]
>
> Lt Col Watherston RE [?] Administrator of the Northern Territory of the Gold Coast said that the district was under a deep debt of gratitude to Dr Horn for excellent work carried out under the greatest difficulty. Drs Sandwith, Low and the President also spoke and on the motion of the latter the Society thanked Dr Horn for his paper and Microscopical demonstration. ...

Twenty Fellows for Election were approved by *Council* on **20 November**, taking the Fellowship to 228. Thirty-three Fellows were present to hear several communications at the following *Ordinary* meeting:

> [FILARIASIS AND INVESTIGATION OF DYSENTERY]
>
> Mr [W] Sampson Handley showed a patient suffering from Elephantiasis, who had been treated by a procedure which he named Lymphangioplasty and which had given excellent results in a somewhat similar condition of the upper limb. Silk threads, deeply buried in the tissues, and carefully spaced out round the limb were inserted for the whole length of the lower extremity. The result had been highly satisfactory so far as it went.[46] Sir Havelock Charles spoke as to the possibilities of the operation, and the importance of considering blood infection. The President thanked Mr Handley for his demonstration and congratulated him on the result.
>
> Dr Sandwith showed casts of two large Vesical Calculi removed by Messrs Milton and Richards, in Cairo [and] a series of specimens illustrative of Bilharziasis, [which had been] sent by Professor Kartulis of Alexandria.
>
> Mr Cantlie read a paper on *'The Sigmoid Flexure and Rectum in Colitis, Dysentery and Post-dysenteric States'*.[47]
>
> Sir Havelock Charles having spoken, a Ballot was taken for three candidates [including Dr C M Wenyon – a future President], all of whom were unanimously elected. ...

The two items of note at a *Council* meeting on Friday **18 December** were:

> The Secretaries stated that owing to an unanticipated increase in expenditure, it had become necessary to inquire into the financial position of the Society, and [they] undertook to bring up a statement at [the] next meeting.
>
> Dr Sandwith stated that he had been appointed a member of the Library Committee of the [RSM] as representative of the Society. ...

The attendance at the *Ordinary* meeting that evening at 8.30, was 36:

> ... Dr W C Hossack read a paper on '*The present position of the Rat-flea theory of Plague; recent observations in Calcutta*' [now Kolkata] in which he contended that the importance which had been attached to the Fleas of Rats as disseminators of Plague was greatly exaggerated.[48]
>
> Dr G Ford Petrie, [a] Member of the Indian Plague Commission contended that the conclusions of the Plague Commission on this point were fully justified by experimental and other evidence.[49]
>
> Sir Patrick Manson, Sir Havelock Charles, Dr Low, Mr Cantlie and Dr [H G] Waters having taken part in the discussion, Dr Hossack replied. A large number of microscopic preparations illustrative of the subject were afterwards shown by Dr Hossack. ...

1909

The first *Ordinary* meeting of 1909 (the preceding *Council* meeting had been largely restricted to approving new nominations for Fellowship), again under Manson's Chairmanship, was held on **15 January** at the MSL; attendance was 36:

> ... Capt W Scott Patton IMS of the King Institute of Preventive Medicine, Madras [now Chennai] read a paper on '*The Parasite of Kala Azar and allied organisms*', in which he claimed that the morphological appearances and life history indicated a close relationship between these organisms and the genus herpetomonas [sic].[50]

Drs Sambon and Low, Sir Havelock Charles, & Dr Wenyon having spoken, Sir Patrick Manson said that the Society was much indebted to Capt Patton for an admirably lucid and clear statement of his views, and for an excellent and interesting paper, and Capt Patton replied.

Dr [F M] Sandwith showed for Dr Creswell of Suez a specimen of a 'Jeddah' ulcer.[51] ...

And on **19 February**, after a very short *Council* meeting, with 22 present:

... Dr H G Waters read a paper [at the *Ordinary* meeting] on '*A new Pathogenic Spirochaeta associated with Bronchitis and fever*'; and demonstrated specimens of the organism under the microscope. [52] Dr C W Daniels and Dr G C Low spoke on the subject [and] Dr Sandwith read a paper for Dr T Fausset McDonald entitled '*Tropical Notes from Barbados*'[53] and Dr G C Low [also] spoke. Dr [E] Ribas, Director of the Sanitary Dept São Paulo, Brazil [also] read a paper on *Yellow Fever*, in which he stated that experience in Brazil completely confirmed the results obtained by American investigators in Cuba. [54] He also gave a lantern demonstration of the statistical aspects of epidemic outbreaks of the disease and their relation to general sanitation and mosquito campaigns. Dr Loudon Strain having spoken of the vast improvement which had recently taken place in the general health, Sir Patrick Manson thanked Dr Ribas for an able and interesting paper, and Dr Ribas replied. ...

At *Council* on **19 March**:

... It was resolved that *Local Secretaries* be appointed [for the first time], and the Secretaries were asked to prepare a geographical list of Fellows residing out of Gt Britain.

A letter from the Secretary of the [ISTM] with reference to the appointment of delegates for the Annual meeting of that Society was ordered to be brought before the next *ordinary* meeting. ...

And at the following *Ordinary* meeting of the Society (with 28 present):

Sir Patrick Manson showed a case of apparent cure of *Kala azar* by atoxyl injection.

A paper by Capt C F Craig NSA on '*Various questions of interest in Tropical Medicine*' was read by Dr Carnegie Brown, and an

Epidiascope demonstration illustrating Dr Craig's conclusions was given. The subjects touched on by Capt Craig were:

- A new species of Filaria, indigenous to the Philippines
- *Entamoeba Coli*
- The Etiology of Dengue
- *Treponema Pertenuis* and the production of yaws.[55]

Dr Low spoke with reference to the species of filaria claimed as distinct by Capt Craig. Dr Sandwith referred to the etiology of dengue fever, and Mr Austen described an epidemic - pappataci [sic] fever, hundsfieber [sic] – akin to Dengue which was conveyed by a species of sandfly – *Phlebotomus Papatassii*. Sir Patrick Manson also spoke.

Two cases of Malta fever both [of] which originated in Northern Nigeria were described by Drs Low and Andrew Foy. ...

At a meeting of *Council* held on **16 April** the first list of Local Secretaries [requested at the last meeting of Council] was announced. This list included 25 geographical locations together with the proposed Local Secretary [the following were included]:

British Guiana	A T Ozzard
The Soudan	Andrew Balfour
Bengal	L Rogers
Ceylon	Albert J Chalmers
South China	Oswald Marriott
Canada	Professor J L Todd

With a mere 15 Fellows present, the proceedings of the *Ordinary* meeting which followed that of *Council*, contained:

> ... A letter from the General Secretary of the [ISTM] (Professor Nuttall) was read, in which he suggested that if any Fellows wished to attend the International Medical Congress at Buda-Pesth [sic], they might be appointed delegates to the meeting of the [ISTM].

[BERI-BERI]

A paper was read by Dr T S Kerr for Dr L Braddon of Seremban [sic] on 'The Etiology of Beri-Beri'.[56]

'*Some notes of observations on Beri-Beri in Sarawak*'[57] was [also] read for Dr A R Wellington by the [Hon] Secretary.

Dr Carnegie Brown, Lt Col Leishman, Dr James Maxwell, Mr Cantlie, Dr Low, and Dr Kerr having spoken on the subject of *Beri-Beri*, Sir Patrick Manson proposed and Mr Cantlie seconded that the remainder of the discussion be postponed until next meeting. This was unanimously agreed to. ...

With the approval of 30 new Fellows at the following *Council* meeting on **21 May** the total of Fellows was about to rise to 300.

Forty-five Fellows and visitors attended the following *Ordinary* meeting; the proceedings of which were:

> ... The discussion on the '*Etiology of Beri-Beri*' ... from the last meeting was resumed, and Drs Daniels, Sir William Treacher, Mr Beddoes, Dr Hartigan , Dr Harold MacFarlane, Professor Ronald Ross, and Sir Patrick Manson spoke on the subject.[58]
>
> Dr [F M] Sandwith brought to the notice of the Fellows a paper (which had been sent home by Dr Stanton of Kuala Lumpur) which was a translation of a work on Beri-Beri written by Dr Jacob Bontius [1592–1631] of Batavia in 1629.[59] The original works of Dr Bontius, which were kindly lent by the [RCP], were also shown.
>
> A communication by Capt [C A] Gill IMS on '*The Epidemiology of Pneumonic Plague*[60]' was read for the author, and Mr Cantlie and Dr Sandwith spoke on the subject. ...

At *Council* on **18 June** at 4.30pm – as usual at 11 Chandos Street:

> ... Professor Ronald Ross moved and Dr Sandwith seconded that Sir Patrick Manson on vacating office should be appointed an Honorary Vice President of the Society. This was carried unanimously. ...

Second AGM

This was held on **18 June 1909** at 5pm. Thirty Fellows and Visitors were present.

... the *Second Annual Report* of Council [see below] with the Treasurer's Report and Financial Statement for the year [to] March 31 1909 was presented and approved.

One of the new Fellows (who was later to take a leading role in the Society) was:

Philip H Bahr [later Manson-Bahr], MB London.

... Sir Patrick Manson introduced Prof Ronald Ross as the duly elected [second] President, and installed him in the Chair. Professor Ross having thanked the Fellows, and the outgoing President for the honour they had done him in electing him President, read his inaugural address [*see* Chapter 3]. ...

Sir Patrick Manson had thus vacated the presidential chair after two years in office – during which he had been present at most meetings. This brought the first two years of the newly founded Society to a close, and it was time for assessment of its future role.

The first two annual reports

The bulk of the *First Report* (1908) has been covered in Chapter 1 and the first part of this Chapter.

... *Finance*

At the end of the first financial year (March 31st [1908]) the income of the Society had been £160 12s., and the expenditure £102 18s 10d, a balance of £57 13s 2d being thus left in hand.

Transactions

A volume of *Transactions*, which will contain a full report of all Papers and discussions up to the end of July 1908, a list of Fellows, and other information [the Report recorded], will be published in the autumn.

Arrangements are now being made by the *Council* for next year, by which [it claimed], *in place of an Annual Volume of Transactions, Reports of the Proceedings of Meetings will be issued and sent to each Fellow monthly* [author's italics].

F M Sandwith
W Carnegie Brown } Hon. Secs.

June 19th, 1908.

The Second Report (1909) contained the following:

Meetings of the Society

The [RSM] being unable to continue the arrangements for housing the Society at 20, Hanover Square, new quarters were obtained from the [MSL] at 11 Chandos Street, Cavendish Square on October 1, 1908; and, since that date, meetings have been held regularly every month at the latter address.

Papers

During the year twenty-four communications have been read, and seven demonstrations ... given on subjects of interest in *tropical medicine* [*see above*]. Among the more important contributions to the work of the Society were papers and discussions on the *rôle* of *Filaria* [sic] in the Production of Disease, the Surgical Treatment of Elephantiasis, Tropical Skin Diseases, Tick Fever, Epidemic Cerebro-spinal Meningitis, the Rat-flea Theory of *Plague*, the Parasitology of *Kala-Azar*, the Epidemiology of *Yellow Fever*, and the Etiology of *Beri-beri*. ...

Transactions

The first volume of the Society's *Transactions*, containing the Proceedings up to July 31, 1908, was published on September 7; and the Council having decided that it would be more advantageous to publish future *Transactions* in parts, five numbers of Volume II (*Transactions* for the year 1908-09) containing full reports of all papers and discussions at seven meetings of the Society, have already been issued to the Fellows.

Finance

During the financial year, which ended March 31, 1909, the Income of the Society (including a balance from last year of £57 13s 2d) was £273 17s 2d [*see below*]. The Expenditure was £218 19s 1d, leaving a balance of £54 18s 1d to be carried forward to next year. The Treasurer's Report and Financial Statement are appended [*see below*].

F M Sandwith
W Carnegie Brown   } Hon. Secs.

June 18, 1909.

Treasurer's Report

The accounts for the year ended March 31, 1909 [see below], show a credit balance of £54 18s 1d, a sum which is almost the same as the surplus brought forward from last year. In view of the fact that the cost of the *Transactions* has been greater than was anticipated, and that the charges for postages on separate issues are considerably more than on a single number, this may be regarded as satisfactory.

As a result of our move to new quarters the items 'Rent' and 'Refreshments' have been much reduced.

The number of Fellows, resident in all parts of the world, is steadily increasing [it then stood at 302], and their subscriptions come in with commendable regularity.

The accounts have been audited and found correct by Mr Beddoes and Dr Bagshawe.

William Hartigan,
Hon Treasurer

June 18, 1909

Financial Statement for the year ended March 31, 1909

	Income			Expenditure			
	£	s.	d.		£	s.	d.
Balance from March 31				Rent	21	0	0
1908	57	13	2	Reporting and Clerical			
Subscriptions	216	4	0	Assistance	26	14	4
				Transactions, Printing,			
				and Stationery	139	1	7
				Postages	14	15	1
				Refreshments, and			
				Petty Charges ..	17	8	1
					£218	19	1
				Balance	54	18	1
	£273	17	2		£273	17	2

W Hartigan

Audited and found correct,

Arthur G Bagshawe

T P Beddoes

May 12, 1909

References and Notes

1   G C Low. A retrospect of tropical medicine from 1894–1914. *Trans R Soc trop Med* 1929; 23: 213–32.

2   *Ibid*.

3   *Ibid*.

4   T Watson. *Lectures on the principles and practice of physic; delivered at King's College, London*. London: John W Parker 1843: 830 + 812.

5   W Osler. *The Principles and practice of medicine for the use of students and practitioners*. 6th ed. London: Sidney Appleton 1905: 1143.

6   A Davidson. *Hygiene and diseases of warm climates*. London: Young J Pentland 1893: 1016. This was without doubt the best and most widely read text on *Diseases of Warm Climates* before Manson's book which was published in 1898.

7   T C Allbutt, H D Rolleston (eds). *A system of medicine by many writers* (part 2). London: MacMillan & Co Ltd 1907: 1055.

8   G C Cook. *Tropical Medicine: an illustrated history of the pioneers*. London: Academic Press 2007: 67–79.

9   M S Dunnill. *The Plato of Praed Street: the life and times of Almroth Wright*. London: RSM Press 2000: 256.

10   *Op cit*. See note 8 above: 145–6.

11   *Ibid*: 145–7.

12   *Ibid*: 103–13. [*See also*: G Williams. *The Plague Killers*. New York: Charles Scribner's Sons 1969: 345].

13   *Ibid*: 219–23.

14   *Ibid*: 153–4.

15   *Ibid*: 197.

16   G C Cook. Tropical Sprue. In: F E G Cox (ed). *The Wellcome Trust Illustrated History of Tropical Diseases*. London: The Wellcome Trust 1996: 356–69. [*See also*: G C Cook. *Tropical Sprue: history of an enigmatic disease* (in preparation)].

17   *Op cit*. See note 8 above: 163.

18   **Robert Thomson Leiper** (1881-1969) was later to play a major role in the establishment of the *London School of Hygiene and Tropical Medicine*.

19   *Op cit*. See note 8 above: 177–82.

20   G C Cook, A I Zumla (eds). *Manson's tropical diseases* 22nd ed. London: Saunders 2009: 1830.

21   **Joseph Chamberlain** FRS MP (1836–1914) who was the British Secretary of State for the Colonies from 1895 until 1903, was very largely instrumental in getting the new discipline launched. [*See also*: P T Marsh. *Joseph Chamberlain: Entrepreneur in Politics*. London: Yale University Press 1994: 724; P T Marsh. Chamberlain, Joseph (Joe) (1836–1914). In: H C G Matthew, B Harrison (eds). *Oxford Dictionary of National Biography*. Oxford: Oxford University Press 2004; 10: 923–34.]

22   G C Cook, A J Webb. The Albert Dock Hospital: the original site (in 1899) of the London School of Tropical Medicine as a new discipline. *Acta trop*: 2001;

79: 249-55; G C Cook. *Disease in the merchant navy: a history of the Seamen's Hospital Society*. Oxford: Radcliffe Publishing 2007: 630.

23 P Manson. Inaugural Address. *Trans Soc trop Med Hyg* 1907–8; 1: 1–12.

24 J W W Stephens. The development of Piroplasma Canis (and other objects of interest). *Trans Soc trop Med Hyg* 1907–8; 1: 13.

25 A Breinl. Demonstration of 'the morphology of Trypanosoma Gambiense'. *Trans Soc trop Med Hyg* 1907–8; 1: 18–19.

26 L Moore, M Nierenstein, J L Todd. Notes on 'the treatment of trypanosomia-sis'. *Trans Soc trop Med Hyg* 1907–8; i: 14–18.

27 J L Todd. Notes on parasite protozoa observed in Africa. *Trans Soc Trop Med Hyg* 1907–8; 1: 297–303.

28 H Johnston. A few notes on sleeping sickness. *Trans Soc trop Med Hyg* 1907–8; 1: 22–24. [*See also*: Anonymous. Johnston. Sir Harry (Hamilton). *Who Was Who, 1916–1928*. London: A & C Black: 560–1; G C Cook. Correspondence from Dr George Carmichael Low to Dr Patrick Manson during the first Ugandan sleeping sickness expedition. *J med Biog* 1993; 1: 215–29.]

29 A R Cook. On sleeping sickness as met with in Uganda, especially with regard to its treatment. *Trans Soc trop Med Hyg* 1907–8; 1: 25–43. [*See also*: A R Cook. *Uganda memories (1897–1940)*. Kampala: The Uganda Society 1945: 415; B O'Brien. *That good physician*. London: Hodder and Stoughton 1962: 264.]

30 P Manson. Demonstration of oriental sore and its parasite. *Trans Soc trop Med Hyg* 1907–8; 1: 44–7.

31 J E Dutton, J L Todd. A note on the morphology of Spirochaeta Duttoni. *Trans Soc trop Med Hyg* 1907–8; 1: 52–9. [*See also*: *Op cit*. See note 8 above: 167–75.]

32 F M Sandwith. A visit to the Tropical School at Hamburg. *Trans Soc trop Med Hyg* 1907–8; 1: 60–7.

33 T F MacDonald. Experiences of ankylostomiasis in Australia. *Trans Soc trop Med Hyg* 1907–8; 1: 68–75.

34 R T Leiper. Physaloptera Mordens: a new intestinal parasite of man. *Trans Soc trop Med Hyg* 1907–8; 1: 76–82.

35 G C Low. The unequal distribution of filariasis in the tropics. *Trans Soc trop Med Hyg* 1907–8; 1: 84–109.

36 W C Brown. Fritz Schaudinn: a biographical sketch. *Trans Soc trop Med Hyg* 1907–8; 1: 110–20.

37 P W Bassett-Smith. Kala-Azar in the Royal Navy. *Trans Soc trop Med Hyg* 1907–8; 1: 121–5.

38 J Cropper. Phenomenal abundance of parasites in the peripheral circulation of a fatal case of pernicious malaria. *Trans Soc trop Med Hyg* 1907–8; 1: 145–8.

39 W T Prout. On the rôle of filaria in the production of disease. *Trans Soc trop Med Hyg* 1907–8; 1: 152–73.

40 W T Prout. Notes on an unusual cause of dysenteric diarrhoea in the tropics. *Trans Soc trop Med Hyg* 1907–8; 1: 194–7.

41 T F MacDonald. Tropical lands and white races. *Trans Soc trop Med Hyg* 1907–8; 1: 201–14.

42 J P Maxwell. The use of quinine during pregnancy, labour, and the puerperium. *Trans Soc trop Med Hyg* 1907–8; 1: 229–35.

43 C F Harford. African tick fever, with special reference to its clinical manifestations. *Trans Soc trop Med Hyg* 1907–8; 1: 241–57.

44 A Castellani. Tropical trichophytosis. *Trans Soc trop Med Hyg* 1907–8; 1: 268–87.

45 A E Horn. An investigation of cerebrospinal fever in the northern territories of the Gold Coast in 1908. *Trans Soc trop Med Hyg* 1908–9; 2: 2–28.

46 W S Handley. A case of Elephantiasis, treated by Lymphangioplasty. *Trans Soc trop Med Hyg* 1908–9; 2: 41–9.

47 J Cantlie. The sigmoid flexure and rectum in post-dysenteric diarrhoea, sprue, and mucous colitis. *Trans Soc trop Med Hyg* 1908–9; 2: 59–71.

48 W C Hossack. The present position of the rat-flea theory of plague: recent observations in Calcutta. *Trans Soc trop Med Hyg* 1908–9; 2: 75–96.

49 G F Petrie. A short abstract of the Plague Commission's work in Bombay with regard to the rat-flea theory. *Trans Soc trop Med Hyg* 1908–9; 2: 97–107.

50 W S Patton. The parasite of Kala-Azar and allied organisms. *Trans Soc trop Med Hyg* 1908–9; 2: 113–21.

51 F M Sandwith. 'Jedda ulcer' and the non-identity of Nile boils with Oriental Sore. *Trans Soc trop Med Hyg* 1908–9; 2: 142–4.

52 H G Waters. Presentation of specimens of spirochaeta believed to be pathogenic to man, causing fever and bronchitis with thin mucoid expectoration. *Trans Soc trop Med Hyg* 1908–9; 2: 145–8.

53 T F MacDonald. Tropical notes from Barbados. *Trans Soc trop Med Hyg* 1908–9; 2: 151–2.

54 E Ribas. The extinction of yellow fever in the state of São Paulo (Brazil) and in the City of Rio de Janeiro *Trans Soc trop Med Hyg* 1908–9; 2: 154–63.

55 C F Craig. Observations of the United States Army Board for the Study of Tropical Diseases in the Philippine Islands upon Filaria Philippinensis, Entamoeba Coli, the etiology of dengue, and Treponema Pertenuis and the experimental production of Yaws in monkeys. *Trans Soc trop Med Hyg* 1908–9; 2: 172–94.

56 L Braddon. The cause of true or tropical beri-beri. *Trans Soc trop Med Hyg* 1908–9; 2: 212–25.

57 A R Wellington. Notes on beri-beri. *Trans Soc trop Med Hyg* 1908–9; 2: 226–31.

58 Adjourned discussion on the cause of beri-beri. *Trans Soc trop Med Hyg* 1908–9; 2: 245–56.

59 F M Sandwith. A historical note on beri-beri and rice, from the writings of Dr Bontius. *Trans Soc trop Med Hyg* 1908–9; 2: 257–9.

60 C A Gill. A note of the epidemiology of pneumonic plague. *Trans Soc trop Med Hyg* 1908–9; 2: 260–8.

Chapter 3

Ross's presidency: 'from a very tender plant to a very vigorous tree' – 1909–11

Chapter 3

Ross's presidency: 'from a very tender plant to a very vigorous tree' – 1909–11

Two years after its foundation, Professor (later Sir) Ronald Ross CB FRCS FRS (*see* Figure 3.1) (*see* also: References and Notes to Chapter 1) succeeded Manson as president. Before introducing him, Manson outlined the progress of the Society which 'from a very tender plant … had grown up to be a very vigorous tree'; the fellowship had in 1909 risen to 306. Like Manson, Ross (although much younger) was then a major national and international figure; his work at Secunderabad and Calcutta, India, which clinched the rôle of the mosquito in the transmission of *Plasmodium* sp infection had captured the public's imagination. The accepted viewpoint prior to this had been that malaria was caused by a miasma.[1] Taken in conjunction, Manson's and Ross's researches had paved the way for the discovery that yellow fever (a viral infection) is also mosquito-borne. However, Ross did not dwell on this theme (*ie malaria*) when he delivered his presidential address '**The future of tropical medicine**' at 11 Chandos Street, Cavendish Square, on **18 June 1909**. Nor did he touch on *clinical* medicine, unlike Manson two years before. Instead, he dwelt on his favourite theme – 'hygiene'. He began:

> Gentlemen, – I had hoped to acknowledge the honour which you have done me to-day in electing me your President by an address which should contain a worthy survey of the wonderful advances recently made in that science and art – nay, rather that family of sciences and arts – which under the name of *Tropical Medicine* we have banded ourselves together to serve. But on attempting the task I found it to be beyond the limits both of my time and my capacity; and I trust, therefore, that you will bear with me if I move towards an easier but perhaps more profitable theme. The past is passed – already shaped and done with; but the future is before us, to be moulded by reason and labour. Will you permit

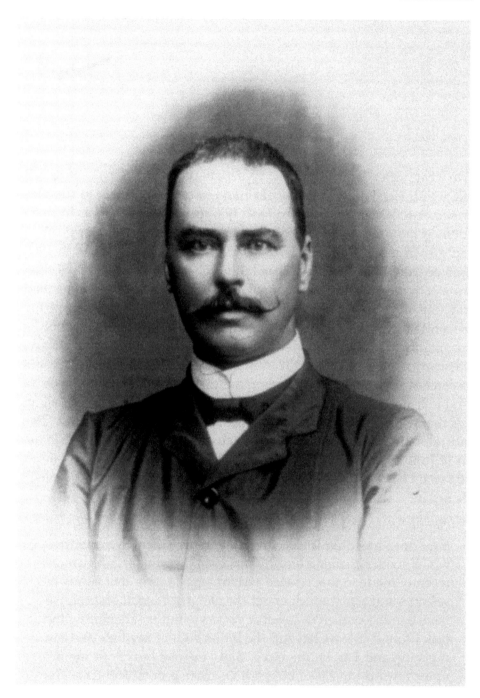

Figure 3.1: (Sir) Ronald Ross KBE, FRS (1857–1932) – second president of the Society (1909–11) (reproduced courtesy the Wellcome Library, London).

me, then, to lay before you very briefly, for your consideration and judgement, some thoughts … on a few points which I believe to be connected with the future of *Tropical Medicine*?

Ross then dealt first with the effect of disease on whole countries – and even continents, as well as on individuals:

> … It would be well if our historical and medical writers would deal more thoroughly with this interesting subject. The work of Mr W H S Jones and Drs G G Ellett and L T Withington on the probable influence of malaria on Greek history is known to you. [2] The failure of nations is often ascribed to many causes, but too seldom to one which may be a predominant cause – endemic disease. Weakness of national character should tend to be effaced by natural competition from outside. The effect of climate – mere heat and moisture – should be met by gradual acclimatization; and many of the most vigorous animals flourish in what we consider are the most enervating countries. Yet we know that certain regions breed strong races and others weak ones. Why, for instance, has that great continent, Africa, remained so long barbarous, in spite of its proximity to Europe, while India and China – countries as warm as it is – swarm with civilized or semi-civilized millions? I hazard the effect of malaria in this case; but in other cases, other diseases – perhaps bilharziasis in Lower Egypt, and ankylostomiasis, amoebic dysentery and filariasis in many fertile areas. Palaeontology tells us of whole races of animals extinguished, and archaeology of whole civilizations wiped out; but the disease factor in such events has probably been more potent than hitherto admitted.

What was it, he asked, that led to 'physical deterioration' in many large cities in the tropics?

> … As a curious hypothesis I may venture to suggest helminthiasis – especially *Ascaris* infection, which is … so extremely common in tropical cities. But we should endeavour to go beyond mere conjectures; and I can hope for the time when pathological maps and surveys will be attempted with the object of finding correlation between the physical state of a people and the prevalence of diseases among them.

This was followed by speculation on the origins of various religious practices in some tropical countries – for example, the Hebrews and Hindus:

> ... Many of these can scarcely be based on moral or even on sacerdotal grounds, and must, I think, have been enjoined for sanitary reasons at times when the priests were also the physicians – such as rules regarding fasting and the washing of hands before food, and segregated cooking and water supply. It would be interesting to examine these anew in the light of our present knowledge of parasitology.

His perceptive remarks concerning medical publication (both contemporary and historical) are as relevant (probably more so) today than they were when he gave the address:

> ... Nothing is more instructive and more stimulating to the intelligent student than the record of the difficulties, the failures and the successes of the human mind in its efforts to gain the truth. A good book on the labours of the early pioneers – written now, before the mist of time has obscured their names and works – would be most welcome[3]; and especially, I think, should it be appropriate for our young Society to encourage such a noble study. But I have another thing to suggest – a new class of monograph. The general text-book on *tropical medicine*, written by a single author [such as Manson's great work of 1898[4]], is now becoming impossible. I will not depreciate any writer by remarking that, whatever may have been the case in the past, the gigantic infant is rapidly growing beyond the control of any sole nurse, wet or dry. A man is fortunate if he knows thoroughly even one item of our subject. Moreover, advance is so quick that many chapters of such text-books become obsolete a few months after publication. Even the monograph, written by the most capable expert of the time, is apt to become wrinkled and old immediately after birth, and is superseded by another a few weeks younger. The kind of monograph which I suggest will at least remain always of value, since it will consist, not of the work of a single individual, but of reprints of classical papers, or of extracts from such, strung together on a historical thread. What more interesting than to have such a book at hand – not to supplement the ordinary

monograph, but to furnish the student with a genuine record of discoveries written in words of those who made them.

On the subject of instruction and *education* in *tropical medicine*, and *sanitation*, Ross had this to say:

> … I do not know what we who are called upon to teach are to do for lack of time. Medicine, sanitation, pathology, parasitology, medical entomology, all in three months. Yet the time for a fuller course cannot apparently be granted. The only solution seems to be that some of our baggage should be unpacked into the general medical curriculum. This has been much widened of late, in order to admit especially the higher departments of professional knowledge. I think, therefore, that the time has come when it should contain much completer instruction in parasitology, and also something of medical entomology. These sciences should be instilled to such a point that the man qualified for general medical practice shall possess the power of identifying all the human parasites and their carriers, generically at least; and that he shall know how to use a microscope for any practical purpose. He ought also to have – in this Imperial country at least – a clearer view of the list of tropical maladies. The degree or diploma certifies that its holder is competent to practise anywhere – in the Tropics as in Britain; but this becomes untrue if the instruction referred to is not given. Certainly the large majority of qualified medical men are called upon to practise here only; but still a considerable number take up work in plantations, mines, ships, and Government services in the Tropics; so that some preparation in the subjects I mention seems to be demanded in the general curriculum. If this cannot be done, the only course will be, I fear, to separate sanitation from medicine in our diplomas, and to give three months to each. I do not like the idea much, especially as practical tropical sanitation cannot easily be taught at home; but what else are we to do?

Clinical practice, he said had advanced, but mostly in the area of diagnosis in which microscopic presence of malaria, dysentery, and the 'blood diagnosis' of typhoid and Malta fevers were important, but he felt that the future lay in therapeutics:

... Already great foreshadowings of this are apparent. The application of atoxyl [*see* Chapter 2] with other agents to trypanosomiasis and, perhaps, several parasitic diseases, the more continuous use of quinine in malaria, correct serum therapy in plague, various radiations in numerous maladies, all point the direction of the coming advance. We are apt to ridicule the old subject of treatment by drugs, but it is by no means exhausted. Rather we should demand much fuller researches upon it – exhaustive researches, chemical and experimental, regarding the effect of drugs on parasitism, animal and vegetable. On the nature, structure, and classification of parasites our investigation has been immense, fundamental and all fruitful, but we have still to find, in most cases, how to drive them out of existence in the human body. We are still ignorant as to how exactly quinine acts in malaria, and we may be able to find even a better cure. Serum-therapy has been a great advance, but our resources are not yet finished. We should ransack our armoury for every possible weapon. I have long thought that we have never made sufficient use of such simple agents as high and low external temperatures, and I hope shortly to commence work on the subject. Of course, much purely pathological research remains to be done, but I do think that the next great chapter in our book will be a therapeutical one.

But, as anyone with a knowledge of Ross's major interest at this time would anticipate, the most extensive section of the address was devoted to 'sanitary practice' (*ie preventive* medicine):

... The first [remark] deals with the housing of the poor, especially in towns – a burning question in all countries, and the basis, not only of sanitation, but of government. For whatever science may discover, the practical prevention of disease will always remain impossible where the poor – the bulk of the people – are compelled to live, like animals, in the midst of filth and squalor, and whatever governments may aim at, whatever high ideals of liberty, law and justice, the man so housed will remain base and miserable. I take this as the first great principle of sanitation. For figure to ourselves what the modern city is: a few fine public buildings, squares and parks, many good dwelling houses, and a wilderness of hovels and kennels, called slums. But it is not impossible to banish slums. Two years ago I met in Berlin a number of members of the Corporation of Liverpool who had been studying the subject in Germany, and who confessed that they had scarcely seen such things there. We can find none in Stockholm, either. But you all know them in other countries, and especially in the crowded cities of warm climates. It is not exactly true that they are produced by poverty – rather, they produce poverty; they make a lower caste of man – degenerates, living, so to speak, on the waste and refuse of the richer classes, like the dogs of Constantinople! A miserable sight, but one which, we trust, the future will banish from our eyes. The statesmen and the artist join us. We know well how to deal with slums – honest and enlightened administration, good building laws, and discipline in enforcing them. For the Tropics – is there really any reason why the natives in towns should be so terribly housed? Bamboo-shelters and mud-huts swarming with vermin, noisome yards strewn with rubbish, unspeakable latrines, broken gutters, and poisonous wells! Our first duty should be [to] try to better this condition of things.[5]

Removal of 'town refuse' was next tackled:

… For several reasons, sewerage is at present difficult in most tropical towns, and we have to fall back upon removal by sweepers and carts. This is not only a noisome process, but one which constantly cripples the sanitary budget of municipalities. After much consideration, I have been preaching that the solution may be found in some development, suitable for houses, of the septic tank principle – some kind of well-made cesspit such as is used in Egypt. But another, and perhaps better, idea will be found in papers by Colonel Haines and Surgeon-General Hamilton in the *Indian Medical Gazette* for 1907 and 1908 – depending upon an extremely cheap and yet quite inoffensive process of incineration. [6] The matter is well worth study by formal investigation; it is only one of several subjects connected with practical sanitation, such as house-construction for the poor and the management of wells in the Tropics, which require more scientific consideration. Pathological enquiry has grown immensely, but the time has come when a number of practical questions like these should receive more attention from our soldiers of research.

Plague and 'other maladies' could not be eliminated, he claimed, by *extermination* of vermin alone; therefore tropical towns 'must be built and so governed that no kinds of vermin can thrive in them'. This could be achieved 'only by science and discipline'. And of 'sanitary organisation' in the tropics:

> ... Scarcely more than half a century has elapsed since any such organization was attempted anywhere. Before that time, even in this country, sanitation was in the hands of town councillors – guided, seldom by experts, but usually by energetic laymen. Special health officers then began to be appointed, and special sanitary diplomas to be given by certain examining bodies. Health Acts were passed, and the present British organizations were established – good in many respects, but by no means perfect. Similarly, in the Tropics, sanitation was generally urged forward by energetic individuals, laymen or doctors. India made the first great advance by the appointment of Sanitary Commissioners and their assistants, and by the institution of the annual sanitary report; and many tropical cities now commenced to employ special health officers. Many of our colonies, however, have not even yet risen to this pitch, their sanitation being mostly in the hands of local medical officers (who are given special allowances for attending to such work), and no adequate special reports are published. Recently, India has appointed a head to its sanitary service, but I gather that he is rather a statistician and inspector than the commander-in-chief of an army. Very rarely do the chiefs, either of the Sanitary or of the Medical Services, have a seat on the local executive council; while in many cases sanitary officers are appointed who possess no special sanitary qualification.

Ross then outlined in considerable detail his practical solution(s) to the problem of sanitation in tropical countries:

> I hope and trust that the future will show improvement in these respects. Every town of considerable size should be in the charge of a whole-time health officer who should possess diplomas

both of *public health* and of *tropical medicine*, and who should be assisted by a proper staff of inspectors and labourers. Every large village and rural area, in countries which are at all civilized, should be in the charge at least of a qualified sanitary inspector … The labourers, sanitary inspectors, and health officers are only the soldiers, sergeants and captains of the sanitary army, and we know what an army becomes without a general. I submit that every tropical country or colony must have a whole-time chief sanitary officer to inspect and direct the units under his command, and that this office should hold a place of proper power and influence in the public councils, not second to that held by the chiefs of other departments – military, judicial, ecclesiastical, educational, financial, and public works. Moreover, for large territories, he should be assisted by a staff corresponding to the general staff of an army – that is to say, by a number of men specially qualified to deal with special branches of his department; let me say, one man for water and food supply, one for drainage, one for conservancy and house sanitation, one for statistics, one for vaccination, one for mosquito-borne diseases and one or more for epidemics. Personally, I should like to have the whole *clinical* side made into one of these sub-departments, in its logical place, as at Panama. Still further, in a large country (like India, for example), I think that each section of the department should be provided with a certain number of men engaged upon research on the work of that section. For smaller colonies, of course, the scheme must be modified according to circumstances.

He further expanded on this theme using analogies in organisation within the Army. Ross then followed this with a few philosophical (and emotional) words on *research* into *tropical medicine*:

… To enter upon research is to stand upon the brink of an infinity where every step leads to other steps and every discovery to a thousand secrets. Endless toil – but every step there is a gain to the whole of humanity, and every discovery a treasure. Of what other class of efforts dare we say so much? When we look round upon the multitudinous labours of mankind we are struck by the fact that most of them end only in personal or local profit. The great masses of men toil for their own subsistence, and that of their families. Others, perhaps less fortunate, spend their lives merely in gathering for themselves unnecessary and indigestible riches, often at the expense of their fellows. Others, again, more fortunate, are able, by doing their duty, to shed some halo of benefaction around themselves – but often how small a halo! Even many of those whose names fill our history books have really helped the world but little – leaders only of intertribal wars – kings of hamlets and conquerors of parishes. Where are now the works of Turenne and Marlborough – the victories of Napoleon? Or take the statesmen who are said to have led the world – I see in them, for the most part, only begetters of petty rivalries.

Ross then introduced a theme which is topical even today in Britain:

… For two centuries we in this country have heard round us everywhere the din of party politics – the dogmatists and demagogues tearing each other's hair amid the tub-thumping of a thousand newspapers. With what result? A cynic might remark with some truth that the net result of British party politics during two centuries has principally been the creation of the British slum. All these are mere intermolecular contentions, generating heat without work.

Far above this noise, those peaceful sisters, Science and Art, sit weaving the real fabric of civilization. The man who discovers a single law of Nature, constructs a single useful instrument, or creates a great work of art, benefits, not only his neighbours his nation and his age, but all nations and all ages. And he gives his gift, not at the cost of the blood or misery of others, but out of his own brain – for nothing. And of all discoveries that can be made, which are so great as those that save our very lives? Think of those mighty pestilences which wander to and fro over the face of the earth, each of them slaying, crippling and disfiguring every year millions of human beings – tuberculosis, cancer, pneumonia, typhoid, malaria, dysentery, cholera, filariasis, and a score of others. Compared with them, what are the little battles, heats, and triumpheries round us? Do we care a jot whether a Whig or a Tory wins in the great tongue-fight of to-day? But we do if our children are snatched from us, or if we are dashed to earth in the days of our strength. A few months ago I was in a great Indian temple dedicated to the Destroyer, Shiva, and saw the dreadful presentation of him in his mood. The face is beautiful, but touched with anger; the upper canine teeth project over the lower lip, the right hand grasps a spear on which a human being is impaled, the left hand gathers the blood in a bowl. That is the allegory of the Thing we have to face. But not only does he destroy the body; we medical men know, I say, that he maims the mind also. We are here wiser than the dogmatists. What would the world be without these subtle poisons penetrating everywhere, secretly corrupting, suddenly assassinating – which we call the infectious diseases. I say, the man who finds the cause or cure of any one of them does the greatest work that a man can do. I say, the very greatest work. Such is medical research, and it is your duty and privilege to undertake it.

The reader can of course, gain an insight into Ross's mind (including his great poetic gifts) from these remarks; he then added, however, a word of caution:

… Do not think that when you have made your discovery, great or small, you have finished the matter. It was not given to you for you to sleep upon it. Medical research is not a mere academical amusement consisting in the publication of elegant articles adorned with coloured plates. The discovery is only half-way up the mountain, and beyond it extends the arduous summit of the practical application. [The theme of application of discoveries to medical practice was pursued by Manson in the discussion which followed the lecture – *see* below]. It is your duty to attain that summit. This is a lesson which our whole profession would do well to consider more deeply. Our theory and our practice are too apt to wander apart; our practice, in fact, to lag far behind our theory – especially our sanitary practice. They should walk hand in hand. And why is this? Because, I think, our profession is not sufficiently well organized; is a body without a head; has no central nervous system. We do not, as a profession, take a sufficiently firm stand with the world on medical and sanitary matters. We do not sufficiently rally together in the battle of life round our great standard. We are apt to take too haughty a view of our scientific superiority – to stand above and apart and to contemplate men as children gathering berries and catching butterflies below us. But in this we do *not* perform our duty. It is for us to descend and save them from the dangers which we know threaten them. It is not enough for us to discover; we have also to teach, beseech, demand and command. Science is above the world; but, also, duty is above science.

And, Ross concluded this *second* presidential address to the STMH – which is in many respects complementary to that of Manson's in 1907 – thus:

> … the past has given us much regarding the theory of our subject, let us hope that the future will give us more regarding its practice. Above all, let us pray that our profession will shortly take, more determinedly than heretofore, its appointed place in the world as the army of humanity against disease.[7]

Discussion then took place on Ross's Address:

> Sir Patrick Manson said that Professor Ronald Ross was one of the poets of science who had the faculty of finding articulation for ideas which occurred to many minds. The opinions expressed in connection with the duty of the profession – not only in the direction of research but the necessity of getting the results of research applied in practice – were very important, and they had not been formulated definitely before. The application of their present knowledge to the benefit of the less civilized communities of the world was the most important problem in the *tropical medicine* of the present day. Of course everyone desired to see these theories applied, but the practical difficulties hitherto had apparently been insurmountable, and the principal reason was that they, as a profession, had not been sufficiently active as apostles of their science. They had not preached their doctrines with convincing eloquence and … had not got the public to accept them. If the public believed that they themselves would be benefited, without doubt the suggestions would be adopted. He had been impressed by a remark made the other day by Lord Morley [1838–1923][8] in a notable speech to the journalists of the Empire, in which he quoted [Oliver] Cromwell as saying:

'Brethren, in the name of Christ, I beseech you to think if it be not possible that you may be mistaken'. Governments were often blamed for not adopting the suggestions of science. The reason for that was, he believed, that Government had been taught by experience not to put their money too freely on scientific recommendations. They had been taken in too often, so to speak. For example, in India millions of pounds had been wasted on the idea that cholera was an air-borne disease, solely in consequence of the profession thrusting on the Government erroneous views. Scientific men must first convince the rulers and the people thoroughly, and when Government really believed what they said their recommendations would be carried out.[9]

Dr [W] Hartigan said he had great pleasure in seconding the vote of thanks to Professor Ross. [He] had called their attention to the fact that they had to place duty before science, and this was an important point which they ought to keep steadily before them. Their duty was to keep on trying, to keep on explaining what was really required, to refuse to be rebuffed, and to do their best to get what they considered necessary for the community carried out.

Following this address and the discussion which followed, Manson moved and Hartigan seconded a vote of thanks from the Society be given to the president for his able and eloquent address. This motion was unanimously carried.

The first of the Society's annual dinners

The first annual *dinner* of the Society was held following Ross's address; *Transactions* recorded:

The first annual dinner of the *Society of Tropical Medicine and Hygiene* was held on June 18, 1909, at the Trocadero Restaurant. Professor Ronald Ross, CB, FRS, presided, and among those present were Colonel Seely, MP, Sir Archibald Geikie, Sir Henry Morris, Sir Alfred Jones, Sir Patrick Manson, Professor Count Mőrner, Sir Havelock Charles, Sir A Haslam, Sir William Treacher, Sir Rubert Boyce, and Mr Ramsay Macdonald MP [a future Prime Minister].

Colonel [later Sir Charles] Seely [1833–1915][10], in proposing
'Success to the Society', spoke of its efforts to abolish the plagues
which oppress the people in tropical climes. What had been the
results of the Society's work? He thought they had been amazing.
From information which he had obtained at the Colonial Office
it was fair to say that half a million people had died of *sleeping
sickness* alone in Uganda, but, owing to the discovery of the
method by which it was propagated, the ravages of that disease
had been, if not stopped, at least reduced to quite one-tenth of
what it was formerly. The public were under a great obligation
to the Society, for its members were vicariously paying the
enormous debt which the white man owed to the black races
in tropical countries for the awful wrongs perpetrated on them
in the past. In conclusion, he said that Lord Crewe [1858–1945]
[11] and himself – and in this matter he felt he could pledge his
successors at the Colonial Office – would do all they could to
further the Society's noble work.

Sir Alfred Jones [1846–1909] [*see* below] said it was a
remarkable thing that the investigation of tropical diseases was
not undertaken earlier. In Liverpool they had spent £100,000 on
the work and £28,000 in sending out expeditions, and it was the
best expenditure they had ever incurred.

Sir Rubert Boyce [1863–1911] said that on all sides they saw
the principles of tropical sanitation, as first enunciated by Sir
Patrick Manson, being adopted. He believed that *yellow fever*
[*YF*] was a disease of the past in the West Indian group. In the
Isthmian [Panama] Canal zone, in the time of M. de Lesseps,
48,000 men employed on the canal works died, but during the
last three years there had not been a single case of [*YF*] in that
zone.

The Chairman [Ross], in acknowledging the toast, said that the
members of the Society were now numbered over 300, most of
whom were doing their duty that night in the Tropics. Mr [Joseph]
Chamberlain [1836–1914] really began this movement, and he
proposed that they should send him a message. He acknowledged
the help given by Mr Lyttelton, Lord Elgin, Lord Crewe, and all
the officials at the Colonial Office, and said that Sir Alfred Jones
had been one of their most generous supporters. This country
had led the way in research in *tropical medicine*, and he hoped

it would now lead the way in the practical application of those researches.

Sir Patrick Manson gave the toast of 'The Guests', which was responded to by Sir Archibald Geikie, Sir Henry Morris, and Count Mörner. The health of 'The Chairman' was proposed by Mr Ramsay Macdonald MP [1866–1937].

The following telegram was [then] forwarded to Mr Chamberlain [*see above*]:

> The *Society of Tropical Medicine* thanks you for the great services to *tropical medicine* rendered by you. Sent at the first banquet of the Society. – Ronald Ross, President.

A reply was afterwards received from Mr Chamberlain expressing his great appreciation of the kind message and of the goodwill of the Society, to which he sent his best wishes for its success.[12]

The Society during Ross's presidency

The Society was therefore by late 1909 (with Sir Ronald Ross now installed as president) in 'full swing'. It was agreed that Cantlie be treasurer, and Carnegie Brown and Harford joint secretaries for the following two years. However, as today, various relatively trivial matters were raised at meetings of *Council*; for example, on **16 July 1909** a minute records:

> Dr Carnegie Brown read a letter from Dr Moss a medical missionary in Madagascar suggesting that some reduction in the subscription might be made to Fellows resident abroad. After … discussion it was proposed by Dr O Baker and seconded by Sir R Havelock Charles [who was to become the fourth President] that, as a provisional measure, medical missionaries when resident abroad might on application have their subscription reduced to half a guinea yearly. This was unanimously agreed to.

At the *Ordinary* meeting (Table 3.1 summarises the subjects and speakers at these meetings under Ross's presidency) which followed at 8.30pm (with 15 Fellows and visitors present), several presentations were made, including ones as diverse as: an amoebic abscess of the spleen, a case of blackwater fever[13], 'Preventable diseases in Siam'[14] and 'Fevers in Rangoon'.[15]

Table 3.1: Ordinary meetings during Ross's presidency

Date	Subject	Speaker
1909		
16 July	Amoebic abscess of spleen Blackwater fever	J Preston Maxwell (Amoy)
	Preventable diseases in Siam	P G Woolley (Ornaha)
	Fevers in Rangoon	J R Forrest (RAMC)
15 October	Recent advances in Sleeping Sickness	A G Bagshawe
19 November	Several epidiascopic demonstrations	H W Thomas
	Guinea worm of Nevis	J N Rat (Nevis, British West Indies).
17 December	Tick fever infection	W B Leishman
	Non-ulcerating oriental sore	A Balfour, D B Thompson (RAMC)
	Linguatulidae parasitic to man	L W Sambon
1910		
21 January	Ankylostomiasis in non-tropical countries	Sir Thomas Oliver (Newcastle on Tyne)
	Ankylostomiasis in Natal	J J Elliott (Rostrevor)
18 February	Dipterus insects	E E Austen
	Calabar swellings	Sir Patrick Manson
	Etiology of beri-beri	H Fraser, A T Stanton
18 March	Latency of malarial infection	O Baker
	Fever with urticarial rash [Katayama syndrome]	A C Lambert (Kin Kuang)
	Typhoid prophylaxis	E I Vaughn (Panama Commission)
	Immunity from Sleeping Sickness	G Campbell (Congo State)
27 May	Functional psychoses in dark races	R Howard (Zanzibar)
	Schistomum japonicum infection	H S Houghton
	Bionomics of helminths	W Nicholl (Lister Institute)
25 June (3rd AGM)	Study of parasitic disease	R Ross
	Blackwater fever/Haemoglobinaemia	J O W Barratt
21 October	Research on sleeping sickness	A G Bagshawe
18 November	Yellow fever in West Africa	Sir Rubert Boyce FRS (Liverpool School of Tropical Medicine)
16 December	Causative agent of yellow fever	H Seidelin (Yucatan)
1911		
20 January	Discussion of Boyce's paper (*see* above) [Subject not stated in minutes]	W T Prout (Liverpool School of Tropical Medicine)
17 February	Eggs of *Schistosoma japonicum*	R T Leiper
	Studies on malaria & sleeping sickness	R Ross (Liverpool School of Tropical Medicine)

Date	Subject	Speaker
17 March	Yaws treatment	R P Strong (Manila)
	Santonin in intestinal infections	J Preston Maxwell (Amoy)
18 May	Zambesi fever	W J Bruce (Zambesia)
	Quinine prophylaxis of malaria	W Carnegie Brown
	Streptothrix of white mycetoma	N F Surveyor (Bombay)
16 June (4th AGM)	Alastrim, amaas or milkpox	E Ribas (São Paulo)
	Leishman's *presidential address* (*see* Chapter 4)	W B Leishman.

The popularity of the Society was clearly on the ascendancy, and at a *Council* meeting held at 8.15pm on **15 October**, also at 11 Chandos Street, no less than 54 candidates were *approved* for election; they included:

> *315* Sir David Bruce CB FRS, Uganda
> *328* A A D McCabe-Dallas LRCP, Liverpool
> *329* Sir Thomas Oliver MD FRCP, Newcastle
> *366* Warrington Yorke MD, Runcorn

> A letter was read from Dr George Pernet [sic] suggesting that the hour of meeting be changed to 5pm. After some discussion it was agreed to send an inquiry to each Fellow as to which hour would best suit his convenience.

And a paper by Dr A G Bagshawe at the following *Ordinary* meeting at 8.30pm, at which 63 Fellows and visitors were present, was devoted to '*Recent advances in our knowledge of Sleeping Sickness*'[16] followed by a histological demonstration of this disease, showing 'lesions of the Brain'. Drs [D N] Nabarro [1874–1958], Low and others took part in the discussion.

Minutes of a *Council* meeting held on **19 November** contained:

> An invitation from *The Liverpool School of Tropical Medicine* for the Society to meet [for the first time] at Liverpool on March 19th 1910 was accepted.

The subjects of presentations at the *Ordinary* meeting that day were: Oesophagostomiasis[17], experimental studies with yellow fever [YF][18], mossy foot of the Amazon region[19], Stimson's spirochaete (in a case)[20] (all presented by H W Thomas) and '*The so-called guinea worm of the Island of Nevis*'.[21] *Transactions* at that time conveyed a verbatim reflection of the content of the *Ordinary* meetings. In fact, this journal (unlike today's version) conveyed the precise content(s) of the *Ordinary* meeting, rather than being a medium for original communications in *tropical medicine* and clinical parasitology.

At the following *Council* meeting on **17 December**:

> Resolutions drafted by Sir Patrick Manson relative to the death of Sir Alfred Jones KCMG, and by Col. Baker to the gift of Mr Otto Beit were approved and ordered to be placed on the agenda of the *Ordinary* meeting to be held [that] evening [*see* below].
>
> The Secretaries stated that several Fellows had asked if papers in French would be received by the Society, and published in the *Transactions*. [It was] Resolved, that if approved by the Council, papers in 'French be published in the Transactions', a précis in English having been read before the Society.

Among Fellows *approved* for election, at that meeting were:

> *398* Albert R Cook MD Lond FRCS, Uganda
> *400* John H Cook FRCS MB, Uganda

And the following were [then] appointed *Honorary* Fellows of the Society:

> Lt Col. W C Gorgas (previously elected, but [had] not replied)
> Professor Raphael Blanchard, Paris
> Professor Robert Koch, Berlin (has accepted. W.I.B)
> Professor Angelo Celli, University of Rome
> Professor J Mannaberg, Vienna
> Professor Shibamuro Kitasato, University of Tokio, Japan
> (previously elected but [had] not replied)

Among the new *local* Secretaries was:

> Philip H Bahr MB, Secretary for Fiji [who had been elected on 18 June 1909 – *see* Chapter 2].

At the *Ordinary* meeting the same day (with 70 Fellows and visitors present) the following minutes were recorded:

> The following resolution proposed by Sir Patrick Manson, seconded by Sir Havelock Charles and supported by Dr Harford was carried unanimously:

> That this Society, recognising the great services rendered to *Tropical Medicine* by Sir Alfred Jones KCMG, desires to record its appreciation of those services, and sense of loss in his death. Further, that the Secretaries be instructed to communicate this resolution to Sir Alfred Jones's family, and to convey to them the sympathy of the Society in their bereavement.

The following resolution proposed by Lt Col O Baker, and seconded by Sir William Leishman was [also] carried unanimously:

> That the President be requested on behalf of the Fellows of this Society to convey to Mr Otto Beit their high appreciation of the great benefit he has conferred on scientific medicine, and the study of disease including tropical disease, by his munificent grant for the endowment of research.

A paper was later read by Sir William Leishman on tick fever,[22] and one by Capt Douglas Thomson RAMC, on non-ulcerating Oriental sore[23] ... taken as read and published in the *Transactions*. Also, Dr Sambon read a note on '*The Linguatulidae parasitic in man*'.[24]

On the two resolutions carried at that meeting, *Transactions* carried the following contributions:

- *Death of Sir Alfred Jones.* Before the business of the meeting [on 17 December 1909] was proceeded with – Sir Patrick Manson said he had a Resolution to submit to the Fellows of the Society. He presumed they were all aware that their distinguished President was not present that evening for a cause which was most unfortunately something in the nature of a calamity for workers in *Tropical Medicine*. Professor Ross that afternoon had attended the funeral of Sir Alfred Jones. Nobody acquainted with the history of the public recognition of the value of *Tropical Medicine* knew better than the Fellows present the important role that Sir Alfred ... had played in the furtherance of this subject, both in this country and abroad. When Mr Joseph Chamberlain [*see above*] first brought to public notice the great importance of *Tropical Medicine* as a factor in colonial development, Sir Alfred ..., with characteristic energy and generosity, came forward with practical assistance.

  He was mainly instrumental in developing and supporting the *School of Tropical Medicine in Liverpool*, but his efforts were not confined to Liverpool. He looked upon the School of Tropical Medicine there as merely a means towards the end, viz., the fostering of *Tropical Medicine* in connection with the developing of the Colonies; and as a consequence of this view he extended his interest to the London School also. He was a generous benefactor of the *London School of Tropical Medicine*, and indeed of any individual who showed a claim for consideration, whether as a leader or as a humble student in *Tropical Medicine*. He (Manson) could speak personally for this. Although at first quite a stranger to Sir Alfred ..., in his (Manson's) visits to Liverpool and elsewhere, Sir Alfred ... had always extended a generous hand, and had always backed him up with his great influence. He (Manson) thought everyone interested in *Tropical Medicine* who came in contact with Sir Alfred ..., experienced the same treatment. It had therefore been suggested, and it was his (Manson's) privilege to warmly support the suggestion, that a resolution should be passed by the Society, and forwarded to the family of Sir Alfred ..., to the following effect [*see above*].

Sir Havelock Charles said that when he saw the death of Sir Alfred Jones reported a few days ago, he was forcibly stuck with a sense of irreparable loss which the *School of Tropical Medicine at Liverpool* had suffered. Sir Alfred ... had been a successful man in life; he was also a successful man in death, in that he had left behind him a reputation of doing good to his fellow men. It had been a great thing (as Manson had just said) that, at a time when *Tropical Medicine* had but a few friends in England, a man with the determination and the good will of Sir Alfred ... had been present to give a helping hand. He desired to warmly second the resolution which had just been moved. Dr C F Harford, in supporting the motion, said he had had the privilege of knowing Sir Alfred ... for the past eighteen years, not only in connection with his work in furtherance of *Tropical Medicine*, but in what he had done for West Africa. He was confident that all the Fellows would recognise the splendid efforts he had put forward in the opening up of that hitherto very much neglected country, West Africa. Dr F M Sandwith, who occupied the chair, said he was sure they would all emphatically agree with the sentiments of the mover and supporters of the resolution. He would formally put to them the resolution which ... Manson had read [*see above*]. He took it that it was their wish that a copy of that resolution should be sent to the family of Sir Alfred ...; but it had also been suggested that a similar resolution should be sent to the *Liverpool School of Tropical Medicine*, who had lost their head and chief ornament – their President: also that copies should be sent for publication in the *Times* and one of the Liverpool papers.

The resolution was thereupon put and carried unanimously.[25]

- *And of Mr Otto Beit's Gift.* [A] resolution, proposed by Col Oswald Baker and seconded by Sir William Leishman [*see above*], was then put to the meeting and carried unanimously.[26]

1910

At a meeting of *Council* on **21 January 1910**:

Professor Angelo Celli, whose nomination as an *Honorary Fellow* was deferred for further consideration from last meeting [*see above*], was finally elected an Honorary Fellow of the Society.

It was proposed by Sir Patrick Manson and seconded by Mr Austen that the *Transactions* be increased to imper. quarto size. This was agreed to come into effect after the present volume is completed.

Fifty-one Fellows and visitors attended the following *Ordinary* meeting when two papers on *ankylostomiasis* were presented.[27]

At a *Council* meeting on **18 February**:

A letter was read from the Secretary of the *Liverpool School of Tropical Medicine* suggesting that the *Annual Meeting* of the Society should be held in Liverpool on the 18th [later altered to 25th] June, and that the proposed meeting there in March be abandoned. It was resolved unanimously that this invitation be accepted and that the Secretaries be instructed to make the necessary arrangements.

A letter was read from Professor Nuttall asking the opinion of the Society as to the advisability of holding a meeting of the [ISTM] in conjunction with the 17th International Congress of Medicine in London in 1913. It was agreed unanimously that [this] proposal be approved, and that he be asked to use his influence with the Committee of the Congress to have a special section for Tropical Medicine and Hygiene.

Also, Sir Rubert Boyce, FRS (440) was among eighteen *approved* for Fellowship.

The following *Ordinary* meeting was attended by 52 Fellows and visitors, and the three papers presented concerned '*Dipterous insects which cause myiasis in man*'[28], the '*Nature and origin of Calabar swellings*'[29] and the '*Etiology of beri-beri*'.[30]

On **18 March**, *Council* minutes record that:

> Dr [C W] Daniels proposed and Dr Low seconded the following Resolution which on being put to the *Council*, was carried unanimously:
>
>> That, in the case of medical candidates, either the proposer or seconder must have personal knowledge of the value of the qualifications held by the candidate, and the conditions of practice in the country from which he comes.
>
> [And] Mr Austen proposed and Dr Carnegie Brown seconded the following Resolution, which was also carried without dissent:
>
>> That Fellows who read papers before the Society shall, if application be made at once, be supplied with 25 Reprints of their paper similarly paged to the *Transactions* without charge.

Thirty-four Fellows and visitors were presented at the following *Ordinary* meeting at 8.30 pm, when the following four papers were presented and discussed: '*The duration of latency of malarial infection*'[31], '*Fever with an urticarial rash - occurring in the Yangtse Valley*'[32], '*A problem in Typhoid fever prophylaxis and the solution of same*'[33], and '*A note on the comparative immunity from sleeping sickness of the Ngombe tribe, possibly due to the Nkusi dye*'.[34] The last was presented by the British Vice-Consul of the Congo State!

Minutes of a *Council* meeting on **15 April** contained the following:

> The Secretaries read the correspondence with the Secretary of the *Liverpool School* [*of Tropical Medicine*]: and it was resolved to accept the invitation of that institution to hold the *Annual General Meeting* of the Society in Liverpool on June 25th. The Secretaries were instructed to make the necessary arrangements.

Dr Carnegie Brown submitted the Accounts and Draft Reports of the Society for the year ended March 31 1910.

DEATH OF KING EDWARD VII

At a *Council* meeting on **27 May**:

The following letter, drafted by the President (Ross), was approved by *Council*:

Sir, I am directed by the *Council* of the *Society of Tropical Medicine and Hygiene* to offer to His Majesty and to the Members of the Royal Family our respectful and heartfelt sympathy on the death [on 6 May] of our late beloved sovereign, King Edward VII [1841–1910], and to assure his Majesty of our loyalty and devotion.

I have the honour to be, Sir, your most obedt. Servant.
(Sgd) R Ross. President
Sir Arthur Bigge GCVO

The President [then] informed *Council* of the arrangements which were being made for the *Annual General Meeting* at Liverpool, and expressed the hope that there would be a large and representative attendance.

Twenty-nine Fellows and visitors attended the *Ordinary* meeting at 8.30pm, when three papers were presented; they were devoted to: '*Functional psychoses in dark races*'[35], *Schistosoma japonicum* infection[36], and '*Biomonics of helminths*'.[37]

Third AGM – Liverpool

This was held on **Saturday 25 June 1910** at 3pm, and was the first AGM to take place out of London.

The President moved and the Vice President seconded that the Society do record in the minutes its sense of the loss which in common with the whole world of Science it has sustained in the death of Professor Robert Koch[38], Honorary Fellow, and that a Resolution of condolence be forwarded to his widow. The motion was unanimously adopted (in silence).

Two addresses followed – the first by the president, Professor Ronald Ross CB FRS, on *'The more exact study of parasitic disease'*[39] and the other by Dr Wakelin Barratt on blackwater fever.[40]

Several matters of interest and/or importance emerged at the next *Council* meeting on **21 October:**

> The *Council* directed that a letter of condolence be sent to the family of Dr John Anderson, [1840–1910] Member of the *Council*, recently deceased.
>
> On the motion of Dr Sandwith, seconded by Dr Harford it was unanimously Resolved:-
>
> > (a) That *Tropical Medicine* and *Hygiene* having now become of such great and world-wide importance, the time has arrived when a special section should be devoted to its consideration at future meetings of the International Congress of Medicine [ICM]. (b) That the Secretaries of the [STMH] be instructed to communicate this Resolution to the President of the Council of the London Meeting of the [ICM].
> >
> > Designs for a Seal of the Society were submitted, and after some discussion, it was recorded that the Secretaries be empowered to decide on a suitable design.

Thirty-eight Fellows and visitors were present for the following *Ordinary* meeting at 11 Chandos Street, at which Dr A G Bagshawe read a paper on *'Research advances in our knowledge of sleeping sickness'*.[41]

A *Special Meeting of Council* was convened on **3 November:**

[KING EDWARD VII MEMORIAL].

Dr Sandwith, Vice President, took the Chair, and said that the meeting had been specially called to consider some correspondence which had taken place with Lord Northcote [1846–1911][42] with reference to an application to the Lord Mayor that some part at least of the Fund which is being raised to provide a memorial to His Late Majesty King Edward VII [*see above*] shall be devoted to the endowment of tropical research. After ... discussion it was decided that a letter should be forwarded to the Lord Mayor endorsing and supporting Lord Northcote's suggestion, and the general terms of the letter were approved. A copy of the letter as it appeared in *The Times*[43] and *Morning Post* on the 5th instant [was inserted]. Copies were also sent to *The Standard, The Daily News, The Daily Telegraph,* and *The Westminster Gazette.* [The letter to *The Times* began:]

> My Lord Mayor, - On behalf of the *Society of Tropical Medicine and Hygiene,* we sincerely beg to endorse the proposal so earnestly urged by Lord Northcote [*see above*], that some part at least of the fund which is being raised to provide a memorial to his late Majesty, King Edward VII, shall be devoted to the endowment of the study and prevention of tropical disease ...
>
> [The letter ended:] In the mind of every thoughtful citizen these facts must necessarily give rise to serious consideration, and we are persuaded that if due regard is had to their importance, the endowment of the study and teaching of tropical disease will no longer be delayed. A remembrance of the late King can take no higher form; it can be devoted to no more noble object, and to no end which gives throughout the Empire so fruitful a promise of speedy and permanent relief of misery and sorrow. The welfare of his subjects – even the lowliest and most remote – was ever a cause of tender and anxious solicitude to his Majesty, and we venture to believe that a memorial fund can be applied to no purpose that would have more fully accorded with his wishes.
>
> We are, my Lord Mayor, yours very obediently,
> R Ross, President
> Patrick Manson, Past President
> C F Harford
>   } Joint Secretaries
> W Carnegie Brown
>
> The Right Honourable the Lord Mayor of London, the Mansion House, E C.

The *Council* meeting held on **18 November** lasted for only twenty minutes, the only business being:

> A letter was read from Sir Thomas Barlow [PRCP] [1845–1945], in which he pointed out that a more elaborate form of request for a separate section of tropical diseases at [the ICM] [*see above*] would have more weight than the letter which had been sent. A

special form of letter signed by the President, Vice President and other officers was accordingly drafted and approved.

Sir Rubert Boyce FRS was the speaker at the *Ordinary* meeting that day (42 were present); his paper was on *Yellow fever* in *West Africa*.[44]

At the next *Council* meeting on **16 December**:

> Sir Thomas Barlow's letter as to a proposed section for tropical diseases at the [ICM] was read and approved, and the Secretaries were requested to offer him the thanks of the Council.

At the following *Ordinary* meeting at 8.30pm, 45 Fellows and visitors were present:

> Dr Harold Seidelin described a protozoan organism which he believed was the 'pathogenic agent' in yellow fever,[45] and later, discussion on Sir Rubert Boyce's paper (*see above*) was resumed.[46]

1911

At the *Council* meeting on **20 January 1911** at 8.00pm, Sir William Leishman FRS was proposed for the third presidency (*see* Chapter 4) by Dr Sandwith, and seconded by Sir Patrick Manson. The continuing discussion of Sir Rubert Boyce's paper was raised:

> The arrangements for the discussion of ... Boyce's paper on *yellow fever* [YF] in West Africa were considered and Dr Daniels stated that if it was limited to an examination of Sir Rubert Boyce's conclusions he would not press his proposed resolution, it being understood however that he did not recede from the position he had taken up. The President agreed that that limit should be placed on this discussion.

And at the following *Ordinary* meeting – at 8.30pm – with 71 Fellows and visitors present:

> A further demonstration of an organism found in cases of [YF] was given by Dr Seidelin [and] The adjourned discussion on Sir Rubert Boyce's paper on [YF] in West Africa was resumed by Dr H E Durham.[47]

A paper by Dr [W T] Prout was read by the [Hon] Secretary, and a letter from Fleet Surgeon Collingwood R N was also communicated to the Society. Sir P Manson, Dr Stephens, Dr Walker (Accra) Capt Skelton RAMC, Dr Carnegie Brown, Dr Seidelin, and the President having spoken, Sir Rubert Boyce showed specimens illustrative of the pathology of [YF], and replied on the whole subject.

At an *Ordinary* meeting of the Society (which followed a very short meeting of Council) on **17 February**, Dr [R T] Leiper spoke on the morphology of the eggs of *Schistosoma japonicum*,[48] and the president spoke on '*Some enumerative studies on malaria ... and sleeping sickness*'.[49]

At a *Council* meeting at 8.10pm on **17 March**, the only items of note were:

> The arrangements for the anniversary dinner ... and a list of invitations approved [and] The price of separate issues of the *Transactions* to non-subscribers was fixed at 3/6ᵈ.

At the following *Ordinary* meeting at 8.30pm (in the absence of both the president and vice-president, Sir Havelock Charles took the Chair), there were 42 Fellows and visitors present, and the contributions were: '*A specific cure of yaws by dioxy-diamido-arsenobenzol*'[50] – read by 'one of the Secretaries' for Dr R Strong of Manila – with epidiascopic illustrations – and a paper on the use of santonin in the treatment of intestinal affections of the tropics[51] by Dr J Preston Maxwell of Amoy. Dr Daniels also exhibited 'slides illustrative of a case of *Leishman-Donovan* infection from the Yangtse Valley'.

At the next *Council* meeting, on **18 May**:

> The Draft Reports of the *Council* and Treasurer and the Financial Statement [for submission to the 4th AGM] were submitted and approved.
>
> The arrangements for the Biennial dinner were further discussed and the Secretaries were instructed to send invitations to the Rt Honble John Burns, Lord Cromer, Lord Lucas and Sir West Ridgeway.
>
> A letter from Drs Melandri and Vincent Dickinson relative to the forthcoming International Exhibition at Rome was considered, and a reply expressing the sympathy of the Society with the objects of the promoters was directed to be sent.

At the following *Ordinary* meeting, 26 Fellows and visitors were present, and a paper on *'the nature of Zambesi Fever'*[52] was read for Dr W J Bruce of Zambesia, B East Africa by Dr Harford, and one on *'… the present position of the quinine prophylaxis of malaria'*[53] was read by Dr Carnegie Brown. Also, *'A note on the Streptothrix of white mycetoma'*[54] was read and cultures and specimens of the organism were shown for Dr Surveyor of Bombay.

A *Special* meeting of *Council* took place on **1 June**, when:

> The arrangements for the dinner [*see above*] were discussed and it was decided to send out the following additional invitations:- Surgeon General Babtie, The Chaplain-General of the Forces, and the Editors of the *Lancet* and *British Medical Journal*.
>
> It was [also] decided to give a personal gratuity of £5 to Mrs Evans, on her resignation after four years work as clerical assistant.

The last *Council* meeting under Ross's presidency was held at 5pm on **4 July**, preceding the 4th *AGM* (*see* below):

> The Joint Secretaries Drs Carnegie Brown and Harford tendered their resignation upon the expiry of their term of office, but at the unanimous request of the *Council* agreed to continue … for a further term of two years.
>
> Dr Harford addressed the Committee on the expansion of the *Transactions*, and after some conversation it was agreed to appoint an Editorial Sub-Committee to consider and direct the publications of the Society:- The Sub-Committee to consist of The President, the Joint Secretaries, Dr Sandwith and Dr Bagshawe.
>
> Correspondence between Professor Nuttall the General Secretary of the [ISTM] and Dr Sandwith delegate of this Society were read, and Dr Sandwith was directed to reply to … Nuttall that this Society agreed with his suggestion that Members of [that Society] should attend the meetings of the [ICM] (Tropical Section) in their individual capacity.
>
> The Secretaries were directed to forward a letter of condolence to the relatives of the late Sir Rubert Boyce and to record the sorrow of the Society at his death. They were also directed to forward a letter of congratulation to Sir Ronald Ross on the honour which [had] recently been conferred on him.

Fourth AGM

This was held on 16 June at 5.00pm, 42 being present, and Ross was to take the Chair (for the last time):

> ... Annual Reports of [both] *Council* and Treasurer for the year ended 31 March 1911 were adopted, and the Statement of accounts for the same period were [all] passed.
>
> The Secretaries announced that as a result of the Ballot, the following officers for the ensuing two years had been elected:-

President	:	Sir William Leishman FRS
Vice President	:	Sir Havelock Charles KCVO
Council	:	E E Austen, Esq, Arthur G Bagshawe Esq MB, Andrew Balfour Esq MD, Fleet-Surgeon Bassett-Smith CB MRCS RN, W Carnegie Brown Esq MD MRCP, James Cantlie Esq MB, Fleet-Surgeon G T Collingwood MVO RN, C W Daniels Esq MB MRCP, Lieut-Col H E Drake-Brockman IMS, C F Harford Esq MD, William Hartigan Esq MD, T S Kerr Esq MB, G C Low Esq MB, Sir Patrick Manson KCMG, FRS, Professor E A Minchin, H B G Newham Esq MRCS, Sir Ronald Ross KCB, FRS, L W Sambon Esq MD, F M Sandwith Esq MD FRCP, Professor W J R Simpson CMG MD FRCP, H Stannus Stannus Esq MB MCS, J W W Stephens Esq MD.

> [After Sir William Leishman had been installed as the third president – *see* Chapter 4] the retiring president [Ross] addressed the Society].
>
> Mr J Cantlie was unanimously elected Treasurer, and Dr Bagshawe and Mr Beddoes auditors for the ensuing two years.
>
> A paper on 'Alastrum, Amaas or milk pox' was read for Dr Ribas[55] of São Paulo by Dr Loudon Strain [and] Dr [C W] Daniels spoke on the subject.

So ended Ross's two year presidency, and the STMH was now four years old.

The third and fourth annual reports

These two reports highlighted the major events during Ross's presidency. The number of Fellows in the two reports totalled 501 and 574, respectively. In the third report, income had been £377 3s 3d (including a previous balance of £54 18s 1d) and the gross surplus on the year, £124 4s 0d. In the fourth report, corresponding figures were: £482 8s 6d (£124 4s 0d) and £189 17s 2d, respectively.

References and Notes

1   C F Oldham. *What is malaria? And why is it most intense in hot climates?* London: H K Lewis 1871: 186; G C Cook, A J Webb. Perceptions of malaria transmission before Ross's discovery in 1897. *Postgrad med J* 2000; 76: 738–40.

2   W H S Jones. *Malaria, a neglected factor in the history of Greece and Rome.* Cambridge: MacMillan and Bowes 1907: 107.

3   G C Cook. *Tropical Medicine: an illustrated history of the pioneers.* London: Academic Press 2007: 278.

4   P Manson. *Tropical Medicine: a manual of diseases of warm climates.* London: Cassell 1898: 604.

5   *See*: G C Cook. *Health-care for all: history of a third-world dilemma.* St Albans: TropZam 2009: 226.

6   H Hamilton. 'Small' incinerators. *Indian med Gaz* 1907; 42: 151–2; H A Haines. Small incinerators. *Indian med Gaz* 1907; 42: 204–6; H Hamilton. Incineration in military stations. *Indian Med Gaz* 1908; 43: 241–3. [*See also*: G C Cook. *Caribbean diseases: Dr George Low's expedition in 1901–02.* Oxford: Radcliffe Publishing 2009: 229].

7   R Ross. Presidential address. The future of tropical medicine. *Trans Soc trop Med Hyg* 1908–9; 2: 272–85.

8   Anonymous. Morley of Blackburn, 1st Viscount. *Who Was Who, 1916–1928* 5th ed. London: A & C Black 1992: 578.

9   P Manson. Discussion [on Ross's paper]. *Trans Soc trop Med Hyg* 1908–9; 2: 285–6.

10   Anonymous. Seely, Sir Charles, 1st Bt. *Who Was Who, 1897–1916.* London: A & C Black: 637.

11   Anonymous. Crewe, 1st Marquess of. *Who Was Who, 1941–1950* 5th ed. London: A & C Black 1980: 265–6.

12   Anonymous. Annual Dinner. *Trans Soc trop Med Hyg.* 1908–9; 2: 286–8.

13   J P Maxwell. Two rare cases from the Fukien Province, South China. *Trans Soc trop Med Hyg* 1908–9; 2: 289–92.

14   P G Woolley. Preventable diseases in Siam. *Trans Soc trop Med Hyg* 1908–9; 2: 299–306.

15   J R Forrest. Fevers in Rangoon. *Trans Soc trop Med Hyg* 1908–9; 2: 308–11.

16   A G Bagshawe. Recent advances in our knowledge of sleeping sickness. *Trans Soc trop Med Hyg* 1909–10; 3: 1–27.

17   H W Thomas. Oesophagostomiasis in man, with specimens and illustrations shown by the epidiascope. *Trans Soc trop Med Hyg* 1909–19; 3: 44–55.

18   H W Thomas. The results of inoculation experiments with virulent blood of yellow-fever cases or by the bites of infected Stegomyia Calopus. *Trans Soc trop Med Hyg* 1909–10; 3: 59–61.

19   H W Thomas. Mossy foot of the Amazon region, with microscopic specimens, and illustrations shewn by the epidiascope. *Trans Soc top Med Hyg* 1909–10; 3: 57–9.

20   A M Stimson. Notes on Stimson's spirochaete, found in the kidney of a yellow-fever case. *Trans Soc trop Med Hyg* 1909–10; 3: 56–7.

21   J N Rat. A skin affection of the Island of Nevis, British West Indies. *Trans Soc trop Med Hyg* 1909–10; 3: 63–70.

22   W B Leishman. Observations on the mechanism of infection in tick fever, and on the hereditary transmission of Spirochaeta Duttoni in the tick. *Trans Soc trop Med Hyg* 1909–10; 3: 77–95.

23   D B Thompson, A Balfour. Two cases of non-ulcerating 'oriental sore', better termed Leishman nodules. *Trans Soc trop Med Hyg* 1909–10; 3: 107–28.

24   M C Vaney, L W Sambon. Preliminary notes on three new species of tongue worms (*Linguatulidae*) 1909–10; 3: 129–54.

25   Anonymous. Death of Sir Alfred Jones. *Trans Soc trop Med Hyg* 1909–10; 3: 73–6. [*See also*: P N Davies. *Sir Alfred Jones: shipping entrepreneur par excellence.* London: Europa Publications Ltd 1978: 162; J G Read. Jones, Sir Alfred Lewis (1845–1909). In: H C G Matthew, B Harrison (eds). *Oxford Dictionary of National Biography.* Oxford: Oxford University Press 2004; 30: 436–8].

26   Anonymous. Mr Otto Beit's gift. *Trans Soc trop Med Hyg* 1909–10; 3: 76.

27   T Oliver. Ankylostomiasis: a menace to the industrial life of non-tropical countries. *Trans Soc trop Med Hyg* 1909–10; 3: 155–75; J J Elliott. Ankylostomiasis in Natal. *Trans Soc trop Med Hyg* 1909–10; 3: 176–95.

28   E E Austen. Some dipterous insects which cause myiasis in man. *Trans Soc trop Med Hyg* 1909–10; 3: 215–42.

29   P Manson. On the nature and origin of Calabar swellings. *Trans Soc trop Med Hyg* 1909–10; 3: 244–51.

30   H Fraser, A T Stanton. The etiology of beri-beri. *Trans Soc trop Med Hyg* 1909–10; 3: 257–67.

31   O Baker. The duration of latency of malarial infection. *Trans Soc trop Med Hyg* 1909–10; 3: 271–7.

32   A C Lambert. Notes on some cases of fever with an urticarial rash, occurring in the Yangtse Valley. *Trans Soc trop Med Hyg* 1909–10; 3: 278–99.

33   E I Vaughn. A problem in typhoid fever prophylaxis and the solution of same. *Trans Soc trop Med Hyg* 1909–10; 3: 303–15.

34   G Campbell. Notes on the comparative immunity from sleeping sickness

of the Ngombe tribe, possibly due to the Nkusi dye. *Trans Soc trop Med Hyg* 1909–10; 3: 318–9.

35 R Howard. Emotional psychoses among dark-skinned races. *Trans Soc trop Med Hyg* 1909–10; 3: 323–39.

36 H S Houghton. Notes on infections with Schistosomum Japonicum. *Trans Soc trop Med Hyg* 1909–10; 3: 342–8.

37 W Nicoll. The bionomics of helminths. *Trans Soc trop Med Hyg* 1909–10; 3: 353–78.

38 **Robert (Heinrich Hermann) Koch** (1843–1910) was a major figure in establishing the 'germ theory' of disease.

39 R Ross. The more exact study of parasitic diseases. *Trans Soc trop Med Hyg* 1909–10; 3: 383–90.

40 J O W Barratt. The definition of blackwater fever. *Trans Soc trop Med Hyg* 1909–10; 3: 391–6.

41 A G Bagshawe. Recent advances in our knowledge of sleeping sickness. *Trans Soc trop Med Hyg* 1910–11; 4: 1–23.

42 Anonymous. Northcote, 1st Baron. *Who Was Who, 1897–1916* 5th ed. London: A & C Black: 530.

43 R Ross, P Manson, C F Harford, W C Brown. King Edward Memorial. *Times, Lond* 1910; Nov 5. This letter attempted (unsuccessfully) to divert part of the proposed memorial to King Edward VII to *tropical research*.

44 R Boyce. The distribution and prevalence of yellow fever in West Africa. *Trans Soc trop Med Hyg* 1910–11; 4: 33–58.

45 H Seidelin. Yellow fever. *Trans Soc trop Med Hyg* 1910–11; 4: 65–9.

46 R Boyce. The distribution and prevalence of yellow fever in West Africa. *Trans Soc trop Med Hyg* 1910–11; 4: 69–92.

47 R Boyce. The distribution and prevalence of yellow fever in West Africa: discussion. *Trans Soc trop Med Hyg* 1910–11; 4: 107–30.

48 R T Leiper. Note on the presence of a lateral spine in the eggs of Schistosoma Japonicum. *Trans Soc trop Med Hyg* 1910–11; 4: 133–5.

49 R Ross. Some enumerative studies on malaria, blackwater fever, and sleeping sickness. *Trans Soc trop Med Hyg* 1910–11; 4: 137–50.

50 R P Strong. The specific cure of yaws by dioxydiamidoarsenobenzol. *Trans Soc trop Med Hyg* 1910–11; 4: 153–8.

51 J P Maxwell. The use of santonin in the treatment of intestinal affections of the tropics. *Trans Soc trop Med Hyg* 1910–11; 4: 161–8.

52 W J Bruce. The nature of Zambesi fever. *Trans Soc trop Med Hyg* 1910–11; 4: 183–90.

53 W C Brown. The present position of the quinine prophylaxis of malaria. *Trans Soc trop Med Hyg* 1910–11; 4: 193–9.

54 N F Surveyor. A few observations on the cultural characteristics of a variety of the streptothrix of White Mycetoma. *Trans Soc trop Med Hyg.* 1910–11; 4: 210–11.

55 E Ribas. Alastrim, Amass, or Milk-pox. *Trans Soc trop Med Hyg.* 1910–11; 4: 224–30.

Chapter 4

The pre-war years (1911–14) and the Royal Society of Medicine's attempt to absorb the STMH

It was now over four years since the Society had been founded, and the first two presidents had arguably been the most widely known of the pioneers of this nascent 'colonial' discipline. To follow these two colourful individuals must have been a somewhat daunting task; nevertheless, Lt Col Sir William Leishman[1] (*see* Figure 4.1), although only 46, assumed this mantel admirably. His major work which had demonstrated (jointly) the causative agent of Kala-azar had been published in 1903[2], although he had made the discovery at the Royal Victoria Hospital, Netley in 1900. The other president during those years in the run-up to the Great War (1914–18) was Maj. Gen. Sir Richard Havelock Charles Bt (*see* below). The Society's calendar was now well established: *Council* meetings being followed by *Ordinary* ones, and the *Annual General Meeting* taking place every June (see Appendix I).

Ordinary meetings (which were *not* always well attended, largely because most Fellows lived abroad and were serving the Empire and Raj) continued with one or more contributions – usually at the Medical Society of London's (MSL) rooms at 11 Chandos Street – which exists to this day. From now, I shall *not* quote *all* contributions, but these can be found in early volumes of the Society's *Transactions*.

The two presidential addresses in the pre-war years

In his presidential address given on **16 June 1911**, Sir William Leishman KCMG FRCP FRS (1865–1926) paid tribute to his two predecessors in that office. Manson, he claimed, was the 'recognised head of *tropical medicine*, not only in our empire but throughout the world'. His Address was orientated *not* on the future of *tropical medicine*, but on the Society:

> … I feel it is not enough to *maintain* a high standard of utility but that we should ever seek one still higher [he claimed], and that

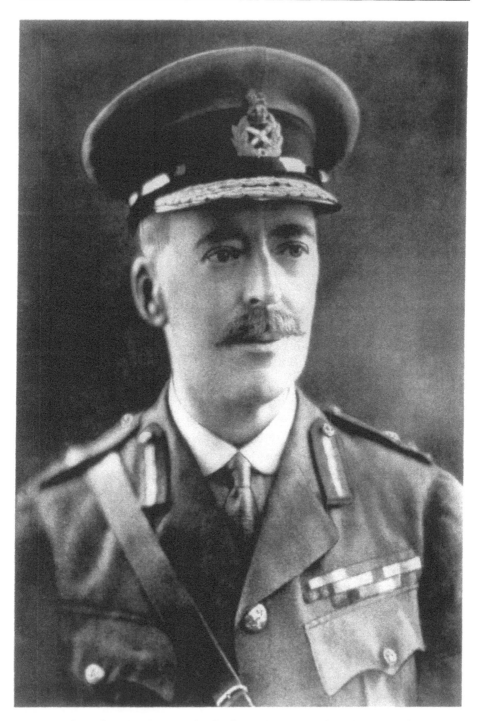

Figure 4.1: Sir William Leishman – the third president (reproduced courtesy the Wellcome Library, London).

no body such as ours can afford to rest satisfied with anything less than constant progress. I may remind you that our position differs widely from that of other medical societies, in that *by far the larger portion of our members are resident abroad* [author's italics] and can only attend our meetings at rare intervals, if at all. It is true that they receive the printed *Transactions* which faithfully record our spoken words, but I think you will agree with me that this is but a poor substitute for attendance at the meetings. For instance, it must at times, happen to all of us that the subject matter of a particular communication may not be one in which we have any great personal interest, and yet that particular meeting may be more helpful to us than the majority by reason of a conversation which we may have had, before or after the meeting itself, with a fellow-worker. It is this opportunity of meeting one another and discussing matters informally which is so great an advantage, and yet this is one from which the great majority of our Fellows are debarred. I think then that we ought seriously to debate the possibility of introducing some scheme by which the interests of our absent members might be better served than appears possible at present.

We may roughly divide ourselves into those who are connected with or interested in research work and those whose busy lives in the tropics limit their energies to administration or to the prevention and treatment of disease; the latter, naturally, form by far the larger group. We ought then to aim at catering for both sections, and I think that each has it in its power to be of the greatest assistance to the other, if only an organisation was adopted which would bring their respective interests into closer touch. As matters stand at present this intercourse is only possible at our monthly meetings, and I do not advocate any increase in the number of these, (few of us could spare the time for more), even if we were successful in obtaining sufficient material in the way of papers and contributions.

It must often happen, then, that a member resident abroad in passing through London may find that there is no meeting which he can make it convenient to attend, although he would probably be glad to have the opportunity of meeting fellow-workers from other countries, and might be anxious to obtain the most recent information upon some problem of etiology or sanitation, or the most recent views on the treatment of some disease which gives trouble in his own district. It is true that the information of which he is in search may be gathered from certain journals or periodicals, but you will agree with me that this quest is not easy, even when one is accustomed to such searches through shelves. A simpler way and a better [one] is to go to the man who has made a special study of the subject and to pick his brains of the latest information. But here, again, the diffidence of the seeker, or the preoccupations of the sought, may prevent the communication of the desired information. We all know that nothing could exceed the courtesy and kindness of the staffs of the two tropical schools [London and Liverpool], and I trust I may add that we are always anxious to help as far as we can in our own College at Millbank [the RAMC College], but after all such meetings are at the best infrequent.

He proceeded to dwell on the theme of other needs of a 'Fellow on his transitory visit to London':

… It may be some years since he was last in England, and he is well aware that things have not stood still in tropical pathology; putting myself in his place I should be anxious to see for myself actual specimens of any new parasites or other material illustrative of recent discoveries which I had only read of or heard of from others. He may not have time or opportunity to go through another course of *tropical medicine* in one of the schools, and his object would be attained if he had the opportunity of spending a few days, or even hours, over good specimens with a text-book beside him.

Again, there is another need, which I know will appeal to all who are connected with either research or teaching, and that is the lack of material with which to illustrate their teaching or with which to prosecute their researches. It is a commonplace that clinical material in the shape of cases of many tropical diseases is exceptionally hard to come by in this country. When cases *are* encountered they are, only too often, chronic or convalescent, and useless for the above purposes. The obvious alternative is that the needful material should be obtained from those whom we know to be stationed in districts where the particular disease is endemic, and, thanks to modern methods of collecting and preserving such material, much may be obtained in this way and usefully employed at home.

As a last instance, it may be that, as a result of investigations at home, some line of treatment or of prevention of a tropical disease may appear worthy of being tested in practice, but it is far from easy to have anything of this sort tried on a scale large enough to allow of judgments being formed as to its value, in spite of its publication in some medical journal. What is wanted is the enlistment of the personal sympathy of some tropical medical officers who are practising in districts which afford the opportunity of a satisfactory test being carried out.

Leishman then put forward three suggestions for improving the Society. The *first* was:

… an alteration in the present character of [the] *Transactions* … I have found that some of the ideas which I had formed on this subject have also for some time been in the minds of our valued Secretaries, Dr [W] Carnegie Brown and Dr [C F] Harford, so I have the greater confidence in presenting them to you. In the first place, I think it would be very desirable to open our columns to *short articles* [author's italics] from Fellows, which need not necessarily have been read at a meeting of the Society. We all know that much valuable observation and information go to waste by reason of the observer being either too busy to commit it to the form of a formal article or paper, or by reason, possibly, of inherent modesty or youth, for I believe that these qualities are neither extinct nor incompatible in the Tropics. Secondly, I would advocate the throwing open of the *Transactions* to *correspondence* [recently abolished] as a means of bringing one's wishes and difficulties to the notice of every other Fellow, with a reasonable hope that one would find in a later number the information of which one was in search. In this connection it should not be difficult, through our Editors, to organise a system by which queries or requests dealing with different departments of our subject should be passed to certain referees who have made those subjects their special study. Through such correspondence columns also an investigator might make his needs for certain material more generally known than [is] possible even to those of us who have generous friends in many countries. ...

Secondly, a small library (which today has ceased to exist) was in 1911 a 'distinct want' in the Society:

> ... I purposely call it a *small* library, for I think it should be strictly limited to publications dealing with the different branches of our subject – *Tropical Medicine* and *Hygiene*. Any attempt to overstep this limit would, I think, be unwise, and also unnecessary, in view of the numerous excellent general medical libraries which are at everyone's disposal in London. In the best of these general libraries, however, it is by no means easy to find all the information of which one is in search, and anyone seeking to study the literature of a particular subject will often have to visit several before he covers the ground satisfactorily. To collect such a technical library cannot of course be a very rapid process, and the means by which it should be started would require very careful preliminary consideration. One of the first things this library would entail would be a room in which to store it and, as you will see from the Report of the Council for this year, this has already been under the consideration of the Council, since the possession of a room of our own as a meeting place for the Fellows is felt to be a matter of some urgency, and I trust it will not be long before we are able to make some satisfactory arrangement in this direction. We should, I fancy, have little difficulty in arranging to have our *Transactions* placed on the exchange list of similar publications, and I feel that we might count on authors presenting reprints of their papers to the Society once they realised how highly this would be appreciated. Books, also, sent for review [also recently largely abolished], would soon accumulate if it were thought well to include reviewing in the programme of our altered *Transactions*.

And *thirdly*, when the Society possessed a room of its own, this might:

> ... also serve to house type-collections of material illustrative of some important branches of *tropical medicine* and *hygiene*. In this I have not so much in my mind a museum of the ordinary kind as the organisation of a series of collections of biting flies and

insects, microscopical specimens illustrating tropical pathology, helminths, etc., which were intended not merely to be preserved but to be used and handled freely by those who wished to study them; the necessary facilities for the examination of such collections should also be provided.

In making this suggestion I have, naturally, had chiefly in my mind microscopical specimens, since it is with them that my personal work is most closely concerned, so I shall illustrate what I mean in connection with this branch alone, although I feel sure that similar collections such as those of biting flies and insects, of helminths and their ova, etc., would also appeal to many of our Fellows, and might be of equal or even greater service to the majority.

Leishman then elaborated on necessary requirements – 'a good micro-scope or two and a few slide cabinets'. He continued:

… What I should like to see would be the development of a custom in the Society that all Fellows who come across interesting microscopical specimens in the course of their practice or their researches should stain and mount extra specimens and forward them, with a few words of description, to the Society, where they would be classified, catalogued and added to the collection. This would not really involve them in much labour, since every worker knows how many specimens he throws away which would perhaps be of the greatest value to others, although superfluous for himself. The collection would be fortuitous at first, but later on, noticeable blanks could be filled in by applying to individual workers, and I have good reason for anticipating that such applications would meet with a most generous response. If this scheme should be taken up warmly I feel sure that it would not be long before we found ourselves in possession of a collection which would be of the greatest value, not only to those who wished to refresh their memories of the appearance of the more usual parasites, but which would also be of incalculable benefit to those engaged in research on many branches of tropical pathology.

I need hardly labour this point, but just think for a moment of the case of an observer who has found what he suspects to be a new haemogregarine or a new trypanosome, if he were able to consult the collection and contrast his parasite with other species, derived possibly from many different sources. The advantages of such a direct comparison over what is more frequent, the study of printed descriptions and more or less accurate plates, need no emphasising. Specimens, also, in illustration of some individual research, such, we will say, as the influence of a certain drug on the morphological characters of a parasite or slides demonstrating the developmental changes which a parasite undergoes in its alternative host or in artificial culture would be of the greatest help to workers on similar lines.

Leishman concluded his lecture:

> ... although the progress of the Society has been almost unprecedented as regards its membership, it cannot afford to stand still, but must aim at an ever-increasing standard of usefulness. I believe that it can best attain this end by endeavouring to stimulate intercourse and mutual help among its members, especially between those resident at home and those who are stationed abroad. In this way we make our Fellowship no vain thing, but the expression of a living and keen desire to help one another, and in this way to forward the cause we all have so closely at heart, the progress of *Tropical Medicine* and *Hygiene*.[3]

From then onwards, presidential addresses focused *not* so much on objectives of the new discipline or the Society itself, but on specific *clinical* problems in *tropical medicine*. In the last address before World War I (1914–18), Surgeon-General Sir (Richard) Havelock Charles Bt GCVO IMS (1858–1934)[4] (*see* Figure 4.2) spoke on **17 October 1913** on **'Neurasthenia, and its bearing on the decay of [expatriates] in northern India'**. Few would be sympathetic to most of his views today, but such opinions were rife in the days of the Raj in the early twentieth century. He began:

> When asked to choose a subject on which to address you, I thought best to take one on which we could have a profitable discussion, which might lead this Society to give its opinion on a matter pregnant to many in this Imperial age – the suitability of the white man for the tropics, and his power of colonizing such lands, together with the effects likely to follow on his offspring from so doing.

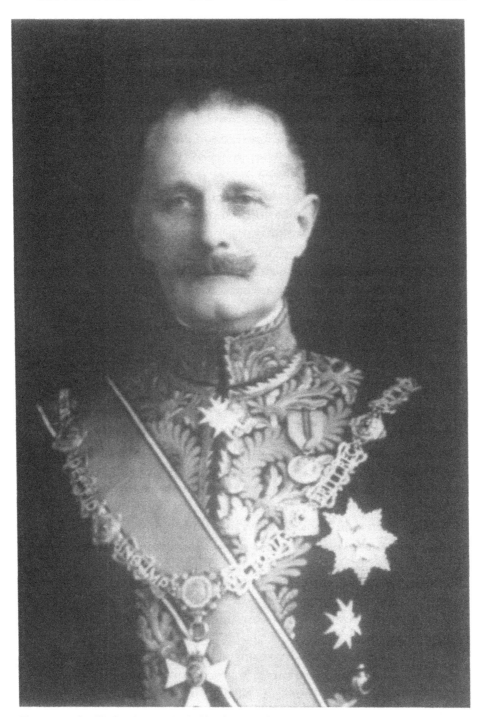

Figure 4.2: Sir (Richard) Havelock Charles Bt – the fourth president (RSTMH archive).

In justifying his choice of subject, he continued:

> … My work on the India Office Medical Board has brought before me –
>
> (a) The unhealthiness from which our countrymen suffer after a long spell of Indian service. All on sick leave come before the Board, and one can see that debility, mental and physical, apart from any special disease, renders a change to Europe every four or five years a necessity. This is the explanation of Government and Mercantile leave rules. It is not a spirit of philanthropy that is at the base of these regulations, but a desire to have the European servant at his best,
>
> (b) The condition of physical fitness of our men going to India – as all recruits are passed by the Medical Board, [and]
>
> (c) The diseases causing ill-health, death, or invaliding – for the Board enquires into such.

Charles then told his audience:

> … In opening a discussion on 'Special Factors influencing the Suitability of Europeans for Life in the Tropics', at the *British Medical Association*, London, 1910, I stated my opinion as to the best health capital to be taken to the tropics, and said that the best kind of man is the good ordinary type of Britisher with a clear head 'well screwed-on', an even temper, not over intellectual, who can take an interest in things around, not unduly introspective, one who can work hard and find pleasure in it, capable of bearing exposure to the sun; one who will practice temperance in all things, with self-control and common sense – meaning that such an [sic] one inherits no *liability* to that neuropathic disposition which requires only a light exciting cause to develop active mental trouble.
>
> In the tropics, normal persons often experience symptoms which, when more strongly marked, are characterised as *neurasthenic*, whilst those of weaker mental calibre become unbalanced. In the former case the condition responds more readily to treatment than does the *neurasthenia* as met with in

Europe, but for its cure a change of climate is absolutely essential. Dr Woodruff[5], in his able work on the effects of light, indeed says that white men in the tropics universally suffer from *neurasthenia*, and his experience in the Philippines was that insanities are more numerous than in America.

Charles continued:

Many years ago, when I began my life in India, stationed in the Punjab, I often heard it said of individuals in the various services, 'Oh! Such and such an [sic] one ought to go to Europe for a bit – he has got, or is getting, *Punjab head*'. On enquiry I found the signs of this peculiarity were – that an officer, otherwise in every way a good fellow, had become short tempered; forgetful of names; troubled with sleeplessness; given to feel his work too much for him; disinclined to take responsibility; given to make molehills into mountains; procrastinating; susceptible on slight exertion, mental or physical, to fatigue; and with a loss of all powers of concentration. In fact an irritable man, more or less unequal to his work, though otherwise fairly fit, save for symptoms said to be due to 'liver'. Subsequently I found that, in Bengal and Burmah [sic], a similar train of symptoms were well known, and designated respectively, *Bengal head, Burmese head*. Those affected were generally such as had been in the country some considerable time without taking furlough, men strenuous at work and valuable as such.

Since then, during much travel in India and Burmah, and twelve years' work in Calcutta [now Kolkata], I recognise that those peculiarities (so manifest to the lay mind as to enable it to label the series of symptoms due to mental fatigue with a special name, and known I believe, to our missionary friends as *brain-fag*) are the commencing signs of an affection which has got the well-known designation of *neurasthenia, ie* 'a complex of symptoms, induced by nerve exhaustion and associated with, if not causing, an alteration in bodily nutrition'.

Amongst Europeans in India it is an affection most worthy of study. It does not directly kill the patient, but it 'hampers his work, interferes with his career, ruins his temper, upsets his friends, and causes him to be unfit for any position of trust or responsibility'.

Cuvier[6] has well said '*the nervous system is at bottom the whole animal, and the other systems are only to serve it*'.

My contention is that the conditions of continuous life in hot countries influence directly the function of the nervous system of the European, or do so indirectly by injuring the systems ancillary to it.

The primary causes leading to this [anomaly] are the humidity, and the sun with its light and heat. Helping these are the parasitic diseases – the causal agents of which owe their vigour to the climate and their preservation to the environment.

An abnormal bodily state is produced by the light, the heat, and the humidity – a change in body temperature, a lowered pulse rate and tension, an irritable heart, a lessened respiratory function owing to deficiency of intake and rarefaction of the air, and a deterioration of the blood. An increasing perspiration causes a lessening of the kidney excretion; with the extra work thrown on the liver there follows a continued congestion, then degeneration; an atonic dyspepsia and impaired function lead to pathological decomposition of protein bodies in the gastro-intestinal canal, and there ensues chronic auto-intoxication and its results. Thus the climatic conditions lower the powers of resistance, and render the individual more liable to fall a victim to the attacks of the specific forms of disease. There is no independence of mind and body, and what influences the one will affect the other.

The predisposing factors to 'nerve weakness' were, Charles considered:

... Heredity. - Neuropathic disposition.
Emotional Disturbances. – Mental over-exertion, worry, disappointments.
Infectious Diseases. – Dysentery, influenza, dengue, enteric [typhoid fever] – all such as bring about exhaustion and prostration by malnutrition.
Manner of Living. – The European hustles – the Native is placid. The latter understands his climate and what suits him best. The former thinks he does, and does not, and insists on having his customs where they were never evolved. He pursues his habits as if he were superior to his surroundings.
Alcohol. – This is a danger. The man, when he begins to 'run down', takes more than his wont 'to keep the clock wound up', and so a

vicious cycle is established (total abstainers, though, also suffer from *neurasthenia*). There is a use and misuse of alcohol. The proper use of it is the difficulty. The counsel of perfection would be, avoid it till over 30 years of age, and then, if taken at all, only take it in moderation, but not till the sun goes down. It is a drug, may be a luxury, never a necessity.

There are certain causes of a more direct nature, and they are those which specially act in India, causing a greater wear and tear on the nervous energy, and making asthenia of the nervous system more common amongst white folks there than in Europe.
Continued Moist Heat. – Producing anaemia, and so weakening vitality by acting on the metabolism.
Imperfect Metabolism. – Predisposed to by bad, or insipid food. Chronic auto-intoxication by impaired digestion may be a cause, or a result of *neurasthenia*. My experience is that the two conditions are oftenest combined. Here again a vicious cycle.
The Sun's Rays. – There is much indeed to be said in favour of the actinic theory that a cause of the nervous collapse of the white man under tropical conditions is due to his white skin. It is true, as Dr Woodruff [*see above*] points out, that the amount of pigment in each individual is in direct proportion to the intensity of the light of the country in which his ancestors have evolved. The continued and excessive heat of the sun lowers vitality and depresses energy. Here it is interesting to quote the paper of Colonel Dawson[7] on the 'Variation of Structure and Colour in Flowers under Insolation'. His experiments began eight years ago, and point to a definite connection between the variations of colour and structure and the sun's altitude, both seasonal and diurnal, and prove that metabolism had been affected, and that changes of colour and structure were produced and could be reproduced in other individuals.

I have met with the subjects of *neurasthenic* troubles during twenty-five years in India, and, in the past six years, on the Medical Board, India Office. In the latter time there have been upwards of 150 cases.

The commonest *symptoms* manifested have been:–

> *Mental.* – A lack of confidence, tendency to introspection, loss of energy, want of power of concentration, phobias, insomnia.

Emotional. – Lack of control of feelings, irritability, depression.
Circulatory and Vasomotor. – Palpitation, headache, sense of giddiness, sweating.
Various Forms of Gastro-Intestinal Trouble. – Gastroduodenal ulcer, colitis, dysentery, diarrhoea, etc.

That is, there was a congeries of mental and sensory disturbances, and signs of defective metabolism were usual in nearly every case. It is a fatigue condition in which one of the most important symptoms, as far as prognosis is concerned, is insomnia. Till sleep returns the patient will not recover.

It has also struck me that a main factor in invaliding of public servants in India is a form of nerve exhaustion which, by lowering their vitality and natural immunity, renders them more susceptible to the onset of various diseases.

There are animals and plants that cannot exist in certain climates, except under special conditions. The growth of man is susceptible, in a degree, to the same natural laws that influence plants and animals. In every part of the world the indigenous inhabitant, adjusted to the climate, has his organism in keeping with the environment. We in the North of Europe have feelings, modes of thought and pursuits, partaking of the character of the climate in which we live, the influence of which, in the course of centuries, is traceable in the working of the brain, and in the natural pursuits and characteristics.

The light-coloured peoples are perfectly fitted to the cold climates, and when they migrate to hot latitudes they are damaged by the conditions to which they are there exposed. This accounts for the fact that though there has been a succession of streams of white races flowing southward to India, they do not there permanently survive *as such.* For it follows that when a race migrates to a strikingly different climate, it must either conform to the necessities imposed by that climate, or, in time, become extinct. Conforming to the climate will probably mean the preservation of a percentage of strains defective in the primitive qualities, and with a liability to nervous weakness. This *liability* is the thing transmitted. In India, owing to the conditions of the life being appropriate, neurotic liability is produced.

> It is the conditions of life which chiefly determine the destiny of a race through their eventual influence on the mentality. I do not say that climate makes a nation, or a nation's customs, but it limits and defines and moulds the characteristics in common with the alteration brought about by the food and soil.

Charles then focused upon the indigenous peoples of India and other tropical countries – residents there for long periods of time:

> To India races have been for ages migrated from the most various quarters, have mingled, and have modified themselves under the new conditions. For whether the invaders were white or yellow, the law has held that when dark and light races have been placed in contact, crossing has taken place between them. The foreigners universally have yielded – Yavana, Scythian, Sakas, Yuehchi, and White Hun – to the wonderful assimilative power of Hinduism. They have been absorbed, have taken on the characteristics of the country. The same soil continues to give the same flavour to the fruit.
>
> Other invaders have disappeared and are forgotten, till someone accidentally finds a coin, or an inscribed plate, which reminds the world that such people have lived there.
>
> Consider what a great people the ancient Aryan invaders of India were! ... What were the influences instrumental in converting the Aryan into the Hindoo? The far-reaching alteration in the manners, physique and notions were due to the exchange of an elevated, cool, unproductive place of abode for the low, warm, rich lands lying on the great rivers where they breathed an air so rarefied by heat that there was less oxygen in a given number of respirations, and being thus an expanded air it was less fitted to dilate the chest. Here they mixed with the conquered peoples and Hinduism evolved. Hinduism, that curious conglomerate of faiths that sprang up after the admission of Dasyus into the Brahminical polity. It is probable that the influence of these half-assimilated Dasyus, while it helped in the acclimatization of the Aryan, worked the great though gradual change from the bright Vedic faith to the highly coloured mythology of the Puranas and the complex beliefs of the modern Hindoo.
>
> In process of time the Honourable and Sovereign Aryan race was, by the effects of climate and social influences, reduced to

a people with energy deteriorated, and with that want of spirit which bends and adapts itself. Becoming inherently lazy, they eventually became possessed of the virtues which are more negative than positive. Exhaustion and anaemia preyed on the people's health, and lowered its vital resistance to disease by a general lessening of natural immunity. They lost their independence, and those who do so end by losing their energy: to such submission becomes a custom and servitude a pleasure.

The dishonoured end of the Hindoo kingdoms of Bengal and Behar points a moral, and shews that had they deserved to exist they would have made a better fight. They fell – because of the nervous exhaustion of the race – a prey to the climate, and corrupted by the departure of the people from the customs and practices of their ancestors. 'The fathers had eaten sour grapes and the children's teeth were set on edge'.

When such a highly civilised society as that of the Moghuls at Delhi disintegrated under the pressure from the surrounding and rising peoples, it was because its energy had been worn out. Those who were left to carry on the traditions of the past lacked the necessary power for a renewed concentration and revival. That power had been kept alive by a continuous stream of fresh blood percolating from Central Asia. This could continue so long as Afghanistan was under the sway of Delhi. When that country was no longer subservient, a dam cut across the immigration, and the deterioration of the Moghul power dates from that time. It is to be remembered also that there was much crossing of the pure blood with the Indian. To us the lesson is: that a similar fate would befall us did the annual fleets of vessels cease to take the young blood from our shores to the coral strands, where each one hopes his fortune calls him.

These examples shew that for a white race to preserve its purity and predominance in a tropical climate, and to keep that vigour, intelligence, and physique which are its characteristics, fresh waves of immigration are essential to make up for the wear and tear due to climatic influences.

… Where in the world can be seen a white race, in a tropical climate, maintaining the original energy of the people that founded the power? The damp heat changes the quality of the blood; the muscular fibre becomes less vigorous; the brain becomes more irritable; the calm reason, the temperate will, the foresight, the strength, the skill, the endurance of the European, become sadly reduced by the tropical conditions; all acting with their depressing effect on the nervous system.

In India the European is in a position of trust and has much responsibility. His work is harassing in nature and entails much mental effort. In the temperate zone many endure strain and mental expenditure, working early and late, and keep their powers unimpaired; but in the tropics the powers of resistance to such strain are greatly lowered, and eventually, *in the predisposed*, the nerve breakdown called *neurasthenia* ensues.

Charles then developed the theme that the strains imposed on the European serving in India were such that only those equal to this stressful environment should be selected for service there:

> … When the normal European goes to India, he first experiences a marked feeling of wellness, his brain is more active and his muscle vigour more marked. He cannot understand either the complaints, or the warnings, of the old residents, for 'all is well with the lad'. He thinks he has an inexhaustible capital of health, but he overdraws, and exhaustion follows. The sleepless nights of fervent heat, noisy with insect life, the food tasteless and unrefreshing, the loneliness of the station, the petty worries incidental to the humdrum of the life, the sun shining in his strength as it were to a perpetual day, bring about tiredness of mind and body. It is this terrible nerve exhaustion which has, in the past, been the most important factor in preventing the northern races settling, and procreating their line, *with a full share of the nerve vigour which the parental stock possessed.* This is why the invaders of India have disappeared, and this is the bar to the settlement of tropical regions by white folk 'bringing forth seed after their kind'. So it has been written of India that there the European struggles during the first, dwindles and degenerates during the second, and becomes extinct, as such, during the third or fourth generation.

Charles continued attempting to silence the sceptics:

> … Some may say, 'Produce your evidence that the white races cannot permanently colonize the tropics and remain white'. I

suggest that the history of the various multitudes of invaders of India, of northern races, and the utter disappearance of many of them, and the absolute change of others, bodily and mentally, is a fact in the case.

… In cold climates chest troubles predominate, in hot climates belly troubles, and for the white man also nerve troubles. Up to this, as far as the plains of India are concerned, it is absolutely certain that it is impossible for Europeans to thrive and continue their race. The native can work in the sun with his head and spine bare – the European, with helmet and spine-pad, withstands it with difficulty, and, as years go by, becomes more and more liable to its influences and likes it less. The nervousness of the children is marked, and physical, intellectual, and procreative degeneration, in the long run, bring about extinction. An infusion of native blood is essential to the continuance of the stock, but the barrier once broken, the remoter descendants partake more and more of the mental and physical characters of the native. The race is ruined. It is the duty of the State to safeguard the individuality of its people so that development will take place along the line of its historic growth. Mixing the white race with the coloured peoples begets another with the virtues of neither; but without the crossing the white race cannot live to colonize tropical regions.

It is true you can to an extent with money enough, *and despotic power*, rectify insanitary conditions, and banish many of the tropical diseases; but you cannot change the heat, the sunlight, the climatic conditions, by either the power of money or the power of knowledge. Neither can you settle a stock of people, evolved to suit the environments of northern latitudes, *so that they retain their characteristics*, in a tropical, or a sub-tropical climate, more than you can cause southern wheat to grow and give its increase on a highland soil.

It can be said that white men of sound constitution can and do live in the tropics; but what of the women and children, and what is the result at the third and fourth generation?

… Prolonged residence in a high temperature, with little range and high relative humidity, with excess of light, will produce not only physical but mental deterioration associated with anaemia. This is quite apart from the onslaught of any parasitic disease –

but the parasitic invasion is rendered easier by the decadence of the victim's vitality.

The application of science to the problems of health at Panama had, Charles continued, in part succeeded, but he did not feel that this could be extrapolated to the sanitary conditions of India. Neither did he feel that there were parallels with experiences in tropical Australia or America. He ended by summarising thus:

> ... 1. I start from Cuvier's [*see* above] axiom:- 'The nervous system is at bottom the whole animal, and the other systems are only to serve it'.
> 2. My thesis is that the constitution of the northern races is developed in temperate latitudes – that its powers are injuriously affected by the climatic conditions of the hot zone.
> The way in which to establish a theory is to advance definite facts in its favour.
> I. If you damage the subservient systems you injure the whole animal, *ie* the nervous system.
> II. Tropical climates injure the various systems of the body apart altogether from the dangers of attack from parasitic enemies.
> III. The characteristics of dwellers in the tropics are distinctive of them and produced by their environment.
> IV. The characters of the northern races are a thing apart and due to similar causes.
> V. Brain power, or the civilization due to it, did not arise in the hot zone, for the seats of this ancient civilization – the old 'culture zone' – were in [latitude] 25°N to 50°N.
> VI. Modern civilization, with higher brain development, has gone still further north than the seat of the 'culture zone', and is now found in the temperate regions.
> VII. The emotional type of brain, when found in the northern peoples, is more peculiar to the races that live in the warmer parts, and they have that in common with dwellers in the sub-tropics.
> VIII. What has happened to the myriads of invaders of India? Have they maintained their power, or have they decayed – Aryan, Greek, Scythian, Hun, Mongol, Parthian, etc? Do the peoples of India preserve the characteristics of these invaders?

Do the descendants of the invaders preserve the powers of the nations from whence they sprung, and are they comparable to the peoples occupying the original homeland?

IX. What has been the effect on the descendants of the European races that have gone to India in old days – Portuguese, Dutch, French, English? To how many generations does the pure blood survive? What is the character of the degenerated stock?

X. How do the heads of the great merchant firms in India answer the foregoing question when employing men for various business posts? The Eurasian gets a certain pay; the country born gets double that; the imported European, with his energy and fresh vitality, gets four times the amount given to the Eurasian, and twice that given to the country born.

XI. The Emperor Babur[8], in his Memoirs, makes an interesting note on the depressing effect of the climate on his followers – a falling off in energy and initiative. For this he gave them permission to return to the cooler regions to recuperate, whilst he himself battled with the discomfort of the sun and the surroundings.

XII. There is a disease – diabetes – which has certain relations to the nervous system. That affection is very prevalent in India, and increasingly so since the Indians have been forced to live more strenuously by their contact with Europeans; the strain being less easy to bear there than in Europe.

XIII. What occurs to the various strains of horses, cattle, sheep, dogs, poultry, and even vegetables, introduced from Europe to the plains of India? Do their distinctive characters remain, or deteriorate?

XIV. Experiment has shewn that metabolism in flowers and changes of colour and structure can be brought about by insolation – according to the altitude, seasonal and diurnal.

XV. What is the meaning of *Punjab head, Bengal head, Burmese head*, and other such terms? (? Warnings of *neurasthenia*).

XVI. The conditions affecting the foregoing are those that have had to do with the formation of races – climate, food, soil – *ie* environment.[9]

This address provoked a very lively discussion.

The Society in the pre-war years

Possible absorption by the Royal Society of Medicine (RSM)

It was during these pre-war years that the Society was first approached by the Royal Society of Medicine (RSM) with an underlying determination to accomplish a takeover![10] The newly created RSM had hoped to include the STMH in the amalgamation of fifteen pre-existent medical societies (*see* below).

The RSM (still housed at 20 Hanover Square) had come into being in 1907, when a supplementary Royal Charter was granted by King Edward VII. The move to Wimpole Street was not to take place until 1912. On the initiative of its first secretary, Mr (later Sir John) MacAlister (1856–1925)[11] (*see* Figure 4.3) the RSM had recently amalgamated with these specialist societies; MacAlister was, it seems very keen to add yet another – the STMH. Sir Francis Henry Champneys, Bt (1848–1930) (*see* Figure 4.4) was president of the RSM from 1912 to 14; he was an eminent obstetrician – the first to use Listerian antisepsis in the practice of this speciality. (His son, Sir Weldon Dalrymple-Champneys Bt [1892–1980], is remembered as an authority on brucellosis.) In June 1912, MacAlister planned to form a 'tropical section' of the RSM and obviously it would have been highly desirable if the STMH could be included!

This matter has been well recorded in the *history of the RSM*, but there it is viewed from the RSM's perspective.[12] The first mention in *Council* minutes of absorption of the Society by the RSM appears at a meeting at 11 Chandos Street on Thursday **9 January 1912**:

> ... after discussion [of the proposed 'take-over'] it was resolved that the question of amalgamation should continue to receive consideration, and that the opinions of those members of *Council* who were unable to be present should, so far as possible, be obtained. A preliminary vote of those present showed them to be unanimously *opposed* [author's italics] to the union of the Societies.

This was followed by a further meeting of *Council* ten days later:

> Some correspondence with Dr Latham, Hon Secy. [RSM] relative to the absorption of the Society by that body was read, in which he asked that a meeting of representatives of the two societies might take place and it was resolved that the Society agree to

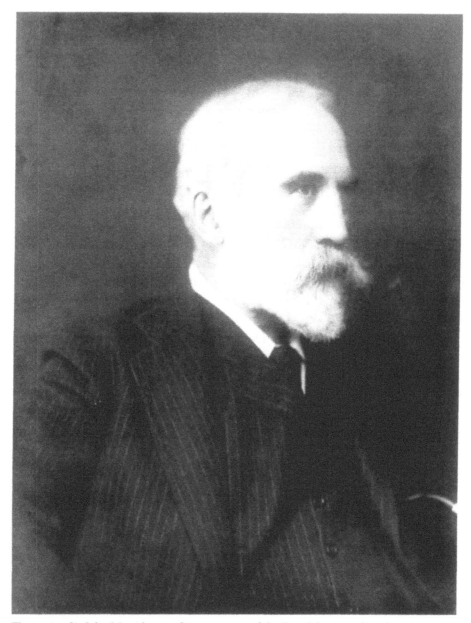

Figure 4.3: Sir John MacAlister – first secretary of the Royal Society of Medicine (reproduced courtesy the Wellcome Library, London).

this, and that the President, joint Secretaries, and past and present Vice-Presidents be appointed … representatives of the [STMH].

A month later, *Council* was updated on the matter:

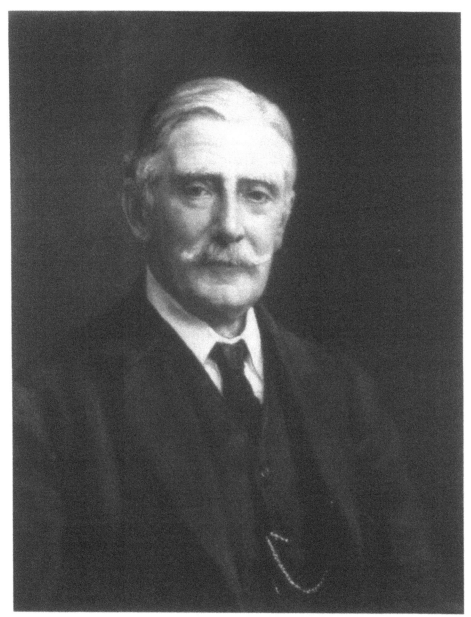

Figure 4.4: Sir Francis Champneys Bt – president of the Royal Society of Medicine (1912–14).

The correspondence having been read which had taken place since the last meeting, it was agreed that the Secretaries be requested to communicate with the Honorary Secretary of the [RSM], and to inform him that the representatives of the [STMH] will be glad to meet with the representatives of the [RSM] at the rooms of that Society at such time as may prove to be mutually convenient.

And at a further meeting on **17 May**:

The joint Secretaries brought up a letter from the Secretary [RSM], in which he stated that the memorandum as to proposed amalgamation which was drawn up at the request of the Council of that Society, had been submitted to the *Council*, but that they did not consider any useful purpose would be served by printing it. The joint Secretary was directed to reply acknowledging receipt of the letter, and to have the memorandum printed for future reference.

But the matter continued to be raised at *Council* meetings; thus on **23 September**:

Dr Sandwith and Dr Harford reported certain correspondence with the Secretary of the [RSM] which they had received concerning the formation of a Tropical section in connection with that Society. It was also reported to the meeting that Sir Havelock Charles [the next President] and Dr G C Low had attended the meeting convened for the purposes of forming that section, and that they had proposed and seconded an amendment to the resolution to form such a section. Their amendment was lost by four votes to three. In view of the fact that the circular issued with reference to the formation of the Section appeared to be misleading, and particularly in view of the fact that the name of Sir Patrick Manson had appeared as if he were supporting the formation of the Section, it was decided to write a letter to Fellows explaining the position and enclosing the memorandum drafted by Dr [W] Carnegie Brown as a result of the recent negotiations. This course was unanimously approved.

The following month:

Dr Low read to the meeting the opinion of several Local Secretaries [of the STMH] from abroad who unanimously opposed the amalgamation with the [RSM], at least for the present.

Communication to Fellows re – [RSM]. The memorandum drawn up in the summer by Dr Carnegie Brown together with a covering letter to Fellows, explaining the negotiations with the [RSM], and a letter from Sir Patrick Manson to the President explaining that the use of his name by the Secretary of the [RSM] was unauthorised were duly submitted to the meeting and approved. Mr [J] Cantlie explained that he had not given leave for the inclusion of his name [either] as supporting the new section of Tropical Medicine of the [RSM], and that he would ask that his name should be removed from the Committee.

However, by **November 15**, it seemed that the whole idea had been abandoned:

A letter was read from Major McCarrison stating that he had agreed to support the Tropical Section of the [RSM] under a misapprehension, and that he had written withdrawing from the Section. Dr [F M] Sandwith stated that he had been informed on good authority that it had [in any case] been decided for the present to give up the idea of forming a Tropical Section of the [RSM].

But the following month:

Dr Sandwith stated that his statement at the previous meeting of *Council* was premature and that the formation of a Tropical Section was still in contemplation.
[Also at that meeting:]
A letter was read from a Fellow stating his intention to resign at the end of the year on account of the decision of the *Council* not to amalgamate with the [RSM] without first consulting the Fellows. It was decided to accept this resignation.

By **17 January 1913**, it was obvious that the matter was still far from being resolved:

Dr Sandwith read a letter from Sir Francis Champneys (President of the [RSM]) stating his desire to have an interview with Sir William Leishman [President of the STMH] with reference to *the recent negotiations between the Societies* [author's italics]. ...

Leishman desired to know the wish of … Council as to whether he should meet … Champneys and it was unanimously agreed that [he] should accept the invitation, but that this should *not* be regarded as the re-opening of negotiations.

At the next *Council* meeting, the result of that interview was made known:

The President [Leishman] reported his interview with … Champneys [who] was most anxious to meet all the difficulties raised by the [STMH]. In particular he would be in favour of granting to the *new* Tropical Section if amalgamation were agreed upon:
- Practical autonomy.
- The right to admit certain non-medical members as at present.
- The right to appoint Honorary members in the same way as the existing Honorary Fellows.
- The admission of Medical Missionaries at half the usual subscription rates.
- The possible remission of entrance fee in certain cases.

After a discussion it was felt that it would not be competent for the *Council* to pass a resolution as to the desirability or otherwise of amalgamation, but seeing that the matter was of some urgency, owing to the expressed determination of the [RSM] to form a Tropical Section, in the event of there being no prospect of amalgamation, it was agreed to appoint a deputation of four Fellows to meet a similar deputation from the [RSM], if such should be appointed. The President [Leishman], and Vice-President [Charles], Dr G C Low, and Mr Austen were appointed as members of the deputation.

Minutes of a *Council* meeting on **18 April** contain the following statement, *ie* a report from this deputation to the RSM:

The report of the deputation which met the [RSM] was then laid upon the table [*see* below]. Copies had previously been distributed amongst members of the *Council* so it was taken as read:

NOTES ON THE MEETING OF DELEGATES ON
APRIL 3rd. 1913.

1. No entrance fee of £2: 2: 0 would be charged to present Fellows
   of the [STMH] joining the Tropical Section of the [RSM] within
   6 months of amalgamation and their annual subscription to
   the new Section would remain, as at present, £1: 1: 0.

   Subsequent to this, new members of the Section would pay
   the usual entrance fee of £2: 2: 0.

   Within 6 months of amalgamation Fellows of the [STMH]
   could become full Fellows of the RSM without entrance fee
   on payment of an annual subscription of £3: 3: 0 (this giving
   membership of all sections the full transactions of the [RSM]
   and the free use of the Library). Later than 6 months the usual
   entrance fee would be charged in addition.

2. To Fellows of the [STMH] joining only the new Section of
   the [RSM], and not becoming *full Fellows*, the Library is only
   available on payment of an annual additional subscript of £1:
   1: 0 if they join within 6 months; *new* members of the Section
   or present Fellows of the [STMH] who join later than 6 months
   after amalgamation will pay the usual Library Subscription of
   £2: 2: 0 per annum.

   The services of the Precis-writer are only available to *full
   Fellows* of the [RSM].

3. Members of the new Section only would receive the
   Proceedings of their Section only, but this would not be less
   full or less completely illustrated than at present.

4. The admission of *Laymen* into the new Section would be as at
   present carried out by the [STMH] and on the same terms as
   ordinary qualified men. They would also be eligible to become
   full Fellows of the [RSM] if approved by the Council of the [RSM].

5. Medical men whose qualifications have not been registered in
   this country, whether British subjects or Foreigners, are eligible
   for Membership of the new Section and also for Fellowship,
   but in their case the personal written testimony of several men
   of authority and position would be required and carefully
   considered by the Council of the [RSM].

6. Medical Missionaries at present Fellows of the [STMH] who
   pay only half subscription might be allowed to continue at this

rate if they joined within 6 months; for those joining later than this the entrance subscription of £2: 2: 0 might be waived, but the annual subscription of £1: 1: 0 would be charged.

7. The *Honorary Fellows* of the [STMH] would become Corresponding Members of the new Section. In the other Sections of the [RSM] these are limited to 20. Future nominations would be made by the Section and approved by the Council of the [RSM], but the latter reserve to themselves the right of nominated Hon Fellows of the [RSM].

8. In the event of amalgamation the funds of the [STMH] would be taken over en bloc by the [RSM].

9. It has not yet been contemplated by the [RSM] that grants of money should be made for research outside this country, but assistance and support has sometimes been given to investigations conducted at home.

10. The [RSM] would be prepared to consider favourably a lenient interpretation of the rules regarding the use of the Library in special cases – eg a reduction in the fee might be made to men coming home to England for short periods of time, but this would have to be decided by the Council of the [RSM] not by the Council of the Section of Tropical Medicine.

Members of the *Council* [who were] present discussed the report.

1. Fleet Surgeon [P W] Bassett-Smith RN said that he considered there were no advantages to be gained by amalgamation. He was therefore strongly against it.

2. Dr A G Bagshawe [Director of the Bureau of Hygiene and Tropical Medicine] said that he thought many of the points in the report were not of primary importance. He thought amalgamation meant loss of position and that if it took place there would be a breaking away again in the course of a few years. He emphasised the fact that Fellows of the [STMH] could use the Library of the Tropical Diseases Bureau at the Imperial Institute free of charge. He also said that there would be a reading room there and further facilities in the near future. He was [thus] strongly against amalgamation.

3. Mr [J] Cantlie thought the [RSM] were throwing a bait to induce the [STMH] to join them. He would not accept the RSM's conditions on any account whatsoever. He did not

think it was worthy of discussion. It would cripple the Society in the future. Fellows would fall off in numbers. Against it.

4. Dr H B Newham [of the LSTM] pointed out that he had been instrumental in getting over 200 fellows for the Society from the Tropical School. 98% of these were going abroad and if amalgamation were proposed the numbers would fall off at once. Men at the School never asked about the [RSM] and shewed no desire whatever to join it. On the other hand they joined the [STMH] with alacrity. Men abroad would get no advantages and the Library was purely a bait. He was certain that of the many men who had joined lately, many would resign at once on amalgamation being proposed and no more would join in the future. There would be loss of growth and the Society would be defunct in a few years. He was absolutely against it.

5. Dr [G C] Low said that the crux of the situation was the increased fees to future fellows, eg £2-2 entry money, a guinea a year for subscription and £2-2 yearly for the use of the Library (£5-5 the first year and £3-3 for subsequent years or if the Library was not taken £3-3 the first year and £1-1 for subsequent years). The Society would lose all future candidates on account of this. He was against it.

6. Professor [W J R] Simpson [also of the LSTM, and a future President] thought that union in some ways was a good thing but after hearing the arguments for and against was decidedly in favour of the latter. Against.

Fleet Surgeon Bassett-Smith then proposed 'that the Fellows of the Society should be circularised on the question of the proposed amalgamation with the [RSM]'. Dr Newham seconded the motion. There was no amendment and the motion on being put to the meeting was carried.

Fleet Surgeon Bassett-Smith thought that the facts should be placed before all the fellows and the reasons why the *Council* were against it. Mr Cantlie thought that the feeling of the *Council* should be put down as a guidance. Dr Newham thought the feeling of ... *Council* against amalgamation should be stated to the fellows to guide them in their decision. Mr Cantle then moved the following motion:

That the terms suggested by the [RSM] and especially the financial proposals should be put before the Fellows of the Society and that ... Council should give an expression of their opinion to guide the Fellows though not necessarily to prejudice them.

Prof Simpson seconded. There was no amendment. The motion on being put to the meeting was carried unanimously.

It was resolved that the Ballot of Fellows should be closed on the 1st of October. A subcommittee, consisting of Sir William Leishman, Dr Harford, Dr Low and Dr Bagshawe, was then appointed to draw up a form to be sent to the Fellows. This form was to be brought before the *Council* at their next meeting, May 16th 1913 for consideration.

Sir William Leishman shewed the members of Council a private document which he had received from the Secretary of the [RSM]. This consisted of Dr Carnegie Brown's old memorandum with the [RSM]'s revisions & suggestions added. These were practically the same, though less full, than that already placed before the *Council* by the Deputation.

On **16 May**, *Council* minutes document that:

The Sub-Committee appointed to draw up a statement for submission to the Fellows with reference to the negotiations with the [RSM], presented their Statement to the meeting and with some slight amendment it was adopted as given below, it being understood that this would be submitted by the President [Leishman] to ... Champneys in order to ensure that the facts there set forth might be agreed upon as correct, the officers being authorised to make any minor changes which might appear to be necessary.

The communication to the Fellows was as follows:

Memorandum concerning recent negotiations with the Royal Society of Medicine

The *Council* of the [STMH] have again been approached by the [RSM] with a view to a reconsideration of the proposal that the former Society should become a Section of the latter. After a Conference between representatives of the two Societies, the *Council* of the [STMH] has decided to put the facts of the case before the Fellows of this Society, and to take a ballot of the Fellows as to whether amalgamation should take place. They hope that every Fellow will record his vote on the special form which is sent herewith. The *Council* have decided that no change should be made unless there is a three-fourths majority of the Fellows who take part in the ballot, which will close on the 1st of October.

Appended to this Memorandum will be found a statement of the terms which are offered by the [RSM], and these will enable Fellows to judge as to the advisability or otherwise of the suggested change.

In forwarding this statement, the *Council* desire to submit the following observations:-

(a) They desire to acknowledge the great courtesy of the President and Council of the [RSM] in the discussions which have taken place in connection with the proposed amalgamation.

(b) They are most anxious that the whole matter should be considered from the point of view of the general interests of *Tropical Medicine*, and from this standpoint they have most regretfully come to the conclusion that it is not desirable to relinquish the present independent position of the Society.

This accompanying document [*Statement of terms offered by the Royal Society of Medicine (April 3rd, 1913)*] was a reiteration of the statement dated 3 April 1913 'laid upon the table' at the meeting of *Council* held on 18 April (*see* above).

On **20 June**:

[This] memorandum … was laid on the table and it was agreed that the date for sending in replies should be November 1st [*not* October 1st] 1913 and that a motion should be brought forward at the *Annual Meeting* [later that day] providing that the decision as to amalgamation should only be carried out by a three fourths majority of Fellows taking part in the ballot.

At the sixth *AGM* that day, a minute states:

> An announcement having been made that it was proposed to take a ballot of the Fellows as to the suggestion of amalgamation with the [RSM], it was proposed by Sir Havelock Charles [the new President] and seconded by Dr Harford that no change shall be made unless there is a three fourths majority of the Fellows who take part in the ballot, which will close on November 1st 1913. This was unanimously agreed to.

And at a *Special* meeting of *Council* in July:

> The Secretaries reported that the Memorandum had been sent out to all the Fellows of the Society in accordance with the decision of the Council.

A meeting of *Council* in October was provided with an update:

> It was announced that the Ballot to date showed 207 against amalgamation and 58 in favour of it.

And on **November 21**, *Council* was provided with the ultimate result:

> The report of the result of the ballot re amalgamation with the [RSM] was read, the figures being 216 votes against amalgamation and 60 for. The *Council* decided that the [Hon] Secretaries should write to ... Champneys, President of the [RSM] acquainting him with these figures, and also announce the result of the Ballot in the *British Medical Journal* & *Lancet*. (The ballot [had been] closed on the 1st. Nov. 1913).

The previous president (Leishman) had apparently written to Sir Ronald Ross in November 1912, indicating that he was glad that he (Ross) had declined the Vice-Presidency of the *tropical section* of the RSM.

Several years later however (well after the Great War [1914–18] had terminated), *amalgamation* of the two Societies was again suggested in a confidential letter to the then president (Simpson) from MacAlister. A *Council* meeting on **21 November 1919** 'was [however] against re-opening the discussion'.

This matter would simply not however 'go away' and MacAlister proved extremely persistent. At a *Council* meeting on **2 January 1920**, Dr

[W T] Prout reported that he had received a letter from the RSM about starting a section of *tropical medicine*. Although the president (Simpson) felt that the Society should 'remain aloof from it', *Council* decided to discuss the matter further at a *Special* Meeting. On **16 January**, they decided that it 'was against taking any action in the matter'.

The matter was still by no means dead, however! At a *Council* meeting on **11 June 1920**, Dr [C F] Harford stated that whether the *tropical section* of the RSM would continue or not would be 'raised on July 5th'. Although he apparently favoured amalgamation, *Council* decided that as *Royal* had by then been incorporated into the title (*see* Chapter 6) 'the question of absorption [by] any other Society was out of the question'. On **18 June**, Harford:

> … made a statement [to *Council*] on his views with regard to the relation between the [RSTMH] and the [RSM]. He thought there should be co-ordination between the two Societies, having regard to the fact that *tropical medicine* [author's italics] was only a part of *medicine in the tropics*.

At a later meeting of *Council* in November:

> Dr [G C] Low called attention to the meeting of the Tropical Section of the [RSM] [to be held] on Nov 30th to arrange for the Election of Officers & for a paper by Dr [F G] Rose.[13] Were Councillors who were also Fellows of the [RSTMH] to attend such a meeting? The general feeling was that Councillors of the [RSTMH] must follow their own leanings as far as attendance was concerned, but that Councillors should not accept any office in the new Section. The Hon Secs were directed to write to absent Councillors, informing them of this expression of opinion.

And on **19 November** came what was considered to be the 'finale':

> Correspondence between Sir John MacAlister, Secy of the [RSM] and Prof Simpson was read [to Council] dealing with the attitude of this Society to the Section of *Tropical Medicine* of the [RSM]; the Councillors present were asked for their opinions. Sir Patrick Manson thought there was not room for two Societies & regretted the formation of a new one & expressed the opinion that this Society should preserve its individuality. Col [S P] James thought

that this Society should provide advantages as an offset against those provided by the [RSM]; he suggested a small laboratory. Dr [W T (later Sir William)] Prout was against any attitude of hostility, & would leave members of the *Council* perfectly free as regards the new Section & would deprecate any resolution of *Council*. Prof [R T] Leiper agreed. He would give a paper at the new Section if asked & thought that there was sufficient material for both the Society and the new [RSM] Section. Other members were strongly against Councillors of the Society being officers of the [RSM] Section.

A further letter from MacAlister was read at a *Council* meeting on **18 March 1921**. In it he indicated that 'the title of the Section of Tropical Medicine had now been altered to *Section of Tropical Medicine and Parasitology*' and he hoped that rivalry between the councils of the two societies would cease and they would feel able to 'work harmoniously together …'. It should be noted however that on 18 February, 'Dr Prout [had *not* been] re-nominated [to *Council* of the RSTMH] on the grounds that he was Secretary of the Tropical Diseases Section of the [RSM]'.

> *Council* on **17 February 1927** considered a letter addressed to the President [Balfour] by … Prout and referring to the 'embargo' which prevented officers of the *Section of Parasitology and Tropical Diseases* of the [RSM] from serving on the Council of the [RSTMH]. … Prout felt that this restriction should now be withdrawn.
>
> It was pointed out by the President, Dr Balfour, Dr Low, Dr Bagshawe and others that at the time of the decision referred to (1920) there was no other course possible and that but for the firm action of the *Council* this Society would have been absorbed by the [RSM], which did not cater for foreign members as did the [RSTMH]. The President, Dr Balfour added that events had proved the wisdom of the line of action taken to preserve the individuality and independence of the [RSTMH]. The establishment of the Tropical Section of the [RSM] had in no way affected this Society adversely.
>
> Dr [A G] Bagshawe agreed that in view of the strong position of this Society it might be well to remove the restrictions but considered it inadvisable that the Society should have on its *Council* anyone who was an executive officer of the other Society.

It was then proposed by Dr Balfour and seconded by Colonel [A] Alcock that members of the *Council* of the [RSTMH] should now be free to take office in the *Section of Parasitology and Tropical Diseases* of the [RSM], but that no member of the *Council* should hold executive office in the other Society. This motion was carried unanimously.

Despite this, however, relations with the RSM continued to be strained. For example, at a meeting of *Council* as late as **20 October 1932**:

A letter was read from Dr Andrew Robertson (Secretary of the *Section of Tropical Diseases and Parasitology* of the [RSM]) making various suggestions calculated to 'prevent' overlapping in the activities of the two organizations.

The first suggestion was that this Society and the Section of the [RSM] should each year hold one joint combined Laboratory Meeting at the R A M College and the London School of Hygiene and Tropical Medicine [LSHTM] in alternate years. In the event of this first suggestion being impracticable the second proposal was that the Society and the Section should hold Laboratory Meetings in alternate years and that each organization should in turn be the guest of the other.

After some discussion the President asked the members of *Council* present for their opinion on the suggestion of holding joint meetings. The majority were *not* in favour of joint meetings.

It was suggested that the Section of the [RSM] might be able to devote itself to joint meetings with other Sections; or to other types of meetings. The *Council* was of opinion that in any case it would be undesirable for the Section of the [RSM] to hold Laboratory Meetings on dates which would interfere with the Laboratory Meetings of the Society.

It was further felt that there ought *not* to be any spirit of competition or antagonism between the two organizations though it was not clear how this was to be avoided. The position was complicated by the fact that officials of the Section of the [RSM] were actually members of the Council of the [RSTMH].

Finally Professor Yorke asked for the minute to be read dealing with the relations of the two organizations. Professor Yorke then gave formal notice that at the next meeting of *Council* he would propose that the minute of 27th [sic] February 1927 be re-affirmed.

At a later meeting of *Council* on **17 November 1932**:

> Professor Yorke having given notice at the previous *Council* [*see above*] that he would propose the re-affirmation of the minute of February 17th, 1927 relating to the position of executive officers in the [RSTMH] and the *Section of Tropical Diseases and Parasitology* of the [RSM], the minute was read.
>
> A general discussion resulted in which various members of *Council* expressed their views. It was noted that all the executive officers of the Society, except the Treasurer [Bagshawe], had, at one time or another, held office or served on the Council of the Section. It was pointed out by Dr Stanton that the *Council* had no authority to make a rule forbidding any Fellow or Councillor of the [RSTMH] to hold office in another Society; the utmost it could do would be to give its opinion in the form of a minute.
>
> It was clear from the discussion that there was no unanimity regarding the situation. The general feeling expressed by more than one member of *Council* was that the minute of February 1927 should not in any case be interpreted as applying to members of the present *Council*.
>
> In accordance with notice given Professor Warrington Yorke then moved the following resolution:-

> > That the *Council* affirms the expression of opinion contained in the Minute of February 17th 1927 namely, that while it is considered that members of this *Council* should be free to sit upon the Council of the *Section of Tropical Diseases and Parasitology* of the [RSM] it is deemed inadvisable for anyone to serve on this *Council* who is holding executive office in that Section (viz President & Hon Secretaries).

> This resolution was seconded by Dr Hanschell and resulted in 10 votes in favour, 6 votes against, while 6 did not vote.

Some two years later, on **17 May 1934**, Dr Manson-Bahr actually resigned from *Council* as he had been nominated president of the *Section of Tropical Diseases and Parasitology* of the RSM!

According to Hunting, a General Meeting of members of the RSM in 1936 voted for a *dissolution* of the *Section of Tropical Medicine and Parasitology*.[14] Thus, MacAlister's dream had come to an end at last!

In the opinion of Low, writing in 1928, this was the first occasion on which the Society had 'passed through troublesome times'. The second was associated with a significant reduction in the number of Fellows during the Great War (*see* Chapter 5).[15]

More accommodation problems

It will be recalled that the Society's first venue had been at the Royal Medical and Chirurgical Society (later the Royal Society of Medicine (RSM), and it had transferred to the Medical Society of London (MSL) on 1 October 1908 (*see* Chapter 2). On **15 November 1912**, *Council* was informed of a letter recently received from the MSL, 11 Chandos Street W., where they were at that time housed:

> ... a letter had been received from the [MSL] with reference to the accommodation of the Society at 11 Chandos Street stating two alternatives – (a) The [MSL] offered to store the Library in the room of the Psychological Association, to allow the desk to remain in the Library where Miss Hooper [the secretary] could work, and to allow Miss Hooper to do typewriting in the big room: Fellows to be permitted to go on using the Library as at present, and accommodation would be afforded for the [Hon] Secretaries to have interviews with the Fellows: for this a charge would be made of £21 per annum, in addition to the charge of £21 as at present for the use of the big room for the meetings and accommodation for Council meetings. (b) The [MSL] were unable to offer a special room for the use of the Society, but if so the total charge would be £63 per annum.
>
> It was decided to agree to the first proposal, it being understood that this arrangement might be modified if it were possible for a room to be placed at the disposal of the Society, and in this case the [STMH] would have first refusal.

At the next meeting of *Council*:

> A letter was read from the [MSL] confirming the arrangement agreed to at the last meeting of *Council*. It was decided to formally accept this arrangement subject to the possibility of securing a special room for the Society, if this was available and suitable and if the conditions were acceptable to the *Council*.

However on **18 February 1913**:

> A [further] letter was read from Dr Carnegie Brown pointing out that the room of the Ophthalmological Society would shortly be vacant and urging that it should be engaged at a rental of £80 per annum, this charge to include the use of the large room for meetings as at present. The honorary Secretaries were instructed to make enquiries from the [MSL] and to secure if possible the refusal of the room pending further consideration of the matter by the *Council*.

And in April:

> ... Dr Low [Hon Secretary] read a letter [to *Council*] from Mr Bethell, Registrar of the [MSL], about the room just vacated by the Ophthalmological Society at 11 Chandos Street. He, Mr Bethell, said the room was now at liberty and could be prepared for the use of the Society, should they desire to take it, early in May. The rent which would include the use of the large room for the meetings would be £80 per annum. An early reply was asked for. The *Council* resolved, that owing to the uncertainty at present existing as to the amalgamation with the *Royal Society of Medicine* [*see above*], the question of the room might be deferred for the present, but that Dr Low might see Mr Bethell and get the first refusal of the room.

The matter did not apparently receive further consideration by *Council* until July of that year.

> It was agreed that the room at 11 Chandos Street should be secured for the use of the Society, in case the vote of the Fellows should be against amalgamation [with the RSM], but the decision was deferred until after the result of the ballot could be declared [*see above*].

And on **17 October**:

> It was agreed that steps should at once be taken to secure a room at 11 Chandos St. and a Sub Committee was appointed consisting of the Vice-President, the Secretaries and the Treasurer to meet with representatives of the [MSL] in order to discuss the terms on which the room could be let to the Society.

At a Council meeting on **21 November**:

> Dr Low read a report from the Sub-Committee who had been appointed to confer with a similar Sub-Committee of the [MSL] with regard to acquiring a room at 11 Chandos Street. This meeting [had been] held on Nov 18th.... The [MSL] offered the room which used to belong to the Ophthalmological Society (*ie* the room [in which] the [STMH] hold their *Council* meetings in) under the following terms:
>
> (1) That the [MSL] be allowed to keep three book cases (not more) containing Lord [Joseph] Lister's books in the room;
> (2) That they should be allowed to hold their *Council* meetings in the room after 5pm when necessary.
>   Roughly speaking these would be as follows:
>   8 Council Meetings per year (on Mondays)
>   2 Library Meetings
>   4 Finance Meetings
> & four meetings of the Metropolitan Branch of the British Dental Association at 8pm on Wednesdays. Outside of these, *no other* meetings were to be held in the room;
> (3) That under the reservations ... they would give the [STMH] complete use of the room, for their book cases, desks, papers &c for £70 per annum;
> (4) That light and fire be included in the £70;
> (5) That the agreement be from year to year with a 6 months notice for termination from either side;
> (6) Ingress to the room to be at once or on the 1st of January 1914, as the [STMH] might desire.
>
> The *Council* agreed to accept the [MSL]'s proposals and directed the Secretaries to notify the Treasurer of that Society (Dr Mitchell Bruce) to that effect. They were also directed to get the necessary agreement drawn up.

But in December 1913, *Council* was informed of yet another letter from the MSL:

> The Secretaries reported that a letter had been received from the [MSL] stating that there had been a misunderstanding as to the terms on which the room could be let on one point, viz that the

[STMH] could not have the use of the room after 5pm except on the days of their meetings or when it was desired to hold Council meetings. On reconsideration of the matter ... *Council* decided to accept the [MSL]'s proposal and instructed the Secretaries to communicate with the [MSL] to this effect, and to arrange for a formal agreement to be signed.

That seems to have been the last negotiation until Manson House was acquired in 1931 (*see* Chapter 8).

Other Society matters

Contributions to Ordinary Meetings

Table 4.1 summarises the subjects and speakers at *Ordinary* meetings during the pre-war years. Discussions on *Sleeping Sickness* (at that time a very topical subject) seem to have been numerous, contributions being made on 20 October 1911 (A G Bagshawe), 21 June 1912 (M Anderson) and 17 January 1913 (G C Low).

Leprosy was covered by no less than five contributions on 16 February 1912.

At a *Council* meeting on **20 October 1911**, the following were identified as suitable topics for discussion: *beri-beri*, *pellagra*, and *filariasis*.

At a *Council* meeting on **16 October 1914**, *ie* immediately after the outbreak of the Great War (*see* Chapter 5):

> In view of the fact that some of the proposed readers of papers were [already] abroad, and that others were unable to take the subjects previously selected, the following Programme was suggested. For the November meeting a paper on Anti-typhoid inoculation, if possible by Sir William Osler or by Dr C J Martin – failing that a paper on Tetanus by Dr MacConkey. Dr [later Sir Andrew] Balfour agreed to give an account of his recent tour ... at the meeting in December. It was also decided to secure a paper during the session upon the subject of Bacillary Dysentery.

There were also numerous demonstrations – often of newly discovered parasites or bacteria.

Table 4.1: Communications at *Ordinary* meetings in the immediate pre-war years

Date	Subject	Speaker
1911 (cont.)		
20 October	Researches on Sleeping Sickness	A G Bagshawe
17 November	Etiology of beri-beri	H Schaumann, A Holst (Hamburg)
15 December	Epidemic dropsy in Calcutta	E D W Greig
	Pellagra in Nyasaland	H S Stannus
	Pellagra in America	F M Sandwith
1912		
19 January	Filariasis in Fiji	P H Bahr
16 February	Cultivation of leprosy bacillus	P S Abraham
	Treatment of leprosy	G Deycke
	Experimental studies on leprosy	H Much
	Recent advances in leprosy	E Marchoux
	Cultivation of leprosy bacillus	H Bayon
17 May	Tuberculosis in primitive races	S L Cummins
	Tuberculosis in Australian aborigines	J Burton Cleland
21 June (5th AGM)	Trypanosomiasis of Nyasaland	M Anderson
18 October	Etiology of blackwater fever	Sir William Leishman
15 November	Ankylostomiasis in British Guiana	W F Law
	Fistulous diseases of the buttocks	J L Maxwell
20 December	Fungi in the tropics	A Castellani (Colombo)
1913		
17 January	Advances in Sleeping Sickness	A G Bagshawe
21 February	Pellagra, a deficiency disease?	F M Sandworth
	Fatal pellagra	C R Box, F W Mott
18 April	Sanitation in the Panama Canal Zone, Trinidad and British Guiana	D Thomson
	Cultivation of malarial parasite and *Piroplasma Canis*	H Ziemann
16 May	Phlebotomus fever and Dengue	C Birt (RAMC)
20 June (6th AGM)	Helminths of man	R T Leiper
	Flagellation in malarial crescents	W M James (Panama)
17 October	Neurasthenia – (*presidential address*)	Sir Havelock Charles
21 November	Mosquito reduction and eradication of malaria	M Watson
19 December	Kala azar in Malta	C M Wenyon
1914		
16 January	Visit to Cyprus	Sir Ronald Ross
20 February	Research on undulant or Mediterranean fever	P W Bassett-Smith
20 March	Research on Sprue in Ceylon 1912–14	P H Bahr

Date	Subject	Speaker
15 May	Surgery in the tropics	J Cantlie
19 June (7th AGM)	Mosquito work in Ceylon	S P James

[NB: Contributions at *Ordinary* meetings during the second year of Charles's presidency are deferred until Chapter 5 (*ie during* the *Great War*).]

Biennial Dinner

Transactions had carried a report of the second 'Biennial Dinner' of the Society (*see* Chapter 3) which was held following the third (ie Leishman's) presidential address (*see above*):

> The [second] Biennial Dinner of the [STMH] was held at the Trocadero Restaurant, under the Presidency of Lieut-Col Sir William Leishman, the [new] President of the Society, on the evening of June 16th, 1911, following the *Annual Meeting*. After the usual loyal toasts had been proposed, the prosperity of the [STMH] was proposed by Sir Thomas Barlow[16] President of the Royal College of Physicians, and supported by Mr [H T (later Sir Henry)] Butlin[17], ... President of the Royal College of Surgeons, and responded to by the President. The toast of the guests was proposed by Mr James Cantlie, and responded to by Sir James Porter.[18] Professor Ronald Ross proposed the health of the President, and with this the proceedings terminated.
>
> Owing to the many engagements in connection with the Coronation [of King George V] season[19] the dinner was not so largely attended as was expected, but those who were present enjoyed the opportunity of social intercourse, which was much appreciated.

Miscellaneous matters

At a *Council* meeting on **16 February 1912** the following was minuted:

> The following resolution ... was proposed by the President [Leishman] ... and carried unanimously:- 'The [STMH], meeting on the day of the funeral of the late Lord Lister [1827–1912], desires to place on record an expression of profound respect for the memory of one, who, in his generation, has contributed

more to the progress of science in its application to the benefit of mankind than any other individual. The Society recognises that the practical connection traced by Lord Lister between micro-organisms and disease, laid the foundation for the work which is now being done by this and kindred Societies in the same direction.

On 23 September 1912, William Carnegie Brown resigned as a joint Secretary on the grounds of ill-health (he died in October 1913), and was replaced by George Carmichael Low.

The *International Congress of Medicine* (ICM) (*see* Chapter 3) (the Secretary of the tropical section was A G Bagshawe) was the subject for discussion at several *Council* meetings (20 December 1912, 18 April 1913 and 16 May 1913); the possibility of combining their annual dinner with the *biennial dinner* of the STMH being a focus of much attention.

In 21 November 1913, *Council* decided to make Sir John Kirk (1832–1922) and Sir William MacGregor (1847–1919) Honorary Fellows of the Society.

The fifth to seventh annual reports

The fellowship rose numerically to 723, 787 and 874 in the three years prior to the war. Finances continued to be on a sound footing; in the year 1911–12, income was £496 1s 6d and expenditure £441 16s 9d. Respective figures up to 31 March 1913 were: £565 16s 1d and the expenditure £589 16s 2d. In that ending 31 March 1914, the income was £667 13s 9d and the expenditure 'much the same as in the preceding year'.

References and Notes

1   **Lt-Gen Sir William Boog Leishman** FRS studied medicine at the University of Glasgow, and entered the RAMC in 1887; after seven years in India he became assistant to Almroth Wright at Netley. When the Army Medical School was transferred to Millbank in 1903, Leishman became Professor of Pathology. In 1923, he was appointed Medical Director-General of the Army Medical Services. [*See:* H D Rolleston, H J Power. Leishman, Sir William Boog (1865–1926). In: H C G Matthew, B Harrison (eds). *Oxford Dictionary of National Biography.* Oxford: Oxford University Press 2004; 33: 283–5; Anony-

mous. Leishman, Lt Gen Sir William Boog. *Who Was Who, 1916–1928* 5th ed. London: A & C Black 1992: 479].

2   W B Leishman. On the possibility of the occurrence of trypanosomiasis in India. *Br med J* 1903; i: 1252–4.

3   W B Leishman. Presidential address. *Trans Soc trop Med Hyg* 1910–11; 4: 214–23.

4   **Maj-Gen Sir Richard Havelock Charles Bt** (1858–1934) qualified from Queen's College, Cork, Dublin, London, Paris, Berlin and Vienna. He obtained the FRCSI, and was later Professor of Surgery at Calcutta. Returning to London, he served at the India Office, and became Dean of the London School of Tropical Medicine. [*See*: Anonymous. Charles, Maj-Gen. Sir Richard Havelock GCVO, 1st Bt. *Who Was Who, 1929–1940* 2nd ed. London: A & C Black 1967: 241].

5   C E Woodruff. *The effects of tropical light on white men.* London: Rebman Ltd 1905: 358. This work hypothesises that skin pigmentation has evolved to protect against the actinic rays of light which 'destroy living protoplasm'. The final chapter (13) is titled: 'Practical rules for white men in the tropics'. [*See also*: Anonymous. Medical News. *Br med J* 1914; ii: 123].

6   **Georges Léopold Cuvier** (1769–1832) was born in Paris and became a major figure in natural sciences research. [*See*: A Sebastian. *Dictionary on the History of Medicine.* London: Parthenon Publishing Group 1999: 233.]

7   Quoted by Charles in his presidential address (*see above*).

8   **Zahir ud-din Muhammad Jalal ud-din Babur** (1483–1531) was a (Sunni) Muslim conqueror from Central Asia who laid the foundations of the Mughal dynasty of India. His memoirs are in fact an autobiography.

9   R H Charles. Presidential address. Neuraesthenia, and its bearing on the decay of northern peoples in India. *Trans Soc trop Med Hyg* 1913–14: 7: 2–15.

10 P Hunting. *The history of The Royal Society of Medicine.* London: RSM Press 2002: 505. [*See also*: Anonymous. Champneys, Sir Frances (Henry), 1st Bart. *Who Was Who, 1929–1940* 2nd ed. London: A & C Black 1967: 237].

11 E Kerslake. MacAlister, Sir John Young Walker (1856–1925). In: H C G Matthew, B Harrison (eds). *Oxford Dictionary of National Biography.* Oxford: Oxford University Press 2004; 34: 1015–6.

12 *Op cit. See* note 10 above (Hunting: 342–3).

13 F G Rose. Report of the Government bacteriologist, British Guiana to the Tropical Diseases Research Fund Committee for the period January 1919 to March 1920. *Proc R Soc Med* (Section of Tropical Diseases and Parasitology) 1920; 14: 1–15.

14 *Op cit. See* note 10 above (Hunting: 342–3).

15 G C Low. The history of the foundation of the Society of Tropical Medicine and Hygiene. *Trans R Soc trop Med Hyg* 1928; 22: 197–202. [*See also*: G C Cook. Evolution: The Art of Survival. *Trans R Soc trop Med Hyg* 1994; 88: 4–18].

16 **Sir Thomas Barlow** FRS (1845–1945) was an eminent physician, who became president of the Royal College of Physicians. [*See*: R Aspin. Barlow, Sir Thomas, first baronet (1845–1945) In: H C G Matthew, B Harrison (eds).

Oxford Dictionary of National Biography. Oxford: Oxford University Press 2004; 3: 933–5; Anonymous. Barlow, Sir Thomas. *Who Was Who, 1941–1950* 5th ed. London: A & C Black. 1980: 57–8].

17 **Sir Henry Butlin** FRCS (1845–1912) was a surgeon at St Bartholomew's Hospital, and president of the Royal College of Surgeons (1909–11). [*See*: Anonymous. Butlin, Sir Henry Trentham, Bart (1845–1912). *Plarr's Lives 1930*: 178–81; Anonymous. Butlin, Sir Henry Trentham 1st Bt. *Who Was Who, 1897–1916* 5th ed. London: A & C Black 1966: 108].

18 **Sir James Porter** KCB (?–1935). [*See*: Anonymous. Porter, Sir James. *Who Was Who, 1929–1940* 2nd ed. London: A & C Black 1967: 1094.

19 The coronation of King George V (1865–1936) at Westminster Abbey took place on 22 June 1911.

Chapter 5

The Society during the Great War (1914–18)

Britain's involvement in the Great War ('the war to end all wars') was to begin on 4 August 1914, and last until 11 November 1918, with the signing of the armistice at 11.00am.

Presidential Addresses

Two presidential addresses were delivered *during* the war. The first was on **15 October 1915** by Dr Fleming M Sandwith MD FRCP (1853–1918)[1] (*see* Figure 5.1). This was to focus on a single disease entity, but he gave an excellent account of an enigmatic disease at that time – *pellagra*. His title was '**Pellagra considered from the point of view of a disease of insufficient nutrition**'; he began by outlining four hypotheses in existence at that time:

> (1) … the disease is in some way associated with maize, and upon this subject [Sandwith began] I have a good deal to say [*see* below].
>
> (2) [It] is a protozoal disease, probably transmitted and propagated by a *Simulium*, or by some other insect. During the last ten years, and especially since 1909 [he continued], this hypothesis has exercised supreme fascination on the minds of many workers, and a considerable amount of time, energy and money has been expended in the praiseworthy and gallant attempt to prove its correctness in several pellagra-stricken countries. Nearly everyone was tired of the fruitlessness of the maize controversy, and consequently turned with alacrity to the possibility of adding another malady to the famous list of insect-borne diseases. But, alas! up to the present there is no more evidence that *pellagra* is insect-borne than there was when [L W] Sambon first suggested the theory in 1905.

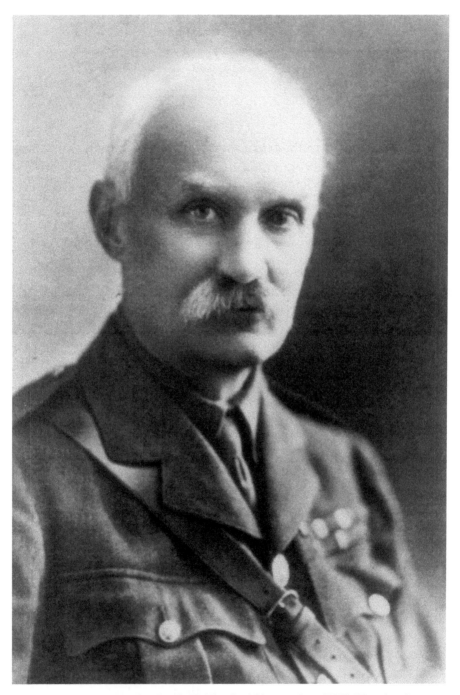

Figure 5.1: Fleming Mant Sandwith FRCP – the fifth president (RSTMH archive).

(3) [It] is contracted in definite zones where the usual drinking water comes from springs arising in argillaceous soil, or from the streams and stagnant pools in a clayey district.[2] This theory, advanced by Professor Alessandrini in 1912, has been provisionally accepted by the Pellagra Commission of the Province of Rome in preference to any theories connected with maize or biting insects. It is urged by ... Alessandrini and Scala, that *Pellagra* is a disease induced by 'chronic poisoning brought about by the silica in colloidal solution in waters of determined composition; in other words, *pellagra* seems attributable to mineral colloids'. Further, that human *pellagra* is an acidosis, and can be cured or greatly improved by administering neutral citrate of sodium to the patients. Doubtless, we shall eventually hear from other parts of Italy what is thought of this chemical theory, but I may perhaps be forgiven for saying that no theory can be considered satisfactory unless it is true for every country (or almost every country) where *pellagra* is endemic. Clay soils derive their character from the aluminic silicate which they contain in a state of mixture, as well as in chemical combination, with other substances. Some soils contain so large a proportion of alumina as 35 per cent, but the Nile water solids analysed in October, when the flood is full of the suspended matter which forms the well-known alluvial soil of Egypt, shew 1.33 grains of silica out of the total solids of 8.59 grains per gallon.

Before passing on from this theory I should like to remind you that all the drinking water in Egypt comes from one source, the Nile, and not from 'clayey districts'.

(4) [It] is due to a strepto-bacillus found in Professor Tizzoni's laboratory in Bologna during the last three years, in blood, cerebro-spinal fluid and faeces during life and in organs after death. But this strepto-bacillus cannot be discovered by other microscopists, and until its existence is a little more recognised we can afford to neglect it.[3]

Sandwith then related his own views on the aetiology of the disease, in the light of personal studies of many hundreds of cases:

> ... In 1890 I was appointed as the first English teacher of *clinical* medicine in the wards of Kasr el Ainy Hospital in Cairo. Many of the patients were suffering from ankylostomiasis, and when some

400 cases of that disease had passed through my hands, I thought it was time to write a paper upon the subject. I had already been struck with the large number of anklyostomiasis patients who exhibited not only bilharziasis, but a symmetrical eruption on the face, chest, and limbs, which the patients themselves believed to be of no consequence, and to be due to sunburn or chapping from the wind. When I noticed that these rashes were most marked between the months of March and May, and that the patients shewed abnormal knee jerks, and a decided tendency to melancholia, and even dementia, I had little difficulty in determining that some of the in-patients were attacked by a group of symptoms for which neither ankylostomiasis nor bilharziasis could be held responsible.

Careful search among the out-patients of the hospital revealed many more unsuspected cases, though the eruption was often disguised by being caked with dirt of black or dark grey colour. I ventured to make the provisional diagnosis of *pellagra*, although neither I nor any of my medical colleagues in Egypt had any practical acquaintance with that disease. Such books as were available were mostly written by dermatologists who evidently had had no first-hand knowledge of *pellagra*. Among the many foreign medical visitors whom I invited to examine a group of presumably pellagrous patients were some Italians, who had no intimate acquaintance with *pellagra*, but who thought that my patients reminded them of *pellagra* seen in Italy in their student days.

Outside my own hospital, one of the earliest converts to the existence of *pellagra* in Egypt, which was so little known that some of my foreign colleagues gravely proposed to call it 'Sandwith's disease', was ... Warnock, the newly appointed Superintendent of the Lunatic Asylum. He soon discovered some certain and many doubtful cases among his inmates, and for many weeks he kindly allowed me to spend part of the Friday holiday in examining his patients. We then were able to determine that *pellagra* in Egypt was confined to the poorest Egyptians, mostly agricultural labourers, with a decided sprinkling of lunatics.

In 1895 I was able to spend a summer holiday in Italy, in order to study *pellagra* in its cradle. I landed in Venice and visited all the hospitals and lunatic asylums, but was disappointed to find that the Venetian doctors knew little, and seemed to care little, about the disease of which I was in search. They referred me to Milan, where I again found that the huge hospital of 1,000 beds was barren of *pellagra*, except one or two doubtful cases in the insane section. Eventually I was passed on to the Pellagrosario at Inzago, near Milan, where I found nothing but pellagrous cases, and a warm reception from Dr Fritz. By his advice I also visited some lunatic asylums, where I saw a considerable number of cases.

The Italian experience was thus similar to that of Egypt. The disease was apparently confined to the poorest peasants sometimes gathered into retreats, and to lunatics – the ordinary private or hospital physician seldom came across the disease. As I wandered about Italy I read the works of Lombroso and other Italians on *pellagra*, but it was holiday time, and I did not succeed in making the acquaintance of many of them, because they were absent from town.

I found that in important respects *pellagra* in Italy was the same disease as in Egypt, though the skin eruptions were better marked and more extensive among the Egyptians, partly because they wear fewer clothes than Europeans, and partly because the sun's actinic rays are stronger in Egypt, and there is more unclouded sunshine there.

I imbibed the belief that good maize could not produce *pellagra* under any circumstances, but that it must be caused by some deterioration in that cereal, due to faulty harvesting, drying, or storage. I now regret that I accepted this theory so completely, because it led to my spending some weary years in trying to puzzle out the cause of deterioration of what the Italians call 'spoilt maize'. For a few years after 1902 I was attracted by the writings of Ceni, who found *Aspergillus fumigatus* in cultures of bad maize and in pellagrous corpses. But these observations were not confirmed by others, and are now seldom referred to.

In 1905 I discovered a case of *pellagra* among [many of] Withington's cerebro-spinal meningitis patients in a hospital at Boston, Mass., but on examination the patient proved to be a recent arrival from Italy. If I had been able, during that visit to the United States, to see the lunatic asylums in the South, I might have recognized some of the pellagrous patients who were discovered there shortly afterwards. I only mention this because I had been long persuaded that *pellagra* must exist in the United States, if the association between that disease and maize were correct, though I was constantly assured by the best American physicians that it had never been seen.

In 1907 I was converted by Braddon's book[4] that beriberi was in some way caused by a one-sided rice diet, though I could not accept all his premises. Soon after, it occurred to me that *pellagra* might be due not so much to deterioration of maize, as to some deficiency of nutrition connected with the maize diet. I began, in fact, to consider that *pellagra* is not caused by what a man eats, but by what he fails to eat. If this view is eventually proved to be incorrect I am prepared again to change my belief, but in the meantime I am of opinion that attention should be drawn to the analogy existing between the historical beliefs concerning beriberi and *pellagra*.[5]

Sandwith proceeded to summarise 'points of resemblance' between beriberi and pellagra, and again alluded to various infective theories; it seems astonishing today that some investigators in 1915 still felt this to be a *communicable* disease:

… I notice that Sir Patrick Manson, in the 1914 edition of *Tropical Diseases*, though now converted to the deficiency belief, still advises that 'in the endemic zone beriberics should be treated as infective and isolated'.

In America, some believe that *pellagra* is found to spread from cases of the disease, but no one else has gone so far as 'Shreveport, Louisiana, Board of Health, which passed an ordinance on May 29th, 1915, designating *pellagra* as a communicable disease. Any house where *pellagra* exists must be placarded and the disease reported to the Board of Health. Children suffering from the disease are excluded from school, and pellagrins are prohibited from selling or preparing food or attending public meetings.'[6]

Sandwith continued:

… if *pellagra* is due to a similar deficiency, why must it always be a deficiency connected with maize? Oatmeal, for instances, might explain some Scotch cases where maize is seldom eaten, and is certainly not the basal diet. If fresh vegetables, fruit, meat and milk are entirely excluded from a sailor's diet, he may in time develop scurvy, but to be certain of the diagnosis we are not obliged to prove that the disease is due to deficiency caused by one particular vegetable.

Perhaps I can put this point most clearly by stating that the association between beriberi and rice is almost accidental. Beri-beri is a deficiency disease, and presumably it may occur after any diet in which the necessary substance is not present. It is this essential substance to which ... Funk[7] has given the name of 'vitamines'. If it can be proved with regard to beriberi and *pellagra* that the 'vitamines' are absent, it does not matter whether the basal cereal diet is rice, maize, or anything else. ... Eijkman[8], since 1890, has pointed out the connection between rice and berberi in man, and between rice and polyneuritis in fowls, and, thanks to the work of several Englishmen in the Malay States, he has lived to see the theory (which he himself only half perceived) accepted, though we still recognise that the pathogenesis of beriberi is not yet fully determined.

The earliest descriptions of *pellagra* associate it with insufficient diet; for instance, ... Casal[9] wrote in Spanish, in 1707, describing pellagra among peasants: 'Their food is maize, milk, chestnuts, herbs and nuts, and the patients have obtained great relief when their food has been replaced by other substances of a more sustaining kind'.[10]

He continued with a brief review of dietary deficiency diseases:

... A group of diseases where some specific diet deficiency is apparently responsible for the symptoms, includes the following: - Rickets, Scurvy and Infantile scurvy, Epidemic Dropsy, Beriberi[11] and Infantile Beriberi, Norwegian Ship beriberi (which seems to be distinct from ordinary tropical beriberi occurring among Orientals in ships), Polyneuritis of birds, and perhaps Lathyrism. If this grouping is allowable, has not the time now come when *pellagra* may provisionally be included in it? It cannot too often be repeated that all early sane cases of *pellagra* can be cured, or apparently cured, by removal of patients from their homes to an institution where they are fed on a liberal diet containing meat, and where, for precaution's sake, all maize is excluded from the diet. There is no exception to this rule, excepting some rare fulminating cases which die in a few weeks. Rest and improved diet seem to be responsible for the change, not the removal of the patient from his home. If necessary, this point could easily be settled, say, in America, by removing 100 patients to an institution and treating another 100 patients in their homes with obligatory rest and a similar improved diet.[12]

Sandwith continued by drawing attention to American experiences of *pellagra*; since the US was not directly affected by the war, he felt that the aetiology of the disease might well be elucidated there:

... Fortunately few States suffer so intensely as Mississippi, where, during the year 1914, with an estimated population of 1,901,882, there were reported the enormous number of 10,954 cases of *pellagra*, with 1,204 deaths. This gives a case incidence per annum per 1,000 of 5.76. After malaria and measles, *pellagra* seems to be the most prevalent disease in that State.

... I should like to draw attention to the view of certain Government officials, ... J Goldberger (Surgeon in charge of *Pellagra* Investigations), ... C H Waring, and ... D G Willets, because their paper appeared in a publication which is not commonly read in this country. They conclude (a) that *pellagra* is essentially of dietary origin; (b) that it is dependent on some yet undetermined fault in a diet in which the animal or leguminous protein component is disproportionately small, and the non-leguminous vegetable component disproportionately large; and (c) that no *pellagra* develops in those who *consume* a mixed, well-balanced and varied diet. ...[13]

After citing an association between *pellagra* and ankylostomiasis which he considered 'noteworthy', he gave an account of 'The criteria of necessary proof':

I cannot do better than quote ... Gowland Hopkins[14], who is the chief authority in this country upon many questions concerned with diet and disease.[15] He says: 'I take it that to obtain satisfactory evidence that a specific diet deficiency is directly responsible for a given complex of symptoms, it must be shewn that the association between the suspected diet and the symptoms is sufficiently frequent, and the occurrence of the symptoms upon normal diet sufficiently rare, to satisfy the statistician; while to obtain rigid proof we must discover what the deficiency really is, and prove that removing it results in prevention or cure of the symptoms .... Our criterion must be this: that the disease is absent from, or rare in, individuals taking a normal dietary, but common among those who are rigidly confined to the diet under suspicion. ... [Samples of] good maize and [also] spoilt maize from the Sharkia Province in Lower Egypt, where *pellagra* is well known [were fed to guinea pigs]. We afterwards found that similar good maize could be bought in this country and, therefore, we were able to replenish the stock of good maize here since January 8th, 1915. The bad maize is often dirty, wrinkled and somewhat weevil-eaten; the germ of the grain is enclosed in a half-empty cavity with powdered débris, and the maize cobs, on arrival in this country, are accompanied by many granary weevils and also by hundreds of moths, which feed on grain and which [Alfred] Alcock has identified for me as belonging to the *Tineidae*, or the clothes-moths family, probably *Gelechia*. ...[16]

Sandwith ended by outlining three experiments on guinea pigs at St Thomas's Hospital Medical School:

... the first experiment was to see whether there was any profound difference when guinea-pigs were fed on good or bad maize. The second experiment was to try and determine the minimum raw cabbage necessary to sustain life when maize was the only other article of diet, and a third experiment was to see, if possible, whether animals already accustomed to a maize diet plus the minimum of cabbage shewed any difference when fed on good ... or bad maize. The maize was invariably given as a sort of porridge by adding water. [From these experiments he concluded]: it is obvious therefore that the best conditions for the experiment have been worked out, but it is certain that 'bad' maize does not produce any deleterious results in short periods of a month to six weeks, even under circumstances most favourable for its action. This throws out of court all the short experiments so prevalent in the literature about *pellagra*.[17]

The presidential address for 1917, the second during the war, was given on **19 October** of that year, and consisted of a lengthy scientific account, again of a single disease: '**Tetanus: analysis of one thousand cases**', by Surgeon-General (later Sir) David Bruce CB FRS (1855–1931)[18] (*see* Figure 5.2):

> [He began] I must apologise to the Society for bringing before it, in a presidential address, the subject of *tetanus*, which can hardly be strictly called a tropical disease, although it is true that it is of more common occurrence in the tropics than in temperate climates. My excuse is that this is a time of war, and tetanus has an important place among war diseases. Moreover, part of my work, since the beginning of the war, has been to supervise the investigation and treatment of tetanus occurring in our home military hospitals. I therefore thought it would be better to address you on a subject of practical importance at the present time. Interest in tick fever, sleeping sickness, and other purely tropical diseases has lapsed for the time being. They seem, in truth, to belong to a past existence.
>
> In this paper it must be understood that only cases of *tetanus* arising in England are dealt with. Many cases have occurred in France among the wounded before their transfer to home hospitals. These have been analysed, at least in part, by … Leishman and … Smallman. An attempt to amalgamate these cases with [those] occurring in England was made, but was found to be impracticable on account of the want of sufficient data.
>
> In regard to the origin of this work on *tetanus* the history may be given briefly. In October, 1914, after returning from Nyasaland [now Malawi], I received orders to report at the War Office on the 1st November, 1914. In his letter of instruction, Sir Alfred Keogh [1857–1936] [*see* Chapter 1], the Director-General, wrote:- 'It is hoped that you will direct your attention specially to the subject of *tetanus*, with a view to elucidating the problems of causation and cure. To this end military hospitals will be instructed to notify cases to you, and send you such particulars as you may require'.
>
> The taking up of this work was, therefore, due to a request from the Director-General. The cases which have been notified up to the present time number a thousand, and form the subject of this paper.

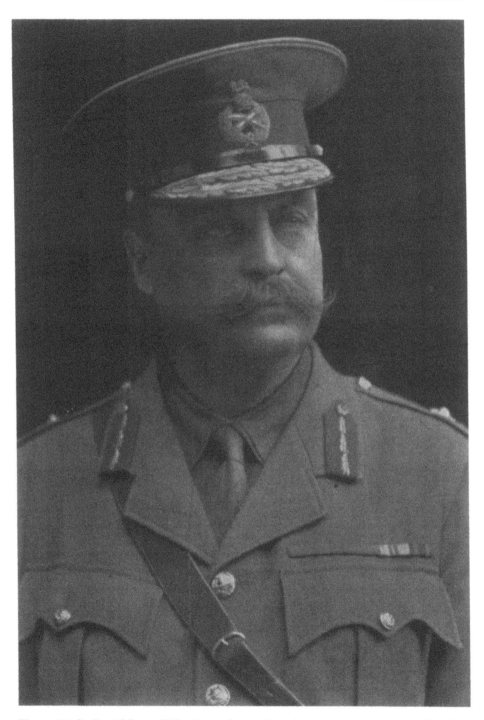

Figure 5.2: Sir David Bruce FRS – the sixth president (reproduced courtesy the Royal Army Medical College, London).

To Lady Bruce fell the work of entering under the various headings the different items of information contained in the Report Forms. This has been a very arduous piece of work, and it is no exaggeration to say that it has taken an average of some five hours a day during the last three years to accomplish. As Lady Bruce is purely a voluntary worker, I am sure you will agree that our heartiest thanks are due to her for the enormous amount of trouble she has taken in this matter.

In March, 1916, a *Tetanus* Committee was formed at the suggestion of ... Waller and Plimmer and ... Golla, and the first meeting took place on the 7th March of that year. A Memorandum on *Tetanus*, which is now in its third edition, was prepared by the Committee and circulated, the *Tetanus* Report Forms were revised, and a new Form for Inspectors of *Tetanus* circulated. At the present there are some forty inspectors in different parts of the country supervising the study and treatment of this disease. It is not possible to mention all of these officers by name, but they also deserve our best thanks for the excellent work they have done. I have already published several analyses of cases of *tetanus* treated in home hospitals, and this paper is merely a bringing together of the previous work, making the figures dealt with up to 1,000.

Members of the Committee have written several papers to the medical journals with a view to giving medical officers the latest developments in our knowledge of *tetanus*. A list of these papers is given in an appendix. The Committee has also instituted original investigations, some of which are bearing fruit. [Both] Robertson [and] Tulloch, ..., have been working at the anaerobic fauna of septic wounds, and especially the *tetanus* bacillus. These researches have been carried out at the Lister Institute.[19]

... [C S] Sherrington [1857–1952][20] has also been studying the effect of the *tetanus* toxin and antitoxin on monkeys at Oxford. The expenses of these various researches are being borne by the Lister Institute.[21]

The published proceedings of this lecture are detailed and contain 11 tables and 16 figures. Bruce analysed: the ratio of the number of cases to the numbers of wounded, the distribution of cases between August 1914 and June 1917, seasonal prevalence, incubation period, rate of mortality, and very importantly, treatment (both prophylactic and therapeutic). On the value of *prophylactic* inoculation, Bruce had the following comments:

> ... the prophylactic inoculation of antitoxin lowers the mortality by more than one-half, namely, from 51.8 per cent to 26.6 per cent ... .[22]

Bruce concluded that analysis of his data on *treatment* did *not* provide any useful deductions; however, he summarised the current situation:

> ... At [the] present [time] the position seems to be this: Antitoxin has no power of neutralising toxin fixed in the nervous system. If a fatal amount has been absorbed, then no amount of antitoxin will save the man's life. If there is any free toxin circulating in the blood or lymph, the antitoxin can neutralise it, and so possibly prevent further mischief. If then a fatal amount has not been absorbed the injection of antitoxin may be of use. By animal experiment it is proved that the intrathecal route is the best. It is believed that the intravenous route is also good, but more dangerous on account of the liability to anaphylactic shock. Therefore the *Tetanus* Committee, in their last Memorandum, recommend intrathecal antitoxin at the first sign of *tetanus*.[23]

The Society during the Great War

In the opinion of Low, this was the second of two occasions when in its early years the Society passed through 'troublesome times'.[24] The first was the controversy surrounding whether or not it should join the newly-formed RSM (*see* Chapter 4). During the war, the fellowship fell sharply in numbers (*see* Figure 5.3) and *Transactions* was greatly reduced in size.

Although meetings of the Society were usually held on Fridays, during the latter War years – from 1916 onwards – most *Council* meetings were held at 5.00pm, and *Ordinary* ones and AGMs at 5.30pm. It was not until late 1919 that pre-war times (8.00 and 8.30pm, respectively) were resumed.

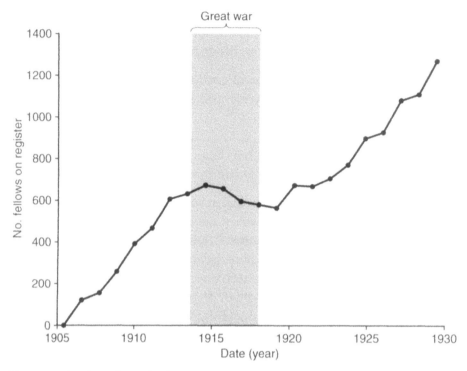

Figure 5.3: Total numbers of Fellows on register before, during and immediately after the Great War (1914–18) (*see* reference 24).

Direct effect(s) of the War

Very shortly after the outbreak of War, an *Ordinary* meeting on **16 October 1914** was told that one of its fellows – Captain Henry Sherwood Rankin – had died 'as a result of wounds received on the field of battle in France'. Later, on **21 May 1915**, *Council* was informed that Dr [C F] Harford (one of the Hon Secretaries) was absent because he had joined the Royal Army Medical Corps. These announcements were amongst many more – either recording further deaths or departure of fellows in the service of the Crown.

The falling numbers of Fellows was the cause of considerable concern; not only was recruitment of Fellows falling, but some (including C W Daniels) had resigned. In order to boost numbers, Col King proposed to *Council* later in the war, on **21 June 1918**, that the Society should gather 'more non-medical men, such as Hygienists, Sanitary Engineers, Entomologists and Agriculturalists etc'. As a result, 'the Secretaries were directed to write [to] the people mentioned on [a list submitted by King], asking if they would care to become Fellows of the Society'. At the following meeting, the Secretaries reported that this had been done and, further, that they had also written to 'several medical men not yet Fellows of the Society'. The question of opening the Fellowship to *veterinarians* had been raised by Dr A G Bagshawe on **15 February 1918**; however, Dr Leiper considered that if the Society started allowing veterinary papers at its meetings 'the veterinary people might be jealous'; as a result, it was decided that only 'individual veterinarians [be invited] to join'.

Soon after the onset of hostilities, the number of *Ordinary* meetings was reduced. It was in fact suggested at a *Council* meeting on **18 June 1915** that 'the Society might only meet once in two months', a move which was subsequently adopted, but during the summer months only. A further move was to change the time of meetings (*see above*) during the winter, viz: the *Council* at 5pm, and the *Ordinary* at 5.30pm; tea to be served at 5pm.

Table 5.1 summarises communications at *Ordinary* meetings during the Great War.

Employment of the Administrative Secretary

Miss Mabel Hooper had served the Society well since 1907, as Assistant Secretary. During the war, at a *Council* meeting on **18 May 1917** however, the Secretary read a letter dated 12 April indicating that she had been offered employment (10–4 daily with Saturdays off) at the India Office 'for three years on work of a tropical nature', and further that unless the Society changed her working hours in order for her to work there as well, she would inevitably have to resign from the Society. It was eventually resolved that her resignation should be accepted, but that she 'should be asked to do part-time clerical work, 1 hour a day and 3 hours on Saturdays ... at a rate of £30 per annum'. Miss Hooper accepted. When the matter was reconsidered after six months, she wrote from the India Office indicating that she wished to return to the Society, but that her salary should be increased to £125 per annum (*see* CM **18 January 1918**]. However, with the Fellowship rapidly declining (due to deaths and resignations – *see* above) this represented an increase that the Society could ill afford. Eventually, R T Leiper proposed a motion (seconded by W Hartigan) that Miss Hooper be offered an appointment as 'Whole time Secretary of the Society [to include work on *Transactions*] at the rate of £125

Table 5.1: Communications at *Ordinary* Meetings during the Great War

Date	Subject	Speaker
1914		
16 October	Classification of African trypanosomes	Sir David Bruce
20 November	Typhoid in War	Sir William Osler (Oxford)
18 December	Tropical problems in 'New World'	A Balfour
1915		
15 January	Bacillary dysentery	H S Gettings
19 February	The War and Cholera	W J R Simpson
19 March	Tropical drugs	F Lee Pyman
21 May	African tick fever in British Somaliland	R E Drake-Brockman (Somaliland)
	Thymo-Benzol treatment of schistosomiasis	C M Ekins (Egypt)
	Ankylosomiasis in Venezuela	C E F Mouat-Biggs
	Leishmaniasis in Paraguay	L E Migone (Paraguay)
18 June (8th AGM)	Malaria on rubber estates	R M C Linnell
15 October	Pellagra (*presidential address*)	F M Sandwith
19 November	Combined vaccinations	A Castellani
17 December	Eosinophilia	G C Low
	Intestinal parasites in northern Siam	W J Kerr (Siam)
	Tropical anaemia	W M Strong
	Glossina morsitans	J O Shircore
1916		
21 January	Aetiology of typhus	W J Penfold
17 March	Syphilis in the Army	H J McGrigor (RAMC)
	Syphilis in African natives	H Bayon
19 May	Cerebro-spinal fever	J M Atkinson (RAMC)
16 June (9th AGM)	Liver abscess	J Cantlie
20 October	Malaria & Sanitary Administration	A MacDonald
17 November	Pathogenic protozoa	H Bayon
	Clonorchis sinensis	C H Treadgold
15 December	Vomiting sickness of Jamaica	H H Scott
1917		
16 February	Beri-beri, scurvy prevention	H Chick, M E Hume
19 May	Yellow fever	H R Carter
15 June (10th AGM)	Yaws in the Belgian Congo	G Greggio (Belgian Congo)
	Yaws treated by tartar emetic	A Castellani
	Helminthic ova	R T Leiper

Date	Subject	Speaker
19 October	Tetanus (*presidential address*)	Sir David Bruce
16 November	Sanitation problems in British Guiana	A T Ozzard (British Guiana)
	Enteromonas hominis	A J Chalmers, W Pekkola
21 December	Geographical distribution and control of disease	J H Tull Walsh
1918		
18 January	Blackwater fever in Eastern Mediterranean	J A Arkwright
15 February } 15 March }	Treatment of malaria	Sir Ronald Ross
17 May	Trench fever – a louse-borne disease	W Byam (RAMC)
21 June (11th AGM)	Treatment of Malaria	J W W Stephens
	Entamoeba histolytica and *E coli cysts* in England	Warrington Yorke
18 October	Filariasis in Macedonia	J G Forbes
	Warfare and sanitation in SE Europe	W J R Simpson

[NB: Contributions at *Ordinary* meetings during the latter part of Bruce's presidency are deferred to Chapter 6 (*ie* after termination of the *Great War*).]

per annum … 10–5 daily, Saturdays 10–1 and to attend official meetings'. This was passed by Council, and was acceptable to Miss Hooper.

However, at a later *Council* meeting in September 1918, it was reported that she wished to return to the India Office with 'part-time' work for the Society, until the end of the war. Council agreed that she should attend the Society 'daily from 4.30 to 5.30pm and on Saturday mornings from 10-1 … for £40 per annum'. Low later reported to *Council*, on **8 October 1919**, that Miss Hooper 'was prepared to come back to the Society as a whole timer'; at the following meeting it was unanimously decided that provided she gave a whole time commitment to the Society 'as in pre war days' she be paid '£150 per annum with a rise of £10 per annum up to £200'.

At a meeting on **14 May 1920**, though, it was reported that she had then been offered £220 per annum by the India Office, and that she wished to 'resign her position with the Society'.

Later that year, at a *Council* meeting in June:

> … It was considered better that Miss Hooper should [indeed] sever her connection with the Society entirely, and *Council* decided that till it was known whether the Society was to remove to Endsleigh

Gardens [as tenants of the Seamen's Hospital Society] or not [*see* Chapter 7], Mr Bethell [Registrar of the MSL] should be asked to carry on [secretarial arrangements] @ £2 per week.

At a meeting a week later:

The following motion was moved by Dr Harford, seconded by Dr Low and carried unanimously that:

The *Council* of the [RSTMH] record their cordial appreciation of the services rendered by Miss Mabel Hooper, who from the early days of the Society has been assistant to the Honorary Secretaries, and whose devotion to the Society's interests has been of great value to the same. They wish her good success in the important appointment which she is now to undertake.

Royal College of Physicians' 'Nomenclature of Disease'

'Nomenclature of Diseases' was first published by the Royal College of Physicians (RCP) in 1869 in an attempt to provide an accurate and uniform system for classification of disease entities which would perfect their statistical registration.[25] On **15 November 1918** (*ie* very soon after peace was restored) *Council* resolved to send a letter to the Registrar of the RCP. The matter had initially been raised by Col Andrew Balfour at a meeting on 18 October. The letter, drafted by the Hon Secretaries, read:

The Registrar [J A Ormerod]
   Royal College of Physicians.   16th November 1918

Sir,
At a meeting of the *Council* of the [STMH] held on 18th October 1918, it was unanimously resolved, as a result of representations made by certain Fellows of the Society, to direct the attention of the [RCP] Joint Committee charged with the revision of the *'Nomenclature of Diseases'* to the following:-

(1) From the point of view of *tropical medicine* there are a number of serious errors in the published List of Diseases.
(2) There are likewise numerous important omissions, especially in the section dealing with Animal Parasites. As examples the *Council* may cite –

(a) The inclusion of two species of *Simulium* and *P. papatasii* (p 234) as intermediate hosts of the malarial parasite.

(b) The omission of *Stegomyia pseudo-scutellaris* as a host of the filarial parasite (p 235).

(c) The employment of the term 'Mediterranean Fever' instead of 'Undulant Fever' in view of the fact that the latter name was officially adopted by the International Congress of Medicine held in London in 1913.

(d) The omission of an important intestinal parasite amongst the Flagellata – viz. *Chilomastix mesnili* (Wenyon) p 322.

(e) The neglect to mention *Schistosoma mansoni* Sambon, a very important human parasite, whereas *Filaria gigas* Prout, which does not exist, finds a place in the list.

Many other instances have been brought to the notice of the *Council*. Attention may also be directed to the Chapter on Page XIII dealing with nomenclature. The Rules there given do not correspond with those laid down in the International Rules of Zoological Nomenclature, nor with those adopted by the International Congress of Botany. Even such Rules as are given are not followed in the examples cited by your Sub-Committee.

The *Council* of the [STMH] consider that it is regrettable that no authorities on *tropical medicine* were consulted on these, and other important points, before such a List was issued, and it trusts that when a further revision is contemplated [*see* Chapter 11] this oversight will be remedied.

David Bruce,
President, [STMH].

Acknowledgement came in the form of a letter (20 November 1918) (*see* Figure 5.4) from Ormerod – it was then too late to rectify the errors in the present edition, but 'alterations [will be made] when that is possible' [*see* Chapter 11].

Other matters

The death of Col F M Sandwith (the fifth and previous president) was announced by Bruce (president) at an *Ordinary* meeting on **15 March**

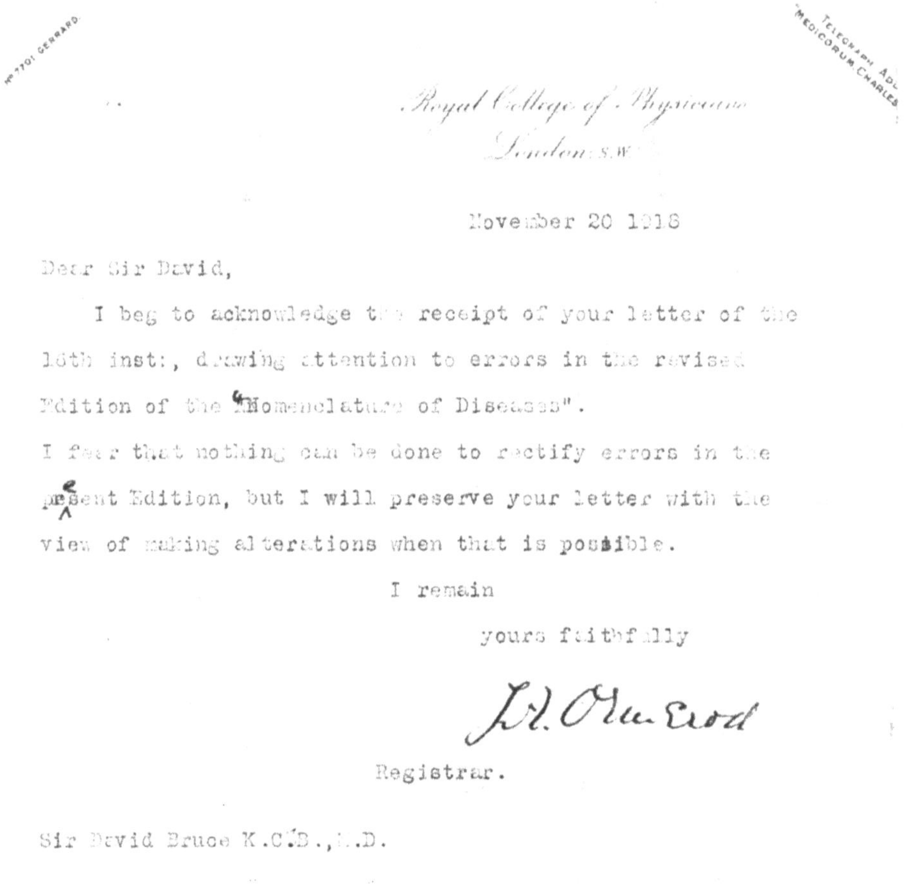

No 7701 Gerrard.

Telegraph Address "Medicorum Charles"

Royal College of Physicians
London, S.W.

November 20 1918

Dear Sir David,

I beg to acknowledge the receipt of your letter of the 16th inst:, drawing attention to errors in the revised Edition of the "Nomenclature of Diseases".
I fear that nothing can be done to rectify errors in the present Edition, but I will preserve your letter with the view of making alterations when that is possible.

I remain

yours faithfully

Registrar.

Sir David Bruce K.C.B.,M.D.

Figure 5.4: Letter from the Registrar of the Royal College of Physicians of London – dated 20 November 1918 – in reply to Sir David Bruce's letter.

1918, *ie* little more than two years after he had delivered his presidential address to the Society, and less than one year since he stepped down from the presidency.

The eighth to eleventh annual reports

The number of Fellows fell sharply during World War I (*see* Figure 5.3); as the eleventh report (31 March 1917–31 March 1918) stated, the 'number [of Fellows] now actually on the books of the Society stands at 585'.

The financial figures also reflect a diminution in numbers: income was reduced to £569 14s 11d, £578 19s 2d, £508 4s 9d, and £510 5s 10d for the years 1914–15, 1915–16, 1916–17 and 1917–18 respectively.

References and Notes

1   **Fleming Sandwith** was educated at Charterhouse and St Thomas's Hospital. After service as a physician at the London School of Tropical Medicine, he worked in Turkey and Egypt, where he became Professor of Medicine at the Egyptian Government School of Medicine. He later served at the Imperial Yeomanry Hospital at Pretoria during the South African War. Anonymous. Sandwith, Fleming Mant. *Who Was Who, 1916–1928* 5th ed. London: A & C Black 1992: 722.

2   G Alessandrini, A Scala. Contribuito Nuovo alla Etiologia e Patogenesi della Pellagra. *Tip naz Bertero, Rome.* 1914; H F Harris. *Pellagra.* New York: The MacMillan Company 1919: 421. *A* Cencelli. New theories and investigations concerning Pellagra. *Lancet* 1914; i: 794.

3   F M Sandwith. Pellagra considered from the point of view of a disease of insufficient nutrition. *Trans Soc trop Med Hyg* 1915–16; 9: 1–15.

4   W L Braddon. *The cause and prevention of Beri-beri.* London: Rebman Ltd 1907: 544; K J Carpenter. *Beriberi, White Rice, and Vitamin B.* London: University of California Press 2000: 282.

5   *Op cit.* See note 3 above.

6   *Ibid.* [*See also: Am J Trop Dis Preventive Med* 1915; 3: 771 cited by Sandwith].

7   **Casimir Funk** (1884–1967) worked at the Lister Institute and was the first to isolate, in 1911, the anti-*beriberi* factor. He was also the first to coin the term: *vitamine.*

8   **Christian Eijkman** (1858–1930) was a Dutch physician who established the cause of *beri-beri,* and proposed the concept of 'essential food factors' – later known as vitamins. He shared the Nobel Prize with Gowland Hopkins in 1929.

9   **Gaspar Casal** (1691–1759) was a Spanish physician who had described *mal de rosa* (pellagra) in 1730.

10 *Op cit.* See note 3 above. [*See also*: Anonymous. Literary notes. *Br med J* 1912; ii: 1067].

11 *Op cit.* See note 4 above.

12 *Op cit.* See note 3 above.

13 *Ibid.*

14 **Sir Frederick Gowland Hopkins** (1861–1947) delineated 'Accessory food factors' required to maintain health, and was a joint recipient of the Nobel Prize for Biochemistry in 1929.

15 F G Hopkins. Diseases due to deficiencies in diet. *Lancet* 1913; ii: 1309.

16 *Op cit.* See note 3 above.

17 *Ibid.* [*See also*: K J Carpenter, W J Lewin. A re-examination of the diets associated with pellagra. *J Nutr* 1985; 115: 543–52].

18 **David Bruce** was born in Melbourne, Australia of Scottish parents and educated in medicine at Edinburgh University. He joined the RAMC at Netley, and his subsequent investigations focused on the cause of Malta fever, nagana and African trypanosomiasis. Returning to England, he was appointed to the Army Medical Services Advisory Board at the War Office and subsequently became Commandant of the RAMC College at Millbank, with the rank of Surgeon-General. [*See*: S R Christophers, H J Power. Bruce, Sir David (1855–1931). In: H C G Matthew, B Harrison (eds). *Oxford Dictionary of National Biography.* Oxford: Oxford University Press 2004; 8: 287–9; Anonymous. Bruce, David. Who *Was Who, 1929–1940* 2nd ed. London: A & C Black 1967: 177–8.]

19 H Chick, M Hume, M MacFarlane. *War on disease: a history of the Lister Institute.* London: André Deutsch Ltd 1971: 251.

20 **Sir Charles Scott Sherrington** (1857–1952) was Professor of Physiology at both Liverpool and Oxford Universities. He made important contributions to neurophysiology and was awarded the Nobel Prize for Physiology or Medicine jointly in 1932.

21 D Bruce. Tetanus: analysis of one thousand cases. *Trans Soc trop Med Hyg* 1917–18; 11: 1–39.

22 *Ibid.*

23 *Ibid*; M Courtois-Suffit, R Giroux, D Bruce, F Golla (eds). *The abnormal forms of tetanus: a clinical, pathogenic, prophylactic, and therapeutic survey.* London: University of London Press Ltd 1918: 249.

24 G C Low. The history of the foundation of the Society of Tropical Medicine and Hygiene. *Trans R Soc trop Med Hyg* 1928; 22: 197–202.

25 Joint Committee appointed by the Royal College of Physicians of London (ed). *The Nomenclature of Diseases* 2nd ed. London: HM Stationery Office. 1885: 431. [*See also*: G C Cook. The College of Physicians in the nineteenth century. *Clin Med* 2001; 1: 234–9].

Chapter 6

Early inter-war years (1919–20) – the Society becomes *Royal*

The Society had survived the four years of war, but only after a considerable amount of trauma. The number of Fellows had declined dramatically due to many factors (*see* Chapter 5). Inevitably, therefore, it would take several years to completely recover from the Kaiser's War.

The second twelve months of Bruce's presidency was well under way when the war terminated (*see* Chapter 5). Ordinary meetings (and also the Laboratory meetings held at Millbank) continued, usually at monthly intervals; Table 6.1 gives details of communications at *Ordinary* meetings of the Society. Meetings were still held at the MSL. *Council* decided on 8 July 1919 to revert to the pre-war time for *Ordinary* meetings of 8.30pm. The twelfth AGM was held, as usual, at 11 Chandos Street, this year on 20 June 1919.

Meanwhile, Professor Simpson had been elected to succeed Bruce as president (he had recently been elected a Corresponding Member of the *Academie des Sciences* at Paris) at a *Council* meeting on **17 January 1919**; he would thus assume office at the AGM in June 1919 (*see* below).

Society activities

A Royal Society?

An attempt to get the Society made a *Royal* Society were initiated at a meeting of *Council* on **10 February 1920**; at the suggestion of Dr W T (later Sir William) Prout (1862–1939)[1]; this possibility was supported by the president (Simpson). Figure 6.1 shows a reply from the 'Home Office' dated 9 June 1920; when the news was revealed to a *Council* meeting on **11 June**, the members broke into applause, and it was decided that the 'letter should be published in the *Transactions*'. The matter was also fully reported in *The Times* under the heading 'The King's Interest'.[2]

Table 6.1: Communications at *Ordinary* Meetings in the early inter-war years

Date	Subject	Speaker
1918		
15 November	Sanitation in Eastern War areas	A Balfour
1919		
17 January	Malaria contracted in England	S P James
21 February	Pathology and epidemiology of 'louping-ill'	Sir Stewart Stockman
	Rickettsia in trench fever, typhus and 'rocky mountain spotted fever'	J A Arkwright
16 May	Fly Sprays	H M Lefroy
	An outbreak of 'itch' in Egypt	F W O'Conner
20 June (12th AGM)	Complement deviation in malaria and influence of malaria on the WR	J G Thomson
	Coenurus Glomeratus in West Africa	R T Leiper
	Prophylaxis of enteric fever in British Guiana	F G Rose (British Guiana)
17 October	Preventable diseases (*presidential address*)	W J R Simpson
21 November	Anti-mosquito measures in Palestine in 1917–18	E E Austen
1920		
16 January	Bacillary dysentery	P Manson-Bahr
	Fleas causing rheumatic fever	J T Clarke (Penang)
	Treatment of malaria and blackwater fever	F Roux (Paris)
20 February	Smallpox and its prevention	W G King
	Malaria in Palestine	N Hamilton Fairley
14 May	Pellagra as a 'deficiency disease'	E J Wood
18 June (13th AGM)	Round-worm infection	F H Stewart
15 October	Trypanosomiasis research	Warrington Yorke
19 November	Tropical fruit foods	G C Dudgeon
17 December	15 Exhibits	[15 Fellows]

Links with the Société de Pathologie Exotique

Now that the war was well and truly over, the Secretaries (Low and Bagshawe) decided to write to the president of the *Société de Pathologie Exotique* congratulating the Fellows of that Society on their newly acquired freedom, and an anticipated revival of *tropical medicine*.

Figures 6.2 and 6.3 show letters to and from its president, Alphonse Laveran (1845–1922) (*see* Figure 6.4), referring to the termination of the Great War; Laveran was, of course, the discoverer of the malarial parasite in 1880.

HOME OFFICE,

WHITEHALL.   S.W.1.

402,819.

9th June, 1920.

Sir,

I am directed by the Secretary of State to inform you

that he has laid before The King your application of the 13th

April last for permission to use the prefix "Royal" in the

name of "The Society of Tropical Medicine and Hygiene" and

that His Majesty has been graciously pleased to command that

the Society shall henceforth be known as "The Royal Society

of Tropical Medicine and Hygiene".

I am, Sir,

Your obedient Servant,

M. Eagleston

ie President,

The Society of Tropical
        Medicine and Hygiene,

Figure 6.1: Letter – dated 9 June 1920 – from the Home Office indicating that King George V (1865–1936) had given his approval to this being designated a *Royal* Society (RSTMH archive).

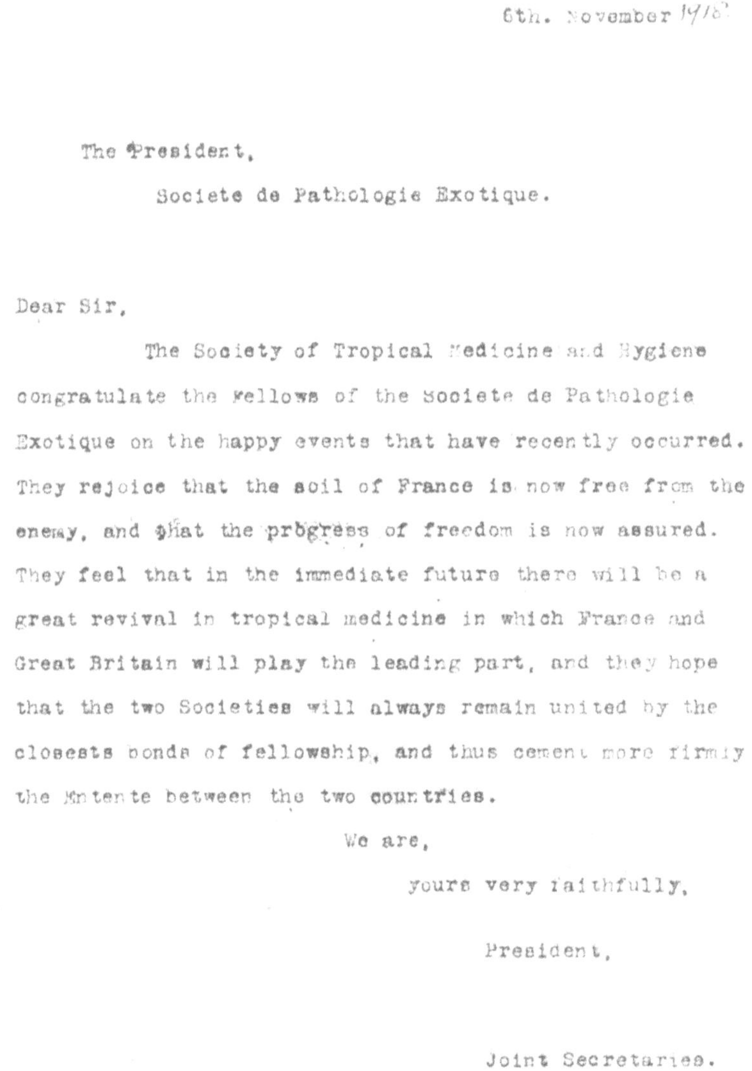

6th. November 1918.

The President,

Societe de Pathologie Exotique.

Dear Sir,

The Society of Tropical Medicine and Hygiene congratulate the Fellows of the Societe de Pathologie Exotique on the happy events that have recently occurred. They rejoice that the soil of France is now free from the enemy, and that the progress of freedom is now assured. They feel that in the immediate future there will be a great revival in tropical medicine in which France and Great Britain will play the leading part, and they hope that the two Societies will always remain united by the closeats bonds of fellowship, and thus cement more firmly the Entente between the two countries.

We are,

yours very faithfully,

President,

Joint Secretaries.

Figure 6.2: Letter to Alphonse Laveran, President of the *Société de Pathologie Exotique* from the Joint Secretaries – dated 6 November 1918 (RSTMH archive).

Is the DTM&H a registrable qualification?

Figure 6.5 shows a letter (dated **28 November 1919**) from the *'General Council of Medical Education & Registration'*. Possible registration of the DTM&H diploma had again been debated by *Council* on 21 November 1919; once again it wished to enquire whether the *General Medical Council*

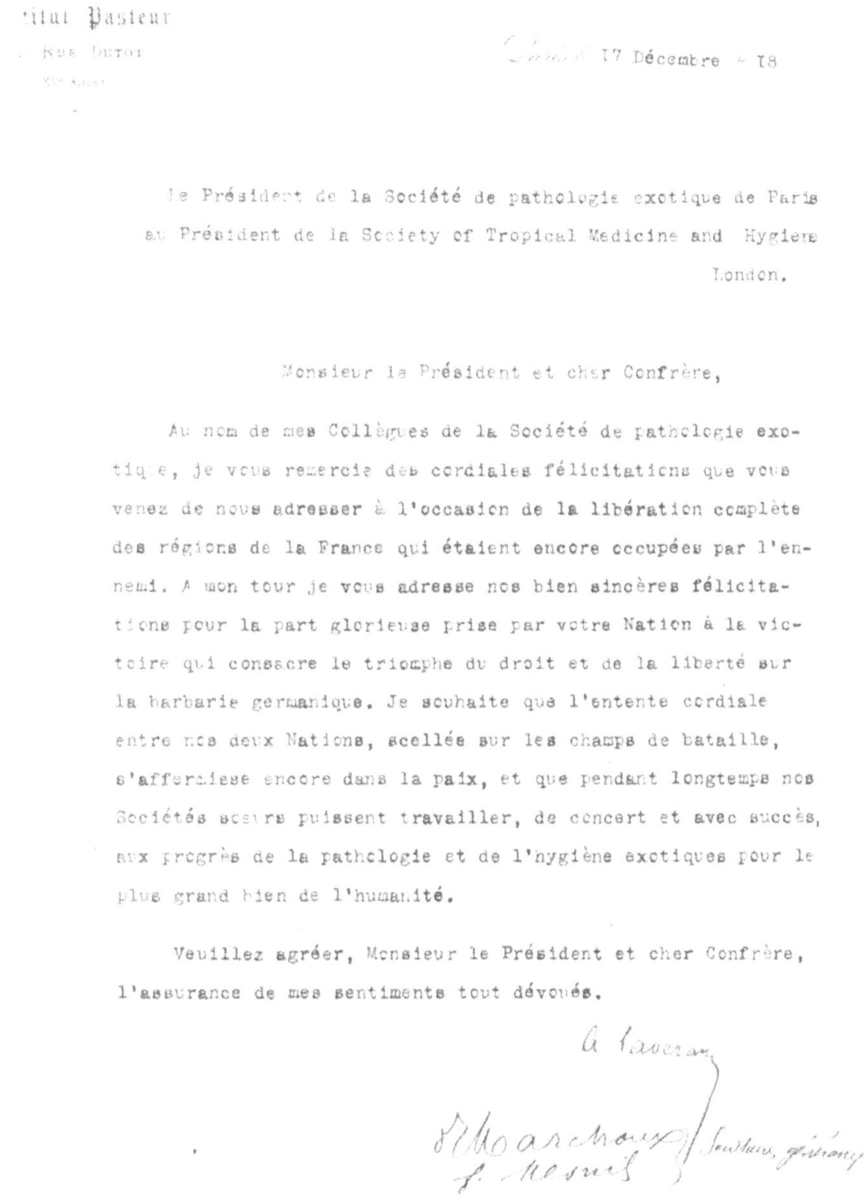

…itut Pasteur
… Rue Dutot

Paris 17 Décembre 18

Le Président de la Société de pathologie exotique de Paris
au Président de la Society of Tropical Medicine and Hygiene
London.

Monsieur le Président et cher Confrère,

Au nom de mes Collègues de la Société de pathologie exotique, je vous remercie des cordiales félicitations que vous venez de nous adresser à l'occasion de la libération complète des régions de la France qui étaient encore occupées par l'ennemi. A mon tour je vous adresse nos bien sincères félicitations pour la part glorieuse prise par votre Nation à la victoire qui consacre le triomphe du droit et de la liberté sur la barbarie germanique. Je souhaite que l'entente cordiale entre nos deux Nations, scellée sur les champs de bataille, s'affermisse encore dans la paix, et que pendant longtemps nos Sociétés soeurs puissent travailler, de concert et avec succès, aux progrès de la pathologie et de l'hygiène exotiques pour le plus grand bien de l'humanité.

Veuillez agréer, Monsieur le Président et cher Confrère, l'assurance de mes sentiments tout dévoués.

A Laveran

Marchoux
F. Mesnil
Secrétaires généraux

Figure 6.3: Letter to the Joint Secretaries from Alphonse Laveran – dated 17 December 1918 (RSTMH archive).

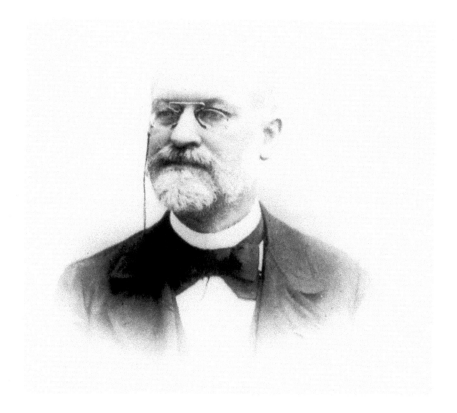

Figure 6.4: Alphonse Laveran (1845–1922), a French microbiologist who first visualised *Plasmodium* spp (reproduced courtesy the Wellcome Library, London).

(GMC) would regard this as a registrable diploma, and if not, why not! This letter, however, from the Registrar of the *General Council of Medical Education and Registration* answered the query in the negative.

The late Dr A J Chalmers

On **29 April 1920**, *Council* was informed of the death of Dr Chalmers (now commemorated by a well established Society Medal). On his way home from Khartoum via India, he apparently contracted 'infective jaundice' from which he died in Calcutta (now Kolkata).

General Council of Medical Education & Registration of the United Kingdom

44 Hallam Street, Portland Place, London W.1

All communications to be addressed to "THE REGISTRAR" and not to any individual by name. In your reply please quote No 58140.

28th November, 1919.

The Joint Secretary,
Society of Tropical Medicine and Hygiene,
11, Chandos Street,
Cavendish Square,
W. 1.

Dear Sir,

In reply to your letter of the 26th inst., I have to say that the Diploma of Tropical Medicine and Hygiene is not registrable as the Council has no power to enter this qualification on the Medical Register without further legislation. The matter was considered by the Council in 1911 and a Memorandum was transmitted to the Lord President of the Privy Council for his information. The Bodies generally were in favour of it, but the Royal College of Physicians of London took exception to this Council having control of the matter under the conditions in Part 3, Clause 21 of the Medical Act, 1886, and consequently no further action was taken in the matter.

Yours faithfully,

Norman C. King

Registrar.

Figure 6.5: Letter from the *General Council of Medical Education and Registration* – dated 28 November 1919 – indicating that the DTM&H would *not* be an acceptable registrable qualification (RSTMH archive).

Renewed accommodation problems

At a *Council* meeting on **14 May 1920**, a letter was read from the Registrar of the MSL (Mr Bethell) indicating an increase in the rent of the Society's room at 11 Chandos Street; this had apparently been brought about by a rise in rates, taxes, gas and electric light.

This development obviously made it more imperative than ever that the Society should acquire its own premises as soon as possible (*see* Chapter 8).

Annual subscription

At the meeting of *Council* in May 1920 also, Bagshawe (the Treasurer) proposed raising the annual subscription for Fellows resident within thirty miles of London to two guineas. However, this was *not* accepted as it stood.

At a special *General* meeting in October of that year, the annual subscription was in fact increased from one to one and a half guineas as from 1 April 1921, and the 'composition fee' was raised from fifteen to twenty-two and a half guineas. Dr Balfour's proposal was thus carried *nem con*.

Dinners

The matter of Dinners was not infrequently aired at this time; thus, minutes of a *Council* meeting on **17 December 1920** contain the following:

> Dr Prout proposed that the Society should have a Dinner with the Secretary of State for the Colonies and other distinguished people as guests. It was decided to hold this event in the second or third week of February, the precise date to be settled when the Hon Secretaries had ascertained when the Secretary of State could attend.

Presidential Address

For the first presidential address after the war, the Society had to wait until **17 October 1919**; Professor W J R Simpson CMG (1855–1931)[3] (*see* Figure 6.6) spoke on: '**Some considerations regarding preventable diseases and their prevention**' (most being based on India's requirements). This lecture emphasised the enormous potential of attention to '*public*

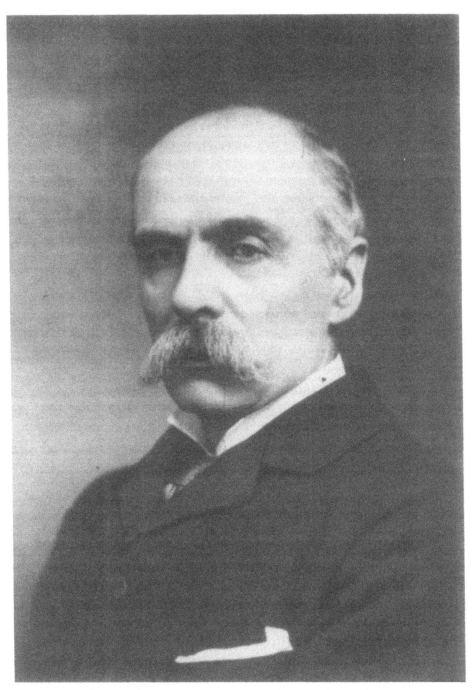

Figure 6.6: Professor William J R Simpson FRCP – the seventh president (RSTMH archive).

health' in the British Empire, at that time dominant in the minds of most of Britain's citizens. He began this wide-ranging 'tour de force' by emphasising how important unravelling the life-cycles of parasites had become in the field of *sanitary* science:

> … The results already obtained bid fair to compete with those of the bacteriological or botanical era which preceded it, and which by its revelation of the causal agents of a large number of infectious diseases linked up man's relationship not only with the vegetable world but also with that of the lower animals. The two have shewn us once more, from different standpoints, how intimate is man's relationship with his environment, and how, even under the most difficult conditions, by the application of that knowledge, protection and safety can be secured. The continuous and systematic application of this knowledge to civil populations in the Tropics is what is now required. The real trouble is that the knowledge we possess is only spasmodically and very restrictedly put into practice. We are familiar with the results of the practical application of bacteriology in epidemic disease in man and the lower animals, both in its detection and prevention. The latest demonstration of its power, when applied on a large scale, is the remarkable freedom of our armies in the West from *typhoid fever*, and in the East from *cholera* and *plague*. Inoculations against these diseases, against *tetanus* and *wound infections*, have removed what were formerly great sources of illness and mortality. …

Of epidemic and endemic disease, Simpson had this to say:

> … Some day, perhaps, as science advances, our descendants will be able to understand the causes of the periodic appearances and disappearances of [the] great epidemics and pandemics … Then they will also be able to explain, apart from the greater supply of food, the causes of the periodic multiplication, swarming and migration of locusts from their endemic homes, and their subsequent limitation to the area from which they came; also of the plagues of caterpillars and agricultural pests, and a host of other puzzling phenomena … Apart from the virulence and diffusiveness gained by the sojourn of the microbe in one or several of these media, what are the factors which combine to form an endemic area for a predominant microbe? The geological

nature of the soil often limits the geographical distribution and kind of animals living underground, and probably the kind of insects and micro-organisms.

Is it in this direction that the explanation may be found concerning the endemic homes of *cholera, plague, influenza, yellow fever* [YF], *bilharzia* and *cerebro-spinal disease*? ... It is the interaction of unusual meteorological conditions on the local fauna and flora of certain limited areas that prepares the micro-organisms for their migration beyond their endemic homes; not by the air, as Bryden and others thought of *cholera*, but by making use of man, the lower animals and insects, and sometimes inanimate objects, as carriers? As regards sudden predominance of a particular microbe, I remember once in Calcutta a pond or tank which contained in its water the ordinary microbes found in others. Suddenly it developed only one kind, the remainder having disappeared. What produced it? ... Was it some slight alteration in the organic or inorganic constituents in the water that favoured the growth of a single organism at the expense of the others? It appeared to me, if this could occur with one kind of microbe it might do so with another, such as the *cholera* bacillus; and if in the water, why not in the soil, where, on the surface of earth drains, the *cholera* bacillus was found?

He then pointed out the necessity for learning more about areas of endemic disease, and highlighted how much remained to be learned about *'preventive medicine'*:

... Although much has been learnt regarding *preventable disease*, there are still vast problems awaiting solution [today]. We require to know more about *plague, cholera, small-pox, leprosy, influenza, cerebro-spinal fever, trypanosomiasis*, [YF], *bilharziasis, blackwater fever*, and many other tropical diseases, and their relation to man's environment, not only in his home but also in nature. Where these diseases most commonly prevail research laboratories are necessary, well equipped with all the modern resources which bacteriology, protozoology, parasitology, biochemistry and geology place at our disposal. The investigations need to be on a comprehensive scale, and not, as I found in Uganda in 1913, where Miss Robertson and Mr Fiske were the only representatives investigating *trypanosomiasis* in a part of the country that, in ten years, had been denuded of nearly a quarter of a million of its inhabitants from this disease and where *rinderpest* was attacking the cattle.

Conditions conducive to the spread of endemic disease were the next area covered:

Once an endemic disease has acquired diffusive qualities there are ample means for its transport and dissemination. Commerce, movements of labour, emigration, pilgrimages in times of peace and the movement of armies and refugees in times of war favour transport, while the insanitary conditions of the locality favour dissemination. The conditions to be found in most countries, even in the twentieth century, are highly insanitary, and even in the best, as in England, there are plenty of slums. The epidemic will find in the huts and houses of the peasants, labourers and poorer classes the fostering conditions for its invasion and spread. If the disease is *plague* or *typhus*, the conditions are ideal where the family live in the same dark and ill-ventilated room or house with the donkey, pig, ox, poultry, rat and insects of each. If the disease is *cholera* the exceptions are few, especially in the Tropics, where a polluted water supply, a primitive disposal of sewage, much filth, numerous flies, and overcrowding are not available conditions for its spread.

In times of war these and other conditions become accentuated by deficiency of food. We realise to-day, better than we have ever done before, what war means to the inhabitants of an invaded country. In previous wars on the Continent, as in the Great War ... it meant the loss to them of their crops, more complete than that sustained by the worst swarm of locusts, the seizure of their cattle and other live stock, the destruction or occupation of their homes, and then hunger, sickness, misery, hardships and the aggravation of insanitary conditions, accompanied with or followed by pestilence. The longer the war lasted the more complete the effects. The population of Germany in the Thirty Years' War [1618–48] was reduced from 17 millions to four, worn down by fighting, famine and pestilence. The world war of 1914–1918, though shorter than many other wars, was on a more gigantic scale, and instead of towns being besieged as formerly, whole countries were blockaded by armies and fleets. Not only did invaded countries suffer, but also those that were blockaded. Epidemics, varying in kind, broke out in both, but in the armies of the West the trained sanitary organisation and adequate food supply were so complete as to immediately check and prevent any considerable extension either in the army or among the civil population over which the military had control. It is an object lesson of importance as to what can be done by good administration. It is also in striking contrast to the failure, in the early years of the war in the *prevention* of tropical diseases in Gallipoli, Mesopotamia, East Africa, Egypt and Salonika, due to the causes explained in my paper on the *Sanitary Aspects of Warfare in South-Eastern Europe*[4] ... In this connection it is only fair to state that great credit is due to the *Mediterranean Sanitary Committee*, whose work did so much to mitigate and remove the conditions which they found inimicable to the health of the troops, and which a short-sighted policy had permitted to arise. There were two diseases which were not checked in the West, and for the same reason in both, viz insufficient knowledge. One was the great prevalence of *trench fever*, whose transmission of infection by the louse was not established until late in the war; and the pandemic of *influenza*, the origin of which is unknown, but which in its intensity and destructiveness throughout the world might, in a slighter degree, be compared with the havoc of the pandemic of pneumonia or influenzal plague [the Black Death] of 1348 ...

Simpson then proceeded to refer to the effects of *influenza*, but soon reverted to historical aspects of the effects of war on *epidemic* disease:

War and epidemics bring out the weak spots in our armour of defence against disease, but their after-effect is generally to set men's minds actively in train to devise means for future protection, and ideas and schemes that have for many years only created a languid interest suddenly get energised into activity and become a reality. This is seen to-day in the creation of a *Ministry of Health* in this country which has been advocated for fifty years, but which the war and epidemic of *influenza* has quickly brought into being. It is seen also in the determination to grapple with the housing question and the problem of the 'C3' men, women and children in the population.

It was the Boer War, with its enormous number of *dysentery* and *typhoid fever* cases, that led to the reinstatement of the *Sanitary Officer* in the Army. There had been a reactionary movement for some ten years before the Boer War, gradually undoing the efficiency of the organisation of sanitary officers which had been the outcome of the Sanitary Commission reporting on the Crimean War. For nearly that period no sanitary officer was appointed at Aldershot, a position formerly held by a Deputy Surgeon-General. The first-fruits of this policy were the large number of officers and men who lost their lives from *preventable disease* in the Soudan [sic] Campaign.

The Navy led the way in protecting her fleets against disease in the tropics. During the wars with France and Spain in 1778, and following years, the West Indies was the principal seat of naval operations, and much greater fleets were then employed in that quarter of the world than in any former period. There was much sickness in the fleet, varying greatly in different ships, and consisting of *dysentery*, *scurvy* and *fever*. Dr Blane (afterwards Sir Gilbert Blane [1749–1834]), when physician to the fleet … had monthly returns sent to the headquarters of the fleet recording the sickness and deaths in each ship, and anything else that related to the health of the ship. He found that the average mortality from disease in twelve months was 1 in 7 of the seamen, and on an average one man in 15 was on the sick list. In 1781 he addressed a memorial to the Board of Admiralty, pointing out the excessive mortality, and expressing his conviction that if certain proposals which he suggested were carried out, more than two-thirds of the seamen who died in that climate would be saved.

These recommendations were similar to those proposed by Dr James Lind [1716–94], a naval surgeon, in 1757, in his essay on the most effectual means of preserving the health of seamen in the Royal Navy, containing cautions necessary for those who reside or visit unhealthy situations, etc. … Blane early recognised the fact that little improvement could be effected in the health of the fleet when left to the initiative of individual officers, and that sanitary rules and regulations, based on scientific knowledge, must be issued by the Admiralty for them to be carried out systematically and efficiently. His recommendations were first put into practice in the West India Fleet with excellent results, and later they were extended to the whole of the Navy. The improvement of the health of the Navy and the reduction in its death-rate contributed to the victories in the revolutionary war [1793–1815]. [Blane] states at a later period, 'that if some new means of preserving the health and lives of seamen had not been discovered and put into practice, the whole stock of them must have been expended before the conclusion of the revolutionary war'. ...

The improvement has continued, notwithstanding the changes in the warships, and average mortality in twelve months [which] is now 1 in 310.

... We are apt to forget [these] lessons of the past. For instance, in the Mesopotamia campaign there would have been no *scurvy* if the history of the Navy ... had been borne in mind and acted upon. It should not have required the valuable and admirable work of Miss Hume and others of the Lister Institute [*see* Chapter 5] to resuscitate the necessity of the supply of vitamines [sic] in the food stuffs supplied to the Army.

One is apt to forget that the use of cinchona bark as a prophylactic goes back to at least the early ... eighteenth century. ... Lind [*see above*] ... mentioned that the continuous use of bark is an effective preservative against a relapse of *malarial fever*, and that 'on the coast of Guinea the factories were furnished with proper quantities of the bark by the late African Company, which was taken by the way of precaution during the rainy and sickly season, and it was attended by remarkable success with such as could be brought to a regular course of life, and refrain from eating such quantities of animal food as they were wont to do in England, which yearly destroyed many on that coast (Guinea)'. One sometimes wonders whether the many relapses of the soldiers from Salonika and other seats of war were due to our preference for the alkaloids of quinine, for which there has been an unprecedented demand, and some of which may have in their preparation lost the complete qualities of the cinchona bark, which itself varies in quality. Are we quite sure that the procedure which destroys the vitamines [sic] of canned food may not affect some of the properties of the alkaloids?

The Crimean War [1854–6], with it[s] tragedies, owing to want of organisation, sanitary and otherwise, and the success which followed the work of the *Sanitary Commission*, of which [Florence] Nightingale [1820–1910] was an important member, led to important sanitary reforms in the Army at home, and in 1859 to the appointment of a Royal Commission to enquire into the health of the Army in India, which in its report published in 1863, disclosed a deplorable condition of things and a death-rate of 69 per 1,000, although in the later years of the *Honourable East India Company*, the conditions in regard to health and the comfort of the soldier had been materially improved, and the mortality had been reduced from 80 to 69. In consequence of this report, remedial measures were at once applied to the Army in India, and were extended to the towns and districts adjacent to the cantonments.

And on to the origins and development of '*Sanitary organisation in India*':

The Royal Sanitary Commission were convinced that if sanitary measures were applied to India under an organised *Public Health Service*, the health of the people of India would in time reach a high standard. It was recommended that such an organisation should be created both in urban and rural areas in India. In 1864 a Sanitary Commissioner was appointed for each Province … for the purpose of improving the sanitary conditions of the people. The Civil Surgeon, ordinarily during peace an officer of the *Indian Medical Service*, temporarily placed at the disposal of a Local Government, was empowered to advise the Civil Commissioner of the district on sanitary questions and later to act as sanitary adviser to municipalities newly formed, for the purposes of local self-government. Gaols were also placed under medical supervision and special health officers were appointed for Calcutta, Bombay and Madras. Later, a very important addition was made by the establishment of *Central Boards of Health* in each province, having for their function the criticism in professional and financial aspects of major schemes of water supply and drainage prior to their sanction by Local Governments. The work which the organisation here described has been able to accomplish is very creditable, considering that a province in India is sometimes about the size of France, and a civil surgeon's district in which he practices is often as large as a third of Scotland. Vaccination, introduced as a protective measure in 1802, was stimulated; then followed the introduction of conservancy, drainage and water supply into some of the more important towns; the registration of deaths, the compilation of statistics, and the regulation of large fairs and pilgrimages, which experience shewed to be always dangerous centres of disease.

The effect of these and subsequent measures has been to reduce the death-rate of British troops from 69 to a pre-war rate (average 1910 to 1914) of 4.51; of Indian troops from 20 to 4.39; and of prisoners from 82.7 to 19.19 per 1,000. Notwithstanding these successes it is obvious that an organisation which consists of a Sanitary Commissioner, Sanitary Engineer and Sanitary Board for each Province, even with the assistance of the Civil Surgeons, is quite unequal to the task of dealing with the sanitary administrations, both rural and urban. It must be remembered that *Civil Surgeons of Districts*, or, as they are called in the Madras Presidency, '*District Medical and Sanitary Officers*' – who ordinarily, during peace, are officers lent temporarily by the Military Department to the Local Government – are expected to attend to the medico-legal work of the district, the medical necessities of civil officials, perform the executive medical and surgical work of all local hospitals and institutions including gaols, and hold administrative and inspecting charge of numerous hospitals and dispensaries scattered throughout their districts. In illustration of the extent of work they are expected to fulfil, I may state that at the Indian Medical Congress of 1894, Dr [Ernest] Hart, then editor of the *British Medical Journal*, made a great point of the absence of research results from the India of that date – there then being only one laboratory specially equipped for this purpose. He had, obviously, fancied that, having regard to the rich possibilities afforded by India, the *Indian Medical Service* men were not workers. After the Congress he was the guest of several Civil Surgeons before his departure to England. ...

Simpson was convinced that until a proper *sanitary service* was formed in India, that country would remain 'defenceless against epidemics'.

… The root of the matter is there is no *Minister of Health* in India, whose duty is concerned solely with sanitation and the health of the population. … No country has waited until its people are educated before it introduced sanitary reforms, and least of all England. Major Justice, the Sanitary Commissioner with the Government of Madras, in his official report for 1911, states that 'to wait till the people are educated will be to indefinitely postpone the evil', and Dr Turner, the late Health Officer of Bombay, remarks that the millennium will have arrived when the people voluntarily carry out sanitary matters. The only education in sanitary matters the people understand is *sanitary laws* and by-laws, and this is the form education should take. It was the form which the wise men in ancient times employed when they included *sanitary laws* in their sacred code. As quoted by Colonel [W G] King [1851–1935], the Education Minister thus defines the position: 'Our first and signal objective is to educate the people as to the value and the necessity of measures for protecting them in their homes and their lives and those dearest to them from the ravages of *plague* and *malaria, cholera* and other communicable diseases, and all the miseries which follow in their train. Fortified by the results of research in India, we can leave the future with confidence to *preventive medicine* and *preventive sanitation*'. When a question was asked in the Bengal Legislative Council what this implied, the reply was that protected water supplies were to be arranged for the people *when they have been taught to appreciate them*. It is difficult to have any patience with such an attitude of mind, and it is no matter of surprise that, with such views, the troops in Mesopotamia were not furnished with the ordinary requisites and organisation to protect them from the ravages of disease and all the miseries which followed in their train. They were left to be educated. …

Research [in addition to poor education] can be made an excuse for doing nothing. My views concerning this in regard to India were expressed some years ago in the following terms: 'We hear a good deal about research, and research is much cheaper than the *application* of sanitary matters. … A few years ago, I urged that sanitary research and administration should go hand in hand. … At the present time a good deal of research has been done [although] I consider that the application of sanitary measures, on the basis of what we already know, is the urgent need of India. ... Supposing the government of India had been asked to construct the Panama Canal, the kind of proceeding they would have introduced with the present *regime* would have been to send out men to make researches; they would not have based their actions on the discoveries already known of [Ronald] Ross and [Carlos] Finlay as the Americans have done. These investigators would have found that the mosquitoes there were a little different from what they were in other places where *malaria* and *yellow fever* existed, and, under the circumstances, the recommendations would have been made to postpone the matter until a further discovery was made. I am convinced that *sanitation* will not receive adequate attention in India until there is a *Ministry of Health*, whose duty is concerned solely with *sanitation* and the health of the population'. Then will the organisation required for urban and rural sanitation be formed, and India will at last be able to throw off the incubus of *plague* and *cholera*, and protect itself against other preventable diseases. ...

He now reverted to cholera in England in 1831 which brought about various *Sanitary Commissions*:

> ... [John] Snow's [1813–58] discovery ultimately, but only very slowly, swept away the time-honoured view – and one which was held in great favour by the Indian Government for forty years afterwards – that the disease was air borne. It was as efficient in this respect as the discovery of Ross ...
>
> Though, compared with the Early Victorian period, there has been an immense improvement in the health and sanitary condition of the population, the problem in England has not been wholly solved, as shewn by Sir George Newman's [1870–1948] recent memorandum and the disclosures regarding the housing conditions ... The same vested interests and ignorance of what is necessary for a healthy community, which obstructed and prevented Sir Christopher Wren [1632–1723], who was the first British *town planner*, carrying out his scheme of making London the most beautiful and healthy city in the world, have marred with ugly and unhealthy spots the cities, towns, and even villages of England.

And next, to housing standards in the tropics:

> The same problem, even in a more acute form, exists in our tropical possessions ... I was particularly struck, on arrival in Calcutta, by the contrast between the airiness of the European quarter and the crowding together on very limited space which distinguished the native quarter. It was very picturesque but exceedingly unhealthy, and I determined to secure a Building Act for the city. It took ten years before a Commission of Enquiry was appointed [and the result] was a Building Act which formed a model for the other towns in India and the Far East. ... Sir Stamford Raffles [1781–1826] – one of the many great Englishmen who have done such magnificent service for their country – laid out Singapore on broad and *sanitary* lines, but those who came after him did not realise the evil that would arise by allowing the Chinaman to cover the whole of his building plot with masonry dwellings. ... The Malay States have taken the lesson to heart, and, in their smaller towns, regulate their buildings so that only a small part of the plot shall be covered. ... Town planning and building regulations [in West Africa] are the forces they are bringing to bear on the question.
>
> In East Africa and Uganda [neglect of attention to sanitary matters] has continued. The Indian Bazaar in Nairobi, and the insanitary conditions in other parts of the town, are [at present a] discredit to all concerned. The result has been that, with African and Asiatic living under conditions which are extremely unhealthy, and where an organised *sanitary service* is only about to be introduced, we have these towns and trade centres constantly affected with *plague, small-pox, dysentery, malaria* and other epidemic diseases. The men are also [significantly] weakened by the large percentage suffering from ankylostomiasis ... The losses from *preventable disease* during the last few years have been exceedingly great. There cannot be the slightest doubt that some of these *epidemic* diseases are capable of becoming even more formidable and destructive as long as existing conditions are permitted to remain, and as long as there is no effective *sanitary* organisation supplied with the requisite funds and powers to take the necessary measures to remove these conditions, to check and prevent disease, and to preserve the native population, which is comparatively small, and ... the chief asset of the country.

We must, Simpson claimed, take a wider and more sympathetic attitude to the native populations from a health viewpoint. 'Next to food and water, the fundamental basis on which a community depends for health is the housing question'. Simpson then told his audience about the progress which had been made in West Africa:

> ... It is [now] ten years since this *Sanitary Service* was created. In that time water supplies have been and were being introduced, drainage was being attended to, breeding-places of mosquitoes were destroyed, extensive marshes were filled up, building laws were enacted, town-planning was engaging the attention of the authorities, laboratories were established, and a special research laboratory was built in Southern Nigeria, and has been carrying out valuable investigations. A Commission on [YF] has been the means of having the circumstances connected with outbreaks investigated, and the disease promptly dealt with. The result has been a healthier life for the European and a greater freedom from disease for the African. ... Much of this success is due to the active and harmonious co-operation of the officials of the Colonial Office with the expert members of the Medical and Sanitary Committee, whose President has been for ... ten years Sir Herbert Read [1863–1949], one of the Under-Secretaries of State for the Colonies, and the interest which the different Secretaries of State have taken in the work. The function of the Medical and Sanitary Committee has been extended to East Africa. ... I should like to see a great *Colonial Medical and Sanitary Service*, the members of which, well trained in tropical diseases and their prevention in our Tropical Schools, should be available after good service and experience in one colony for transfer to others if required. Associated with this service should be a local service of native medical men and sanitary inspectors who have been trained locally, and whose knowledge of their compatriots would be of great assistance to the hospital physician, sanitary officer, and Government in their health administration and their campaign against disease.
>
> I should like to see a league of Local Governments of the Crown Colonies having, through their representatives, conferences on health matters, from time to time, with the object of improving the conditions of life of the inhabitants under their charge.

And lastly, he favoured the setting up of an imperial Institute for Research and an Empire Health Museum:

> When his Majesty King Edward VII [1841–1910] died, I wrote to the Lord Mayor of London [*see also* Chapter 3] – who was chairman of a committee to consider a suitable memorial to commemorate his reign – I pointed out that His Majesty had always taken an active interest in the health of his people at home and in the Tropics. When Prince of Wales, he had been a member of the Royal Commission on the Housing of the Working-Classes. He had interested himself in the Commission to India to enquire into Leprosy, and he had been President of the International Congress of Hygiene, held in London in 1891. I ventured to suggest an *Imperial Health Institute for Research* with an *Empire Health Museum* [which] would contain models, plans and other arrangements for illustrating the causes of *preventable* diseases, the conditions under which they spread, and the methods by which they can be prevented; the diseases communicated by animals, insects and vermin; the diseases of occupations liable to occur in different industries, manufactures, trades, foundries, workshops mines, plantations and large works, and the known methods of prevention. … There would be tropical, industrial, domestic, personal, housing urban and rural, and preventable diseases sections. The museum would be open to all. … There should be sections to represent not only the British Isles, but also Canada, Australia, South Africa, India, Burmah [sic], and our Crown Colonies and Protectorates. Lectures and demonstrations, illustrated by models and the cinematograph should be given, and there should be attached a *Bureau of Information*, on a similar or larger scale than that of the British Museum or the Victoria and Albert Museum. My suggestion was not accepted at the time. Now that there will be an Empire War Memorial, worthy of the far-reaching victory which has secured safety for us all, I would suggest that, in addition to the War Memorial, there should be a Peace Memorial, in the form of an *Empire Health Museum* in London, worthy in every respect to illustrate the means by which we can triumph over *preventable disease*, which, in the long run, is far more destructive to human life and to health than even the greatest war.[5]

The twelfth and thirteenth annual reports

The number of Fellows 'on the books' stood at 566 and 674 for 1919 and 1920, respectively.

The Society's income in the years 1918–19 and 1919–20 was £558 14s 00d and £645 4s 3d, respectively.

Dr G C Low had 'stepped down' as a joint Honorary Secretary in May 1920, and was succeeded by C M Wenyon.

References and Notes

1 Anonymous. Sir William Prout. *Br med J* 1939; ii: 1165; Anonymous. Prout, Sir William Thomas. *Who Was Who, 1929–1940* 2nd ed. London: A & C Black 1967: 1109.

2 The King's Interest. *Times, Lond* 1920.

3 **William Simpson** was born in Glasgow and educated at Aberdeen University and King's College London. He became the first full-time Medical Officer of Health for Calcutta (now Kolkata), and was subsequently appointed to the Chair of Hygiene at King's College, London in 1898, where he became a pioneer of tropical hygiene. Simpson was a founder of the LSTM and also the Ross Institute & Hospital for Tropical Diseases at Putney [*See:* G C Cook. Aldo Castellani FRCP (1877–1971) and the founding of the Ross Institute & Hospital for Tropical Diseases at Putney. *J med Biog* 2000; 8: 198–205; G C Cook. A difficult metamorphosis: the incorporation of the Ross Institute & Hospital for Tropical Diseases into the London School of Hygiene and Tropical Medicine. *Med Hist* 2001; 45: 483–506]. He also undertook several research investigations in tropical countries. [*See*: P Manson-Bahr. In: *History of the School of Tropical Medicine in London (1899–1949)*. London: H K Lewis 1956: 136–7; Anonymous. Simpson, Sir William John Ritchie. *Who Was Who, 1929–1940* 2nd ed. London: A & C Black 1967: 1240; M Watson, M P Sutphen. Simpson, Sir William John Richie (1855–1931) In: H C G Matthew, B Harrison (eds). *Oxford Dictionary of National Biography*. Oxford: Oxford University Press 2004: 50: 719].

4 W J R Simpson. The sanitary aspects of warfare in south-eastern Europe. *Trans Soc trop Med Hyg* 1918–19; 12: 1–10.

5 W J R Simpson. Presidential address: Some considerations regarding preventable diseases and their prevention. *Trans Soc trop Med Hyg.* 1919–20; 13: 31–44.

Chapter 7

The 1920s: consolidation of the Society, but still no *permanent* base, and an unfortunate episode involving the Colonial Office

---

During the 1920s the Society had five new presidents. At the beginning of the decade, Simpson was of course still occupying the position. Dr G C Low was in fact elected towards the end of the decade, but since he is so closely associated with the move to Manson House, his lengthy presidency (1929–33) is related in Chapter 8.

Presidential Addresses

On 20 October 1921, Sir James Cantlie KBE FRCS (1851–1926)[1] (*see* Figure 7.1) delivered a presidential address on the perhaps unusual but highly relevant topic: '**Life insurance in the tropics**'; he began:

> … I have interested myself in the matter for some twenty years, and published several articles and read several papers on the subject. As far back as 1897, a paper was published in the *British Medical Journal*[2]; I addressed a meeting of the Life Assurance Medical Officers' Association in 1903; and, further, read a paper before the *Royal Institute of Public Health* at one of their Conferences.
>
> The question before us seems to resolve itself into – Does residence in the tropics impair the health of the individual to such an extent as to justify the imposition of an extra premium being demanded by insurance companies. In insurance prospectuses I see that a dangerously warm country is regarded as one situated within 33° north of the equator and 30° south of the equator.
>
> … within the area specified we meet with climates of widely different characteristics, varying between climates of an equatorial, a tropical, a sub-tropical and a temperate character; climates, some with an insular and some with a continental type

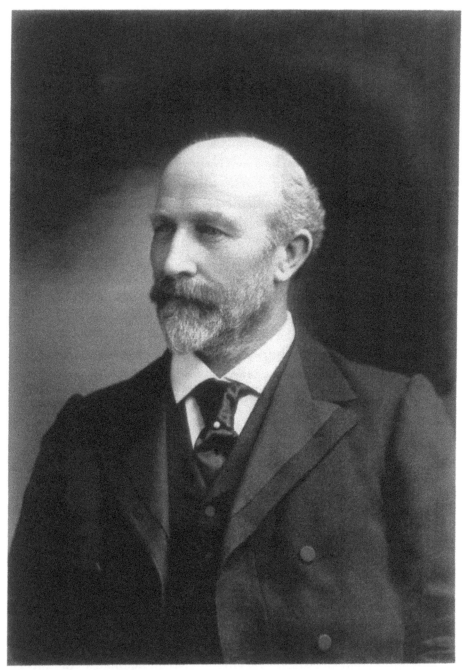

Figure 7.1: Sir James Cantlie FRCS – the eighth president (reproduced courtesy the Wellcome Library, London).

of character. To slump these together, as some of the companies say they do, is perhaps an inevitable method of dealing with such a huge subject as tropical insurance, but it is hard on individuals proceeding to a 'good climate' area within the specified longitude and latitude, and one wonders how the rules appertaining to the amount of extra premium demanded were drawn up. Was it from statistics of the percentages of deaths published by the local governments in Crown Colonies, etc, or was it from information received from travellers? If not, one cannot conceive what were the sources from which the knowledge was derived – say fifty years ago.

I have described the tales we hear of these distant tropical lands as ship captains' gossip gathered from the common talk of those lands when the ship goes in harbour. On the way out in 1887, the officers of the ship – whether sailors or engineers – spoke of little else than the fate of the passengers whom they had taken out on previous voyages, how they were dead in twelve months or sent home wrecks after a few years. When again one's friends and relations at home heard one was to go to the eastern tropics, one was deluged with letters, cuttings from reports, callers beseeching one to give up the idea of going out to a death-trap, a 'white man's grave', and so forth, until one wondered how any Briton ever went out at all.

The difficulties of getting insurance in those days was then recalled:

No wonder some of the Insurance Companies of that date said they would have nothing to do with insuring the lives of persons going to the tropics on any consideration whatever. Were the extra premium charges founded on the local government reports, here, again, the information was faulty in a superlative degree. None of our tropical colonies produces its own labour; the white population is imported from Britain and the native labour from the neighbouring countries, or brought from overseas: Tamils, etc, to Ceylon [now Sri Lanka], Chinese to the Malay States and to the Straits Settlements [Malaysia and Singapore], Indians and Chinese to the West Indies, and so forth. They come as young adults as a rule without their wives and children; without, in fact, the part of the family which swell the death-rates in home countries. The white population consisted of bachelors for the most part, who, on being carefully examined, were sent out in perfect health; often taught by lectures how to avoid diseases; re-vaccinated against *small-pox*, inoculated against *typhoid*, and occupying dwellings – often of a better class than they were accustomed to at home.

When they get ill they are carefully attended to, sent for a change or sent home on sick leave. What are the diseases that give the district a bad name? *Malaria* is the chief, but malaria kills but a small percentage of those attacked. It is a disease that incapacitates, and the loser is the employer or the firm in which they work – not the insurance office, whether the insurance is for a period of years or for life. Besides malaria, its cause, prevention and treatment is so well known at the present day that its danger is fractional. Compared to that of pre-Laveran-Manson-Ross days, it may be said that if a man gets malaria in modern times the fault is with the man, because he did not follow the precautions now so well known.

'... there is now no reason why one who uses the mosquito-net properly should contract *malaria*', he claimed, and the importance of *dysentery* and its sequelae is 'greatly lessened today by the emetine treatment of Rogers'.

What, then, is an extra premium charged for, as other diseases are but on a platform with home ailments? These facts I have brought forward on several occasions, and whether in consequence of my speaking and writing I know not, but several companies now advertise world-wide policies. In a short time all companies must follow suit, otherwise the world-wide policies will kill out the still perverse companies.

The great diseases of the tropics affect, for the most part, the young men – the unacclimatised, as they are called. It is during the first two or three years of tropical life for young men going out that the tropics is dangerous, and the younger they go out the greater the danger. Time was when men went out at a younger age than now. Sixteen or seventeen was a common age to send out young men some thirty years ago. Gradually the advantages of sending young men out at about twenty became apparent, and for a man to go out before twenty-one is looked upon to-day as inadvisable and dangerous. Twenty-three is the better age, and twenty-five the best. This fact, that the earlier the age the more the danger, affects insurance. Before going out the young man is likely to be insured by his parents or guardians; and as the younger the age the better the terms of the policy for home life, he may be insured, say, in the office at home when seventeen.

When, however, he goes overseas to the tropics, the extra-premium question arises. Abroad, his salary barely keeps him, and he has £10 or £20, or in some cases even £40, charged him, over and above the home premium, He is now free from parental help and control, and the extra charge falling upon him either runs him into debt or he lets the policy lapse, and the money he paid is lost to him and given to the benefit of the company, 'for the risk they have run'.

Cantlie then outlined plans for 'lessening ... the policy to lapse':

> I have brought forward more than one plan whereby this dropping of policies may be prevented. Of these attempts to lessen the chance of the young man allowing the policy to lapse, I suggest the following scheme as one which would accomplish this:-

>> Supposing a young lad of seventeen is insured, whilst working in an insurance office at home, for £1,000. When he is twenty years of age he is sent overseas in the company's service. Up to then his father paid his insurance, but when he goes abroad an extra premium is imposed and his father expects him to pay the premium on his life. He finds after a year or two the premium, plus the extra premium imposed, is more than he can meet and he allows it to lapse.

> To avoid this occurring, I would suggest that instead of the company charging the extra premium, that the company reduce their liability, and that, instead of being liable for the £1,000 originally taken out, the liability of the company be reduced to, say, £500 in case of the death of their client, or it might be to £750 if the climate is a 'good' one. This should hold good for say five years, that is to say, until the insured has passed through the

'dangerous period' of his tropical residence. If at the end of the five years, and if the client can produce a doctor's certificate to the effect that he is quite well I suggest that the extra premium be abolished altogether, or at least reduced by half, and their full liabilities of £1,000 be restored. Instead of these hard and fast lines being followed, the restoration might be graded. If it is reduced, to begin with, by £500, after a period the liability might be raised to £700, and, after a few more years be graded up to £1,000.

He continued by claiming that *doctors* should be the 'sole ultimate authorities' and not the actuaries:

When I read my paper before the Life Insurance Medical Officers' Association in 1903, Sir Dyce Duckworth [1840–1928] was in the chair, and he, in commenting upon my paper, said, 'Mr Cantlie's plan of dealing with extra premiums for young men would free the young man from increasing his payment, and at the same time diminish the risk of the company satisfactorily. I do not know if business men would accept the principle, but to me it seems feasible and fair. I happened to see the manager of my own insurance office to-day, and I put this to him. He said it was nonsense on the face of it, and that no insurance office would contemplate such a matter as sound business. He went on further to repudiate several of the assertions of Mr Cantlie throughout this paper, which he had read, and to say that these matters do not, as Mr Cantlie says, rest entirely on the *dicta* of the doctors'. He says, 'I would recommend British insurance offices to reply for advice as regards the value of the lives of tropical residents on the medical officers of their companies, and not on their actuaries. The actuary cannot know, he had no means of knowing, the effect of climate or the local state of heathfulness in any individual colony'. Then he goes on to say that 'the actuary's figures are misleading, and his statistics of no use to him there. To-day I was told that that was not the case. I was told there was a great deal of mathematics in these cases, and that it is not merely an opinion on mere climate which the person goes to, but there are actual matters of great importance which we doctors are not supposed thoroughly to understand'. Something wants doctoring, and it is not the doctor …

This was followed by an intriguing section entitled:

The Insurance of Natives. – The question of insuring the lives of natives remains a vexed one. British offices, for the most part, do not push this business; American insurance offices do. I am not prepared to give you a statistical table of the expectancy of life of, say, a Hindoo, Malay, Chinaman, or negro: no statistics are available; but I am in a position to express an opinion in regard to the matter. The question narrows itself down to a very fine point. It is only the more advanced and intelligent of the natives of any Asiatic country who take out insurances on their lives. It is the natives who have become 'Anglicised' to a greater or less extent that usually come forward for insurances. But in the process of becoming Anglicised they have acquired more than an imperfect knowledge of English and British habits in business.

They affect British ways of living to some extent, and especially do they take to the food and drink which they see supplied to the British table. Beef or mutton take the place of fish or fat pork in the diet, and European wines, especially champagne, are the constant concomitants of, say, the Chinaman who takes to European 'chow'. A rich Chinaman who affects the European mode of living has his Chinese 'chow' with his family, and European 'chow' (it may be immediately afterwards) with his Anglicised *confrères*. The excess of rice at one meal, with beef, etc, and sweet champagne – the sweeter the better he likes it – in time tells its tale. Gout, kidney and liver troubles supervene, and his days are shortened. It is from this very class that most native lives are insured, and they are the very worst lives of the land they belong to.

The ignorant and simple living native might be as good a life as any European – as a matter of fact he seldom is – but when he departs from his simple habits, and takes to 'foreign' ways of eating and drinking, his life is not a good one. I saw much of American methods of dealing with the Chinese in regard to insurance. At one time, in Hong Kong, the Chinese insured largely in American insurance offices, but during the last years of my stay there they almost ceased doing so. Perhaps they have taken it up again, but I hope on a different footing to that which was in vogue when I knew the methods followed.

And lastly:

> *Insurance Anomalies.* – The insurance offices say, 'Well, we slump the risks, and what we lose by the younger men we gain on those of more mature years'. Many hardships are, however, incurred therefrom. But yesterday I saw a nurse proceeding to one of our colonies, a healthy woman of forty, who had to pay an extra premium of £10 a year; her actual salary amounting to about £60. I know also of *patients* who, on being recommended to go to a warm climate by their physician, had to pay an extra premium to their insurance offices – a most anomalous state of affairs. They were being sent to the only place in the world where health could be obtained and where their lives could be prolonged, yet they are asked to pay an extra premium for their doing so.
>
> I have known men who, after long residence in a warm climate, find they cannot keep their health at home, and go abroad again to live. They have paid an extra premium on their life assurance whilst abroad; this has been rebated when they came home, but again enforced when, in order to live at all, they have gone to the part of the world which suits them best; the insurance office in this instance remitting the extra premium in the only place where their client could not live, namely, at home.[3]

The presidential addresses to the Society in the 1920s certainly did not lack variation. That delivered on 18 October 1923 by Surgeon-Rear-Admiral Sir Percy W Bassett-Smith (1861–1927)[4] (*see* Figure 7.2) was entitled: '**The relation of food to the causation of disease in the tropics**'. After praising the former eight presidents, Bassett-Smith began by stating that 'Errors in dietetics ... are fairly common and lead to many cases of *preventable* disease'. He began by giving an historical background to his topic:

> ... We know from history how the want of a sufficient food supply has always had a tendency to culminate in conditions of general and political unrest, that have gone on to mutiny and rebellion, and often overthrown monarchies. In the time of George III [1738–1820] the chief cause of the mutiny in the Fleet was the extraordinarily bad supply of necessary food on board ships filled with pressed men. In the 18th century scarcity of food was a very potent factor in the French capital, and gave rise to the outburst of fierce feeling culminating in the 'Terror'. As an

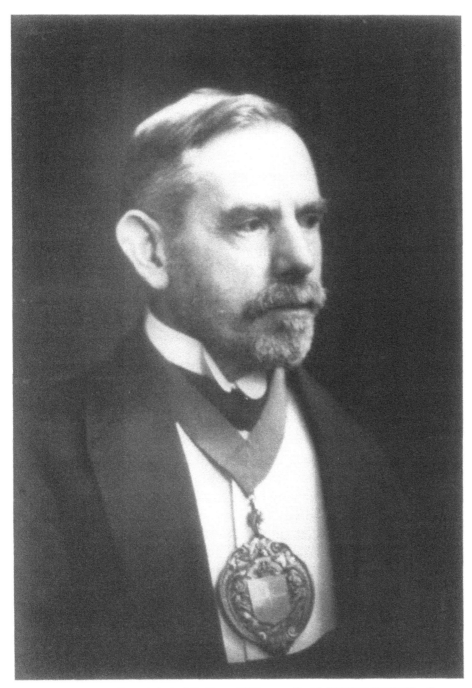

Figure 7.2: Surgeon-Rear-Admiral Sir Percy W Bassett-Smith KCB FRCP FRCS – the ninth president (RSTMH archive).

aftermath of the late war [1914–18], particularly in the eastern part of Europe, famine and distress have had a most disastrous effect, bringing out the brutal characteristics of a selfish and badly educated class; but the brighter side of the picture shows how it has also given an opportunity for unlimited altruism and charity, with a great advance in our scientific knowledge of food deficiency diseases.

Following adverse seasons, in peace, famine brings on conditions of starvation and destitution. Who among us that have ever been in India and across the country in famine times, can ever forget the sad sight of the crowds of attenuated limbed, pot-bellied or sunken bellied, almost naked men, women, and children who crowd the stations and towns in search of food? And we all know that under these conditions of inanition and reduced resisting power infective diseases are rampant. Food, and the sufficient supply of food, is one of the great administrative problems of all countries, particularly of those under conditions of change, or in process of civilisation.

We know that in tropical climates the tendency is for the people to depend more particularly on one kind of food – rice in the orient, maize in South Africa and parts of America, bananas in tropical Africa, manioc, figs and dates in other hot areas; in sub-tropical regions and temperate climates on various cereals and potatoes, so that this very dependence on the particular products tends, from time to time in periods of scarcity, to the causation of, first, malnutrition, then often definite disease. It is important to remember that natives who live in favoured lands, where nature almost unaided provides an abundant and nutritious food, should this food supply fail, are much more helpless and much less able to resist disease than others who are in the habit of fighting for their existence; also the diet in these ideal homes is mostly vegetable and the people are less robust than meat-eating races.

He proceeded to outline the basis of a healthy diet:

For the maintenance of health it is necessary that the food supply shall be such that it is able to provide all those substances that are required to make good wastage, to insure growth, and to supply energy for carrying out the functions of the body. This has been ably set forth in many valuable books, and the number of calories required has, from time to time, been a subject of much discussion; such diet must have its quantity of proteins, carbohydrates, hydrocarbons, salts and water properly balanced, and also contain those accessory food factors [vitamins] of which so much has of late been written, but *I am convinced that the subject of dietetics is the one which is at present woefully neglected in the ordinary course of medicine* [author's italics], and very few newly qualified men have more than touched the fringe of the subject. It is only the result of later observation, and often hardly acquired clinical experience, that has brought home to the practitioner the great importance of this subject. One of the great lessons of the war has been the enormous value of giving the hygienist the control of the food supply. To Surgeon General W W O Beveridge is due the credit of having held out against the tendency to cut down, for economic and administrative reasons, the full dietary of the soldier during the war, when under conditions of abnormal stress. The Italians and other nations attempted such an economy greatly to their discomfiture and discredit. ...

In my Naval experience, in early years, the great conservatism of both the Service and the wishes of the men themselves, led me into constant controversy with regard to the dietary of our crews in the tropics. For many years the old custom of supplying the excessive amount of highly nitrogenous food, taken in the heat of the day with a minimum opportunity of exercise in such places as the Persian Gulf and the Red Sea, led to deficient metabolism and retention of effete products, with often disastrous results.

In the tropics, where the diet adopted under instinctive guidance contains less proteins and fats, with more carbohydrates, than that of the inhabitants of cooler climates, we have indications of what is required. Dr Ziemann says the problem of climate is largely the maintenance of the proper balance between ... intake and ... output of heat. Theoretically the problem could be solved by a diminution of the amount of food taken, or by an increase of muscular activity, but these methods, carried to an extreme, lead to the ruin of the white races.

The amount of food supplied can, it is true, be diminished to some extent, and the nature of the food may be chosen to suit the climate with the utmost advantage, but it is found that the amount of protein taken by a white man cannot safely be less than 100 grams per diem; on the other hand, fats (of which 1 gram equals 9.3 calories) and alcohol (1 gram equals 7 calories) are both to be avoided.

Buckle says – 'Among natives, where the coldness of the climate renders a rich, animal diet essential, there is, for the most part, a bolder, more adventurous spirit than among other natives whose ordinary vegetable nutriment is easily obtained'. A diet rich in protein makes for physical and mental energy, and it is animal not vegetable protein that is most wanted. It is animal protein which is the true food of the brain and nerves, hence all the more energetic races of the world have been meat eaters.

The working classes in England have all adopted … a diet [containing] not less than 3,000 calories containing 120 grams of protein.

The value of a protein depends largely upon the amount and kind of the amino-acids it contains; there are eighteen of these, of which tryptophane [sic] and lysine are indispensable for life. The greater the similarity of the protein supplied to the tissue which is required to be built up, the higher will be its value. The biological protein value of meat and milk is 3.4 times as great as that of maize. …

Bassett-Smith then summarised diets in the US, Japanese, French and British navies; all showed a high calorie value, but those for the French and Japanese were lower in fat when compared with the others – 'more in conformity with a tropical diet'. He continued:

… The subject of diet for the soldier in the tropics is one of very great interest. Food that excessive heat will spoil, or which cannot be easily preserved, must be avoided. The ration should be so arranged that it may be changed accordingly to the climate. It has been abundantly proved, in the United Sates and the Philippines, that men living quiet lives in the tropics eat less than they would in a cold or temperate climate. This difference is particularly marked in the consumption of meat and fatty substances. If, however, on very active service, with excessive labour and resulting fatigue, the meat allowance will have to be correspondingly increased to make up for the wear and tear of the muscular system.

Major Keen, Surgeon-General of the US Army, states that a tropical diet, as compared with one suited for a colder climate, should have less fat and more carbohydrate, less stimulating proteins in the form of meat, a greater variety of food both of meat and carbohydrate, with fresh vegetables and fruit, and lastly a liberal supply of ice. His argument for the substitution of carbohydrates for fats is that the digestion is weakened in hot climates and the liver is inclined to be torpid, while ingested fats are prone to be split up into butyric, caproic, and other irritating acids, which the diminished secretion of the liver is unable to neutralise. As the intestinal digestion cannot proceed in the presence of acidity, the condition known as biliousness is established, with putrification of the intestinal contents and the production of various alkaloidal substances. A catarrhal inflammation of the bowel results, followed by diarrhoea, which is at first an advantage in eliminating the harmful substances but which, under continued irritation of unsuitable diet, is liable to progress and become aggravated. As to the lessened use of meat, he cites the dietary customs of the inhabitants of hot climates, who get their proteins less from meat than from the legumes. The appetite is lessened by long continued heat and becomes capricious; it craves variety, especially in vegetables and fruit.

Ghosh, he continued, had described a suitable diet for ordinary work in the tropics, which had a calorie value of 'about 2,500 calories, with a minimum of fats, high carbohydrates, and good protein value'.

> ... Sugar is a most valuable article of diet in the tropics, especially for men doing hard labour. I have been much struck by the descriptions of the great value placed on, and craving for sugar by those climbing the mountains of the Andes in Peru. It is not only a heat producer but also a saver of proteins. Tropical heat has thus, undoubtedly, a great determinating action upon many physiological processes ...
>
> The digestive powers are less vigorous than in cold climates, and large quantities of food cannot be well borne .... The food given should be such as to produce the minimum of heat, but

... sufficient nourishment. Proteins ... stimulate metabolism and ... produce heat, and naturally are physiologically less required; if, however, much physical labour is taken the requirements of a greater supply of protein are evident.

But what of the diet of the native?:

Woodruff [*see* Chapter 4] states that 'all natives in the tropics are in a condition of partial nitrogen starvation and need much more nitrogen than they can get'. To say that in the tropics we should live like the natives is quite wrong, and examples of certain enthusiastic, but misguided, missionaries could be quoted. He also states that the destructive effects of the concentrated actinic tropical rays on protoplasm cause the necessity of more nitrogen than at home (which is a debateable question), and he thinks that it is untrue that fat is not needed in the tropics. It is evident that in arranging a dietary the conditions of work and the varying states of life must be taken into consideration.

He then digressed and described his own experience as a naval officer, and that of others; despite unsatisfactory diets (often consisting of *tinned* foods) he could only recall a single case of frank *scurvy*. In the tropics, he observed, 'cow's milk and buffalo milk are often deficient in quality, but they rarely contain tubercle bacilli'; however, the latter was a possible source of [*Brucella*] *melitensis* infection. He followed this with a few words on vitamins:

... The view that these vitamines [sic] have a drug-like action on the digestive tract, and may be used for therapeutic purposes, has received some confirmation from recent observations of Murlin and Mattell in their paper 'On the Laxative Action of Yeast'. ...

The value of yeast has been recognised in many tropical diseases, and I have always found it advantageous in the chronic stages of undulant fever [brucellosis], as it increases the leucocyte count and favours phagocytosis.

Recently I have carried out some experiments with guinea-pigs on a diet enriched with 'marmite', a yeast compound rich in vitamines [sic]; the animals with controls were then infected with lethal doses of tubercle bacilli. ... The infecting dose was prepared by Dr S R Gloyne from a well-tried pathogenic strain ...

The [outcome was] that:-

- The duration of the infection was relative to the dose injected and there was a parallelism between the two.
- In the marmite-fed animals there was a distinct prolongation of life. ...
- The gain in weight following the inoculation [was followed by a] sudden fall.
- The high leucocyte count during part of the course [was] probably due to secondary infections.

... it is [therefore] good practice to reinforce the diet of early *tuberculosis* cases and to recommend cod liver oil, marmite and fresh fruit to all cases. It may be that with slight infections ... the addition of these vitamines [sic] would be protective. This is all the more important, as *tuberculosis* is becoming more widespread among native races.

Bassett-Smith proceeded to summarise those 'tropical' diseases which he considered were directly associated with diet (*see* Table 7.1); however, the precise aetiology of beriberi[5] remained controversial.

He then introduced more history:

[It] has been wittily remarked [that] anti-scorbutics were recognised in the most ancient times, for did not Eve give Adam an apple, and Nebuchadnezzer go out to satisfy his craving by eating grass? From a naval point of view, the beneficent action of eating 'scurvy grass' was recognised by Captain [James] Cook [1728–79], but it was due to [James] Lind [1716–94] and Gilbert Blane [1749–1834] that the great preventives, lemon and lime juice, were supplied and regularly issued [to prevent scurvy] when at sea. ... As originally prepared, the lime juice was made from sweet limes, *Citrus medica*, and with lemons, imported chiefly from Spain. In 1793 war stopped these supplies, but in 1802 delivery was resumed, and *scurvy*, which had obtained a temporary hold, was again almost eliminated. About 1860, by the development of the cultivation of limes in the West Indies, a large quantity was made available, and the contract for the Navy caused the sour lime, *Citrus medica* var. *acida* to supersede the sweet limes and lemons formerly in use, and for a time this new lime juice was

Table 7.1: Tropical diseases directly due to diet

Over supply:
- Gastritis
- Diarrhoea
- Hepatic congestion

Deficiency of certain necessary constituents:
- Oriental *beriberi*
- Occidental *beriberi*
- Ship *beriberi*
- Rand *scurvy*
- True *scurvy*
- Pellagra
- Rickets

Bacterial or protozoal infection of food:
- Cholera
- Dysentery
- Sprue (?)
- Undulant fever
- Enterica [typhoid fever]
- Tuberculosis
- Botulism, etc

Introduction of parasites with food:
- Helminths and amoebae
- Larvae

Poisons in food:-
- Animal
- Vegetable
- Chemical

believed to be better than the old. This has been proved not to be the case, both by results of arctic expeditions under Sir George Nares [1831–1915], and by much recent laboratory experiment. …

On to *infections* conveyed by food (both bacterial and protozoal):

… undoubtedly, the first place is taken by undulant fever [brucellosis], for this is almost always contracted through the ingestion of infected milk or the products of milk, and has, in the Services, by the elimination of these, been practically eradicated, thanks to the memorable work of the British Commission under the chairmanship of Sir David Bruce [*see* Chapter 5] …

… the indigenous Boer goat of South Africa was free from [*Brucella*] *melitensis* infection; but, between 1838 and 1880, shipments of the Angora breed were imported, and these brought infection with them and [when] interbred with the Boer goats, [this] infection spread. In 1896, Swiss goats, free from infection, were introduced for their superlative milking properties; these now also have been infected, and, should this spread through want of proper inspection, the Swiss goat industry of the country will be severely affected. It is important that all goats introduced into towns should be proved to be free from infection, and steps should be taken to prevent … introduction of infected goats into herds, more particularly of the Swiss variety. We may go further, and say that the same care should be taken in other countries where goats' milk is much used. … In the Soudan [sic], cases are reported from Khartoum, and, probably undulant fever [brucellosis] is fairly widely distributed in North Africa. In the Soudan area bovine abortion does not occur; the infected goats are probably brought from Arabia. The disease is now known to be [highly] prevalent in Persia [now Iran], and has been proved to be due to the use of goats' milk infected with the Micrococcus.

In *cholera, enterica [typhoid fever], dysentery* and *tubercle* we have organisms which, undoubtedly are directly conveyed to man through food, either by mechanical transference through flies or human carriers, or by the addition of infected water. … Sir William Hamer [? – 1936], in a Presidential address to the Medical Officers of Health, brought forward strong reasons for believing that not only *typhoid*, but also *cholera*, in England, was spread through the agency of oysters.

Ingesting parasites in contaminated food also did not escape him:

… Practically everyone in the Far East is a host for some of these parasites, often of many. Experience teaches us that we cannot use too many precautions to avoid the contamination of fresh vegetables from ova-infected sewage. It is also possible that the infection of endemic haemoptysis [paragonimiasis] may be conveyed by eating uncooked crabs. The infection of meat by *Taenia saginata, T solium*, and the Echinococcus are so well known that they need only be mentioned, but whether *Hymenolepis nana*, Davainea, and Sparganum are contracted through food is not known. *Dibothrocephalus latus* is, undoubtedly, ingested in raw fish in Madagascar and South Africa. It is probable that most forms of *Entamoeba* may be swallowed and infect man through food, as they have been proved by Wenyon, Sellards, Brumpt, and others to be able to infect animals in this way; indeed Walker and Sellards, in the Philippines, have infected men by feeding them with *Entamoeba histolytica*.

The larvae of flies may be swallowed in [the] food on which they have developed; at least twenty species of dipterous larvae have been found in, or expelled from the human intestinal canal, and these when found are a great source of concern to the patient.

And finally to *poisons* – of animal, vegetable and chemical origin:

> … in the tropics quite a number of cases of direct poisoning due to the consumption of fish which may, even when perfectly fresh, give rise to violent symptoms. In certain islands in the West Indies, some forms of the *Carangidae* are definitely believed to be poisonous at all times; others are only poisonous at the times of spawning. Some of the *Clupeidae*, such as *C. humeralis* of the West Indies, *C. longiceps* of Ceylon [now Sri Lanka], and *C. tryssa* of South Africa are always to be avoided. With regard to the latter, there is a saying 'If you begin at the head you never finish the tail'. The symptoms are pain, prostration, convulsions, and unconsciousness followed by death, sometimes in a quarter of an hour, but generally in from two to three hours. A few of the 'Barracudas' of the West Indies are, occasionally, intensely poisonous. Practically all the hard-toothed coral-eating fish are unfit for food. … In the Navy, the old view is still commonly held that fish without scales are not generally wholesome.

Vegetable poisons (when not given for criminal purposes) Bassett-Smith recalled, could also produce health problems:

> … Lathyrism [occurs] in Abyssinia, Algeria, and India, namely, when [a] particular kind of vetch, *Lathyrus sativus,* and allied species, form an article of diet. The disease is very chronic [but] rarely fatal, causing ataxic and spastic paraplegic symptoms. [The] seeds are pathogenic to ducks, pigs, and horses but not to bullocks and buffaloes. 'Loliismus' is another condition found in India due to contaminated bread. In China, an intoxication is caused by eating the leaves of *Atriplex littoralis*, the symptoms of

which are itching, oedema, blebs, and cutaneous haemorrhages, but cyanosis and gangrene of parts may occur. In Jamaica, [Henry] Scott [*see* Chapter 11] was the first to determine that the 'vomiting sickness' [was] found in localised epidemics in rural districts, [and] was due to eating the fruit of *Bhighia sapida*, ... 'Ackee'. The tree is very common on the island and is much in demand. When the fruit is matured and in good condition it is quite wholesome, but if gathered unripe, opened while on the tree, or from an injured branch, or if opened after falling on the ground, it is poisonous. ... the water in which the ackee has been cooked is much more toxic than the cooked fruit. The disease is known to have caused over 5,000 deaths in Jamaica since 1886 ... This is one of the best examples of a tropical disease caused by the ingestion of a food usually considered to be wholesome.

Bassett-Smith concluded this address:

... it is true that we naturally develop certain habits, and on entering new conditions in the tropics we generally carry our food habits with us. A great many vegetables common in colder regions do not grow in the tropics, and we are inclined to use tinned foods instead of adjusting ourselves to the new conditions, and using the vegetables and fruits which grow there, but the ill effects of an excessive starch and sugar diet, deficient in meat and green vegetables, are often very apparent. We need food from animal sources for the growth and maintenance of our body tissues. ... fats and carbohydrates for our body heat and energy, inorganic salts to help to build up our tissues and perform physiological functions, and lastly 'vitamines' [sic] ...

People may remain well for a long period in the tropics on an inadequate diet, but will eventually succumb to some form of constitutional disease, insidiously initiated. Therefore, if you want to live long and keep healthy, a well selected mixed diet, properly balanced, is required, containing all the essentials, and avoiding, as far as possible, the specially prepared foods so common on the market.

[In] recent years, a great improvement of the health of the white man has taken place, by the application of modern knowledge and greater care in providing education in hygiene and food problems before going out and after arriving there, but it would have been impossible to have reached our present state of advancement without the aid of animal experiment, [and in] the words of Lord Moulton [1844–1921], in 1907:-

> No man who knows anything of science has any doubt whatever that the right way to advance knowledge is by experiment. You can take the whole range of the sciences, and I would challenge an opponent to name one in which advance, if it has been rapid and striking, has not been through experiment. When we are reduced to observation, science crawls. Where and in proportion as you can use experiment, the science advances rapidly ... . As soon as you can bring experiment to bear upon a subject, you are free; but as long as you can merely observe, your progress is very slow. The reason is that experiment is like cross-examination. You can put the question you want, and Nature always answers it.

But it must be remembered that our scientists and clinical workers do not stop at animal experiment; the crucial test is on man himself, and this method of trial has been more and more employed, after the basic facts have been demonstrated on animals ... .'Man cannot live by bread alone' – he wants a good deal more – but in its selection a knowledge of the dangers that are ever present must guide him, so as to eat neither too much nor too little, to suit his diet to his environment, and to make use of facts gained by the experience of people who have lived in the various tropical areas.[6]

On 15 October 1925, the tenth president (Sir) Andrew Balfour FRCP (1873–1931)[7] (*see* Figure 7.3), (first – and last – *Director* of the London School of Hygiene and Tropical Medicine), and a leading hygienist, gave what must have been one of the longest (if not *the* longest – forty pages in *Transactions*) of all presidential addresses. His lecture seems in fact to have impinged upon 'refreshment time'! His title was: '**Some British and American pioneers in tropical medicine and hygiene**'. He began:

> ... There is nothing to compare with the historical perspective as a means of adjusting our ideas, of clarifying our conceptions, of stimulating our flagging energies. In addition, a survey of those who have led the way in almost any branch of scientific work,

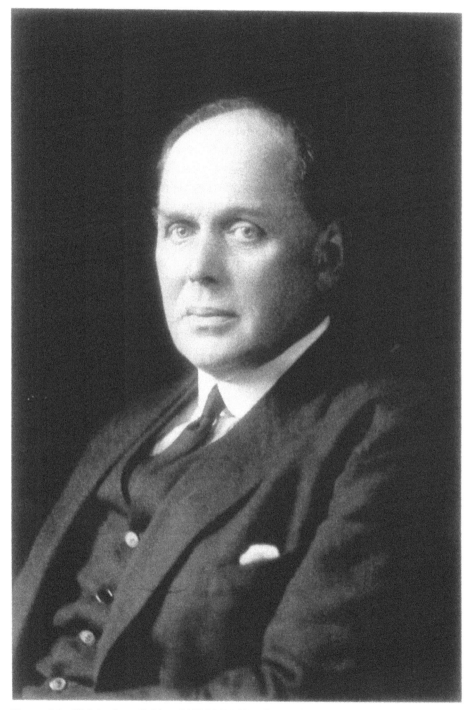

Figure 7.3: (Sir) Andrew Balfour KCMG FRCP – the tenth president (reproduced courtesy the Wellcome Library, London).

and a consideration of what they accomplished, cannot fail to impress useful lessons on the receptive mind. One of these lessons is very likely to be that of humility, and this is specially true in the case of medicine. When we consider all the aids to knowledge which now exist, the extensive armamentarium at our disposal, the valuable literature to which we are the heirs, we cannot but wonder at some of those clinicians of former days who, relying mainly on 'the seeing eye and the understanding heart', grappled successfully with intricate problems and handled disease in a manner which, to this day, commands respect. Indeed, I very much doubt if, in certain directions, the modern doctor, with the laboratory at the back of him and his brain often crammed with scientific or semi-scientific knowledge, is as good at the bedside, or can use his remedies so effectively, as those who had to trust to their powers of observation, to their reasoning faculties and to that intimate acquaintance with the *materia medica* which they usually had gained in the pursuit of their studies and during their careers as apprentices in practice.

Balfour's was a scholarly *historical* lecture, illustrated with many 'lantern slides' of numerous pioneers in this field:

What is true of general medicine is true also of what is called *tropical medicine* although, owing to the nature and severity of many of the maladies commonly encountered in hot climates, the efforts of the physicians in olden days too often failed to avert a fatal issue. Still, the following note, kindly supplied [to] me by Colonel W G King [1851–1935], to whom I am also indebted for some valuable information regarding India, is likely to surprise you. In 1838, John Murray, Deputy-Inspector-General, used warm saline enemata in *cholera*, apparently with satisfactory results, in preference to the formerly-employed method of injecting salines intravenously.[8] The criticism of the period was as follows:

The previous method was 'to inject saline solution into the vein from its having been discovered by chemical tests that the serum of blood in cholera patients is deficient in some of its natural saline ingredients; and the operation was certainly attended with astonishingly restorative effects; but, situated as we generally are in this country, this plan is impracticable.

He alluded to the long history of monographs which described many of the diseases now encompassed beneath the umbrella of *tropical medicine*:

Where symptomatology, gross pathology and prognosis were concerned, the training and experience of the physician in the tropics stood him in good stead. This is clear from a study of the literature, for, let it not be forgotten that, long before the days of Laveran and Manson, a vast deal of work was done upon diseases of the tropics, and numerous papers and treatises were written, many of them by men whose names are now forgotten. Some ... are doubtless familiar with the books of [James] Johnson [1777–1845] and [William] Hillary [1697–1763], but I wonder how many of you have come across [William] Cockburn's [1669–1739] volume on "*Sea Diseases*', dated 1736, or have heard of [Colin] Chisholm [1747–1825]'s '*Essay on the malignant fever introduced in the West Indies*', published in 1801, or have studied [William] Hunter's '[*An essay on the*] *Diseases incident to Indian Seamen, or Lascars, on Long Voyages*', which saw the light in 1804. Then there is [Richard] Reece's '*Medical Guide for Tropical Climates*', 1814, Boyle's '*Letters*' on diseases peculiar to hot climates, 1823, McCave's *Military Medical Reports* of the same year, on similar diseases, and a host of others, some of which, but by no means all, figure in the long list given by Castellani and Chalmers in their 'Manual'.[9] I have twenty quarto sheets of typed references to such publications, ranging from 1568 to 1894, chiefly in English and French, the great majority of which I have never seen. It is by no means complete, but the mere mention will serve to show you how busy were men's brains and pens with tropical problems or ever the new pathology came into being. It is, in my opinion, quite wrong to speak of Patrick Manson as the 'Father of *Tropical Medicine*'. He was the Father, most undoubtedly of *modern* 'Tropical Medicine', but he would have been the last to relegate the other term to himself, for he was well versed in the ancient writings and knew, none better, that many men had laboured devotedly to throw light upon those problems in which he was so interested, and some of which he solved or helped to solve. Possibly an Egyptian priest, steeped in the lore of the temple, pondering upon the mysteries of life and death, grappling with sickness and misery, may have deserved the title, but we may with safety merge it in that of the Father of Medicine and hail Hippocrates as the progenitor. After all, *there is in one sense no such thing as tropical medicine, and in any case many of the most erudite writings of Hippocrates are concerned with maladies which now-a-days are chiefly encountered under tropical or sub-tropical conditions* [author's italics].

What is true of *tropical medicine* is true of *tropical hygiene.* The two are, of course, inextricably mingled, and long ago medical men concerned themselves with the preservation of health in hot climates and laid down rules about it, and fought about it very much as they do to-day. Here, again, Hippocrates gave us a lead, for the great Greek was a hygienist as well as a physician.

In the *British Medical Journal* for 1913[10] there appeared a paper on 'The Knowledge of Tropical Diseases in 1813', a paper to which I will again refer. Its writer relates that the study of tropical diseases was obviously in its infancy in 1813. It may have been in one sense, but certainly it was not if judged by the attention which had been devoted to it and the amount which had been written about it. *Tropical medicine* was a very well-grown stripling two years before Waterloo was fought.

Balfour could not cover *all* of the pioneers from Hippocrates onwards:

... I propose to confine myself to men of our own race and lineage, men who, one and all, their work accomplished, their labours at an end, passed to their rest. Moreover, I commence at a time not very far distant, but a time of stress and difficulty which, as ever, in the case of a virile people, brings out the best that is in them and spells, in some directions at least, progress and development. War means a sword at the throat of the nation, and serious war demands special efforts in every direction. War wipes out the amenities of civilization and drags man closer to Nature and the primitive. War herds men together and favours filth and vermin. In our island story war usually meant service abroad, frequently in hot climates, and hence it is not surprising that I should begin with a period when this country and much of Europe was convulsed, and take, as the first of my pioneers, the great army physician, Sir John Pringle [1707–82]. ...

Balfour then proceeded to give short biographical descriptions of some 73 pioneers in chronological order – finishing with Manson. Clearly it is impossible to summarise these in this text and the reader is thus referred to the original lecture published in *Transactions*. He summed up with the following words:

> [The review is] incomplete, because though the majority of medical men entitled to the title of pioneer have been considered, nothing has been said about the lay community save for Mr Bacot and the three women who have claimed attention. And yet, just as the lawyer, [Edwin] Chadwick [1800–90], laid the foundations of sanitary reform in this country, just as the good Lord Shaftesbury [1801–85] was the prime mover in remedying the appalling conditions of factory labour, so laymen have played a great part in the advancement of *tropical medicine* and *hygiene*. What of Joseph Chamberlain [1836–1914], what of Sir Alfred Jones [1845–1909], to mention only two of them? Not infrequently neither the laboratory worker nor the hygienist could make much progress were it not for the administrator, the merchant prince, or the philanthropist.
>
> The same is true also of men in other walks of life. Now and again, not so often as might be wished, the engineer has led the way in hygienic advance. Let me mention one only, Major Baird Smith [? –1951] and his work on irrigation in Italy and India, which, away back in the middle of the nineteenth century, had an important bearing on *malaria* in its association with rice fields. Again, there must have been some, if not many, who conceived and put forward ideas in advance of their time, but which attracted little or no attention, and passed into the limbo of forgotten things. Of this order was Surgeon-Major T E Demster [1799–1883] of the Hon East India Company, who, as Colonel King [*see* above] has told me, introduced, in 1848, the 'spleen index' test as a guide to the prevalence or otherwise of *malaria*, estimated its value both in children and adults, and defined its limitations. Here is another case in point. Robert Christison [1797–1882], the famous medical jurist and Professor of Materia Medica in the University of Edinburgh, gave an address on public health in 1863 and, amongst other subjects, spoke of ague in Scotland. Incidentally, we may note that he pointed out how prevalent *malaria* was in the colonies and said: 'It can scarcely be that a successful enquiry into

the agencies by means of which ague has been extirpated from Scotland should fail to be of service to our countrymen towards freeing also from that scourge the lands of their adoption'. That is interesting, but the special point I wish to make is that Christison quotes the opinion of a Scotch country doctor to the effect that the *chief* factor in diminishing ague in Scotland was, not *drainage*, but improved living among farm labourers. There is little doubt that this now unknown surgeon was correct, though even if his view had been accepted, it is very unlikely that any light would have been thrown upon the transmission of the disease.

My review is incomplete, and it is also imperfect, for how can a bald narrative of lives and labour, even if enlivened somewhat by the exhibition of portraits, bring home to us the reality and the romance of our subject? We talk of [James] Lind [1716–94] and [Thomas] Trotter [1760–1832], but it is only faintly we can picture them working and reasoning and writing in the bilge-smelling bowels of battleships. Those of you who have been on the 'Victory' at Portsmouth, will recall the conditions between decks, and that was in an empty ship in harbour. Again, consider the difficulties with which some of those pioneers had to grapple in India and elsewhere. Sir Ronald Ross [1857–1932] has given us a graphic picture of his trials when solving the *malaria* problem, but many of our pioneers lived in the olden days in India when, though there was, doubtless, a certain measure of comfort, there were few facilities of any kind for scientific investigation. Timothy Lewis [1841–86] must have worked under numerous disadvantages, [Patrick] Manson [1844–1922] was far from help and advice in China. Knowing the discomforts, disappointments, isolation, ill-health, and other disabilities under which many such devoted men laboured, we can only marvel at their courage, tenacity and success.

It is not for me to point the lessons accruing from this study. Each one of you must lay them to heart according to your lights, according to your necessities, according to your temper. Yet there is one thing which strikes me, and which I would like to mention, even it if be already in your minds. So far as I can tell, few, if any, of these pioneers worked wholly, or even chiefly, for selfish ends. In the case of many, no doubt a laudable ambition was present – a man without some ambition is usually an unsatisfactory type of animal – but the true motive power in most instances was a love of science and desire for knowledge, a devotion to duty, or an anxiety to help humanity or the country to which they owed allegiance. In some also, as in [David] Livingstone [1813–73] and Mary Slessor [1848–1915], religion played a part but, truth to tell, every form of this zeal for research and high sense of duty was of the nature of a religion. These pioneers consecrated themselves to their work and, scorning delights, lived laborious days and passed the torch one to another. That torch, still alight, still glowing, is now in our hands and in the hands of those who are working overseas. It is our duty, it is our privilege, to cherish that light, to tend it carefully, to hand it on to those who will succeed us, so that now and for all time this Society may live up to the proud motto which it bears and which it has earned through the labours of our pioneers: '*Zonae Torridae Tutamen*'.[11]

The Address for 1927, on 20 October, marked a significant change in content of the orations; Professor J W W Stephens MD FRS (1865–1946)[12] (*see* Figure 7.4) chose as his title: '**The functions of the spleen**' – an organ-related and far narrower topic than previous addresses. His portrayal of the anatomy and physiology of this organ summarised contemporary knowledge. The subject he felt was a suitable one because 'the spleen is an organ which almost every Fellow has daily to examine in the pursuit of his profession'. After a detailed pathophysiological account of splenic function, there followed a section on splenomegaly, and finally one on splenectomy. This was well referenced – unlike many previous addresses – and marked the genesis of more *scientific* lectures.[13]

Relations with the Colonial Office

Dr (later Sir Andrew) Balfour, tenth president announced to *Council* on **15 October 1925** that the Colonial Office had agreed to recognise the Society as 'an authoritative body which would be consulted on matters relating to tropical diseases, such as sleeping sickness'. It was hoped that this recognition 'would increase the influence of the Society and add to its usefulness'.

Not all dealings with the Colonial Office had, however, been so straightforward. The seventh president (Simpson – *see* Chapter 6) had, while still in office in early 1921, precipitated an unfortunate scenario:

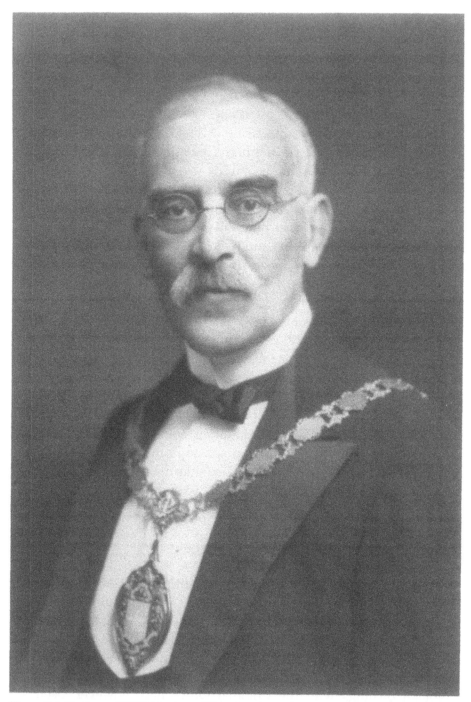

Figure 7.4: Professor J W W Stephens FRS – the eleventh president (RSTMH archive).

The following letter (written on RSTMH headed note-paper) had been sent by Simpson (seventh president) to Sir Herbert Read (1863–1949) the day after a paper on a new treatment for *African trypanosomiasis* had been read to an *Ordinary* meeting by Dr C H Marshall of Uganda.[14]

May 21st 1921

Dear Sir Herbert Read

As President of the [RSTMH] I have the honour of forwarding to you for the information of the Secretary of State for the Colonies a copy of a resolution which was unanimously passed at a meeting of the Fellows of the Society on Friday May 20th after hearing and considering the results obtained by Dr [C H] Marshall with his new treatment of *Trypanosomiasis*. In doing so I desire to state that the experimental observations presented by Dr Marshall, if amply confirmed by further observations, have a very important bearing on the health of the African people, not only from the point of view of treatment but also of prevention of sleeping sickness. Such confirmation would result in measures being adopted which from the humanitarian aspect would confer an inestimable benefit on the African population and would at the same time be of the greatest economical value. The resolution is as follows:

> That in the opinion of this meeting of the [RSTMH] the widest facilities should be afforded for a thorough investigation, on a large scale, of the remedial measures put forward in the very interesting paper read tonight by Dr Marshall of Uganda.

I have the honour to be
Your obedient servant
W J Simpson

The following letter (dated 25 May) is probably from A G Bagshawe – one of the Hon Secretaries:

Dear Professor Simpson.

I was a good deal surprised on receipt of your note this morning and the copy of your letter, dated May 21st, to Sir Herbert Read. This seems to me to be a letter which should not have been sent without consultation with the Hon Secretaries, as it commits the Society to certain opinions which are expressed in the first part;

indeed the sending of it conflicts with the Rules of the Society, number 16 of which reads 'The Secretaries shall conduct all correspondence except in so far as the *Council* shall otherwise direct' [*see* Rule 19 *original* laws – Appendix I].

Had you consulted Dr Wenyon and myself we should have pointed out that the resolution passed was *ultra vires*, it being clearly laid down in Rule 36, sub section ix that 'The Chairman may ... allow any Fellow to propose a motion or resolution ... of which previous notice has been given to the *Council*'. In this instance no notice had been given and the resolution consequently will not appear on the Minutes unless the *Council* decide otherwise. I regret that I did not realize this when the motion was put but it was proposed and passed so quickly that there was little time to think out the proper course.

We are putting down the subject for discussion by the *Council* on June 3 at 4.0., because we feel that the *Council* should have considered this resolution first and decided what action should be taken.

If resolutions were to be suddenly sprung on the meetings, the Society might find itself committed to something which after reflection the *Council* might regret.

I regret having to question what you have done but the Hon, Secretaries would be failing in their duty to the *Council* if they took no action.

Yours sincerely
[This letter is *not* signed].

The Hon Secretaries duly wrote to Read on 6 June indicating that Simpson 'was unaware that the resolution ... on May 20th was *ultra vires* as previous notice had not been given'. They ended their letter by stating that the following resolution [which had been proposed by Dr Newham, seconded by Major Austen, and passed by *Council* at their meeting on **3 June**, and had been passed by 4 votes to 0, was]:

That members of the *Council* who dissent from the resolution put to the meeting of the Society held on May 20 and from the opinions expressed by the President in his letter of May 21 to Sir Herbert Read hereby record such dissent and resolve that a copy of this Minute be sent to Sir Herbert Read.

This brought forth a reply from Read himself to the Hon Secretaries of the RSTMH, as follows:

Downing Street
15 June 1921

Gentlemen,

I am directed by Mr Secretary [Winston] Churchill [1874–1965] to acknowledge the receipt of your letter of the 6th of June forwarding a copy of a Resolution passed by the *Council* of the [RSTMH] dissenting from the Resolution put to a meeting of the Society on the 20th of May and from opinions expressed by Professor W J Simpson in his letter to the Colonial Office of the 21st of May.

The Society will no doubt be interested to learn that Mr [later Sir Winston] Churchill has given careful consideration to proposals which have reached him from more than one quarter as to the dispatch of a Commission to Central Africa for the purpose of effecting measures for treatment of *trypanosomiasis* on a large scale on the lines recently followed by Dr C H Marshall in the case of a European official in the Uganda service and in a number of native cases in that Protectorate. He has however come to the conclusion that the matter is one in which observation for a prolonged period of a limited number of cases in which the treatment has been adopted is required rather than the examination or treatment of a very large number of cases; and he hoped to be able to arrange for work to be carried out on these lines in Tropical African Dependencies where *trypanosomiasis* is prevalent, *eg* Uganda, by Government Medical Officers with the assistance of the government Bacteriologists.

I am,

Gentlemen,
Your obedient servant
H J Read.

The following undated, hand-written note is to be found in minute book 2 (*see* Appendix III) and was initialled by Simpson himself:

Professor Simpson [President] said he was sorry that the Colonial Office held the view that an investigation, on a large scale, into

Dr Claude Marshall's new treatment [for *trypanosomiasis*] was not needed and that it would be sufficient for a limited number of cases to be treated by Dr Marshall and the Medical Officers in Uganda and the effects of the treatment could be watched for 2 or 3 years and tested by the local bacteriologist.

This was tantamount to shelving the question which was of the highest importance to the African people from a health point of view, as well as from an economical aspect. Dr Marshall had already shown the results of the treatment on a small or limited scale. Some of the cases had been treated over a year and some more than 2½ years previously. It was now asked and very reasonably that a Commission should be sent out to make further investigations on a large scale. The larger the scale on which such an inquiry was based provided it was carried out under good supervision & inspection, the more definite would be the result in 2 or 3 years in favour or against the treatment. As to the suggested method of treatment by the Colonial Office, it would be a waste of time and lead to no better results than already achieved by Dr Marshall.

Professor Simpson knew the state of Uganda at the present time. It was suffering from a great prevalence of epidemic diseases which it was impossible for the medical staff to cope with. This was due to the paucity of Medical Officers in Uganda. Lately a severe epidemic of pneumonic plague had broken out and was causing much alarm. There was not a sufficient number of medical officers to deal with it. The Bacteriologist was also overloaded with work and it was absurd to suppose that he could pay proper attention to this problem of Sleeping Sickness. To Professor Simpson the attitude of the Colonial Office, custodians of the health of the Uganda people was simply incomprehensible.

WJS

This matter was thus closed, and a less contentious positive note was later recorded, at a *Council* meeting on **17 October 1929**:

A communication had been received from the Colonial Office in reference to various suggestions regarding the treatment of syphilis and yaws with bismuth and arsenical preparations. Lord Passfield [1859–1947 – Secretary of State for the Colonies] in referring the question to the Society said he would be grateful for any observations on the matter. Copies were enclosed of certain correspondence on the subject from the Governors of Tanganyika [now Tanzania] and of the Straits Settlements*. The Secretaries had previously received copies of other correspondence dealing with the same matter.

After some discussion the *Council* unanimously decided to appoint a Sub-Committee to consider the matter and report to a later meeting. The following were invited to serve on this Committee: Dr H H Scott, Dr H M Hanschell and Dr H S Stannus.

Council on 16 January 1930 accepted the report of the Sub-Committee – a copy of which would thus be sent to Passfield.

The Society's other activities in the 1920s

Accommodation and administrative staff

At a meeting of *Council* on **11 June 1920**, it was decided that 'till it was known whether the Society was to remove to Endsleigh Gardens (*see* Figure 7.5) or not, Mr Bethell should be asked to carry on [the secretarial work] @ £2 per week'.

The House Fund

In October 1923, the ninth president, Surgeon-Rear-Admiral Sir Percy W Bassett-Smith, announced that 'an attempt to start a fund for providing a house for ourselves' (*see* Chapter 8) was to be made; the amount so far collected amounted to £547. He welcomed further contributions, because the MSL (where he incorrectly said they had met since the Society had been launched) were to hold their premises for a further thirteen years *only*.

Secretary

At a meeting of *Council* with the president (Simpson) presiding on **20 May 1921**:

---

* Between 1867 and 1946 this was a crown colony consisting of Penang, Malacca, Singapore and Labuan. They had all been either established or acquired by the East India Company.

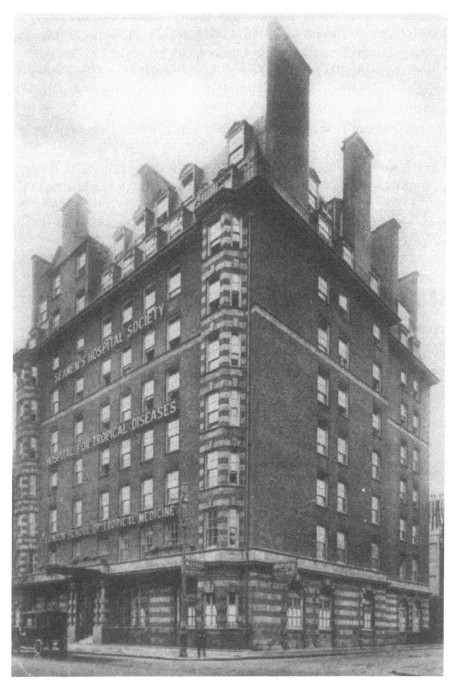

Figure 7.5: The London School of Tropical Medicine and the Hospital for Tropical Diseases at Endsleigh Gardens (23 Endsleigh Gardens WC1) in the early 1920s. Both remained at that time under the aegis of the Seamen's Hospital Society.

A letter was read from Mr Bethell. It was agreed that [although his] service had been of value to the Society [it] was now desirable that it should have a whole-time Assistant Secretary.

Dr Bagshawe recommended the selection of Miss [Mildred] Wenyon as Assistant Secretary. Several candidates had been seen and the Hon Secs [felt] she was the most suitable for the purposes of the Society. Dr Wenyon [her brother] retired during the [following] discussion ... Some [members of] the *Council* thought that the appointment should be given to a person who was entirely dependent on earnings; others appeared to doubt whether Miss Wenyon was the most suitable. Finally Sir David Bruce proposed [and Dr Dobell seconded] the appointment of Miss Wenyon. An amendment that the *Council* should hold a special meeting to interview candidates was put [but] lost. It was [ultimately] agreed to appoint Miss Wenyon at a salary of £180 increasing by 2 yearly increments of £10 to £200.

On **15 May 1924**, *Council* agreed to increase the Assistant Secretary's salary to £230 per annum from 1 April 1924; a pension scheme was also started by *Council* the following month. The matter of Miss Wenyon's salary was further discussed by *Council* on **20 May 1926**; since her appointment in 1921 her salary had been increased from £180 to £230. It was raised to £260 at the following meeting, when it was decided to increase this by £20 annually to £300. *Council* also decided to appoint a Sub-Assistant Secretary (Miss J N Carpenter), at a salary of £130 annually. Her salary was increased by £12 per annum on 15 March 1928. However, at a meeting of *Council* on **17 October 1929** it was agreed to raise her salary to £156 per annum. *Council* decided the following month that Miss Wenyon should be titled *Secretary*. This of course meant a change in the Laws – and this was agreed at the next meeting. Miss Wenyon's salary from 1 April 1930 was again raised from £300 to £350 per annum, and the Society would pay £35 per annum towards her pension (*see CM*, **19 June 1930**).

Improving the Society

Professor Stephens doubted, at a meeting of *Council* on **19 November 1920**, whether the RSTMH 'was fulfilling its [proper] functions'. He thought that 'neither the meetings or [sic] the *Transactions* were attractive. The papers were too long [and] the discussions [required] censoring'.

Probably as a result of this comment, *Council* decided at their next meeting to form a Sub-Committee recommending improvements to the Society, and to make the meetings 'more attractive'. *The Sub-Committee to recommend improvements to the Society* reported to *Council* on **21 January 1921**. Its recommendations (which were discussed) were:

TRANSACTIONS

- To revert to the larger type with the commencement of the next volume in May.
- To report appointments and movements of Fellows-arrivals in the British Isles, departures, change of station &c.
- To revive the Questions Section, which was formerly instituted.
- To publish for the benefit of foreign Fellows, suitable extracts from the *Tropical Diseases Bulletin* in small type to occupy not more than 4 pages in each number. (Col [J] Cummins undertook to edit these.)
- To publish papers either in full or in précis read at local branches of the Society.

MEETINGS

- To have one or more demonstrations, or a microscopical display, at each meeting, the latter preferably in the Society's room.
- To secure short papers, two or three of which could be taken in an evening.
- To edit the discussions, printing only a short abstract of the remarks made by each Speaker for a discussion.
- To adhere strictly to the rule that not more than half an hour is to be occupied in the presentation of a paper.
- Chairman to insist strictly on relevance of discussion and a maximum period of 10 minutes for each speaker.
- To appoint a Sub-Committee before each Session, to meet at intervals through the Session and arrange for papers and demonstrations at each Meeting, by circularising Fellows or otherwise. This Sub-Committee to be responsible for the editing of the discussions.
- To have two laboratory meetings in each Session.
- To commence the meetings at 7.45pm and to have refreshments at 10.0; microscope display from 7.45; paper at 8.15.
- To improve the lighting for microscopes.
- To alter the day of meeting from Friday to Thursday.

OFFICE

To obtain a good permanent whole time Secretary, trained in the keeping of records and accounts. It was considered that a suitable person with these qualifications could be obtained for £200 per annum. This step to be taken as soon as the Hon Secretaries can arrange. An attempt to be made to secure an ex-service officer.

GENERAL

To obtain a larger proportion of papers dealing with the *Public Health* side of the Society's activities, and to have exhibitions at the Laboratory Meetings of apparatus and chemical products of sanitary and industrial import, raw and prepared foods, plans, models, &c, from manufacturers and others.

To draw up and circulate instructions for Local Secretaries, to include the following:-

- To report at the end of each financial year on the position of the Society in their districts.
- To state in the Report the number of Fellows, with their names and addresses, and the number of persons eligible for membership who are not Fellows, and to inform the Secretaries of the movement of Fellows as far as possible.
- To give an account of the proceedings at any meeting of Fellows held locally.
- To induce Fellows coming home on leave, who have been engaged on work of interest, to offer papers and demonstrations to the Council.
- To convey any suggestions for the improvement of the Society.
- On request of the Treasurer to make personal application to any Fellow in their districts whose subscriptions are in arrear.
- To report promptly their arrival in England that they may receive notice of the dates and business of meetings of Council.

At *Council* on **15 January 1925**, the current president (Bassett-Smith) felt that to make the Society more *international*, 'a *foreigner* [author's italics] should be invited to address the Society at one of its [*Ordinary*] meetings'; Professor R Strong of Harvard University was to be invited.

The fellowship and officers

At a *Council* meeting on **18 February 1921**, Cantlie was elected the eighth president *see* Appendix 2); he had defeated Sir John Rose Bradford Bt (1863–1935) by 10 votes to 2.

Minutes during the 1920s make rather gloomy reading. Many men associated with the Society from its early days (*ie* since 1907) were ill or dying.

At a meeting of *Council* on **18 May 1922**, the following resolution was approved unanimously, and later that day it was endorsed at an *Ordinary* meeting:

> The President [Cantlie], *Council* and fellows of the [RSTMH] desire to express to Lady Manson and the members of the family of the late Sir Patrick Manson their sincere sympathy with them in the loss and sorrow they have sustained by Sir Patrick's death, and the deep regret felt by the Society in losing one who had done so much for the cause of Tropical Medicine and Humanity, and who was also first President of the Society.

At a later *Council* meeting (**22 June 1922** – the day of the 15th AGM), Col A Alcock FRS had consented to contribute an article about Manson for the *Transactions*, and later at that meeting a letter from him was read on behalf of the London School of Tropical Medicine (LSTM) inviting *Council* 'to undertake the management and award of the Manson Medal'; this was accepted. The first recipient was Sir David Bruce, to whom the medal was presented at the 16th AGM. *Council*, on 20 March 1930, discussed the possibility of obtaining a copy of the painting of Manson presented by Manson-Bahr to the HTD; it was agreed to inaugurate a Manson Portrait Fund, and the painting would ultimately be hung in Manson House.

The death of both Cantlie and Leishman (both past-presidents) was reported to *Council* on **17 June 1926** and also at the following AGM. Bassett-Smith's death was also announced to *Council* and an *Ordinary* meeting on **19 January 1928**.

Council, on **15 October 1925** was made aware of Harford's death; he had been an Hon Secretary for eight years, and was also a Trustee. Major E E Austen was appointed to succeed him as a Trustee. The death of Camillo Golgi (an Honorary Fellow in 1907) was announced to a *Council* meeting on **18 February 1926**.

At *Council* on **15 November 1928** the death of Robert McKay was announced (although neither a former president nor *Honorary Fellow*, the obituary was, it was decided, to be published in *Transactions*); he had been Laboratory Assistant at the LSTM & Albert Dock Hospital for 25 years.

Dr G C Low's long association with the Society was referred to by the retiring president (Stephens) at the 1929 AGM when Low was elected twelfth president. He had been a founder, original Fellow, Hon Secretary (1912–20), Treasurer, Vice President and Trustee.

Gifts to the Society in the 1920s

At the AGM on **21 June 1923**, the retiring president, Sir James Cantlie had presented the *president's chain* and badge of office … inscribed with the names of past presidents (*see* Figure 7.6).

The Chalmers bequest

At a *Council* meeting on **21 January 1921** it was announced that Mrs Chalmers had given £500 to the Society, which she 'desired should be invested, the interest to pay for a gold medal to be awarded periodically for *Tropical Research* …'. (She also offered to pay for a special number of *Transactions* 'to contain an account of Dr [A J] Chalmers life …'.) This became known as the *Chalmers Memorial Medal*. The cost, design, and conditions of award were delineated at meetings on 18 March and 16 April 1921. The 'motto' on the (memorial) medal was finally decided upon by *Council* on **28 July**: '*Zonae torridae tutamen*'. The first recipient was M E Roubaud of the Pasteur Institute, to whom the medal was presented at the 16th AGM.

Dinners

Society dinners were considered important events in the 1920s. It was reported to *Council* on **21 January 1921** that Lord Milner (1854–1925), Mr Austen Chamberlain (1863–1937), and Col Emery had *not* accepted an invitation to a Society dinner, and that if the latter declined 'it would be better to postpone the dinner till the summer'.

Council decided on **22 June 1922** (the day of the 15th AGM) to organise a dinner in the autumn of that year, to which Mr Winston Churchill, Lord Milner, Lord Ronaldshay, Earl Grey, Lord Buxton and Lord Selborne

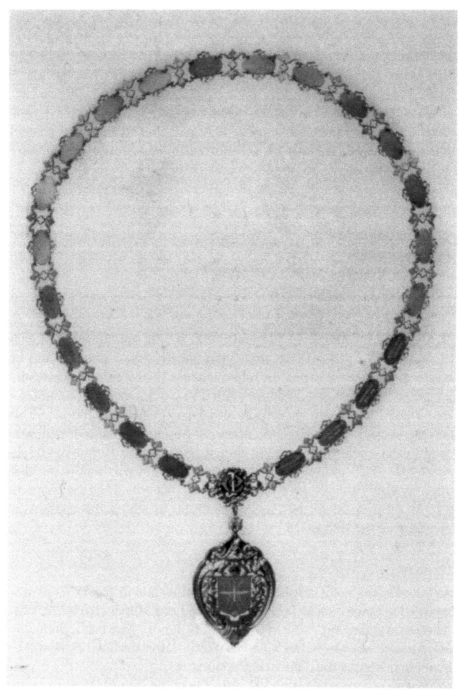

Figure 7.6: The presidential chain and badge of office – presented by Sir James Cantlie on 21 June 1923 (RSTMH archive).

would be invited. At the October meeting, however, it was reported that Churchill had declined and therefore the dinner was again postponed.

On **20 May 1926** the suggestion for a dinner in the autumn to raise money for the *House Fund* was put and that the Prince of Wales (or failing that the Duke of York) be invited; also that the Society should host a biennial dinner on the accession of each new president.

The autumn dinner, it was announced on **21 October**, would be held at the Hotel Victoria, Northumberland Avenue, on 22 November 1926, when the Earl of Balfour (1853–1945) amongst other distinguished guests would be present; this event was apparently a great success (*see CM*, **9 December**) – 184 Fellows and guests being present (*see Times, Lond*, 23 November for a full account).

On 10 May 1928, the Society celebrated its 21st anniversary, and it was suggested by *Council* on **16 June 1927** that a dinner to commemorate that event be held in May/June 1928. A Sub-Committee later reported to *Council* that the chief guest should be the Rt Hon L S Amery, Secretary of State for the Colonies (and failing that, Lord Chelmsford); lady guests should *not* be invited. The dinner was in fact held on 20 June.

At *Council* on **13 December 1929** it was decided to invite Lord Reading as principal guest at the 1930 biennial dinner to be held on 22 May 1930 at the Mayfair Hotel; *Council* agreed that lady guests should on this occasion, be invited. *Council* was told on **20 February 1930** that Lord Reading had accepted (but he later withdrew, and was replaced by Sir John Rose Bradford), and that Lord Ronaldshay, Sir Austen Chamberlain, Sir Leslie Wilson, Sir Robert Williams, Lady Manson, Mrs Chalmers also be invited (*see Br med J* 1930: 31 May).

Council decided on **22 March 1932** that in view of the opening ceremony (*see* Chapter 8) etc, a dinner would *not* be held in 1932.

Royal matters

At the Laboratory meeting of the LSTM (Endsleigh Gardens) on **13 December 1923**, the president (Bassett-Smith) read a letter – dated 11 December – from Sir Frederick Ponsonby (*see* Figure 7.7) informing him that the King (George V) would become Patron of the Society. According to the Society's minutes: 'This announcement was received by the Fellows with a hearty expression of their loyal appreciation'.

It was agreed by *Council* on **13 December 1928** that the following message be sent to Buckingham Palace:

PRIVY PURSE OFFICE,
BUCKINGHAM PALACE, S.W.

11th December 1923.

Dear Sir,

I have submitted your letter of the 8th

inst., to the King, and, in reply, am commanded to

inform you that His Majesty is graciously pleased

to become Patron of the Royal Society of Tropical

Medicine and Hygiene.

Yours faithfully,

Keeper of the Privy Purse.

Surgeon Rear-Admiral
    Sir Percy W. Bassett-Smith, K.C.B., C.M.G., R.N.
            President,
        Royal Society of Tropical Medicine & Hygiene.

Figure 7.7: Letter (11 December 1923) from Sir Frederick Ponsonby indicating that King George V had consented to become patron of the RSTMH (RSTMH archive).

The *Council* and Fellows of the [RSTMH] have followed with deep anxiety the prolonged illness of their Patron, His Majesty the King [George V], and most respectfully and loyally express their hope for His Majesty's speedy recovery.

This was endorsed at an *Ordinary* meeting later that day. A letter of acknowledgement (dated 15 December 1928) (*see* Figure 7.8) was received from Buckingham Palace, and it was read to *Council* at their next meeting.

Announcement of Ordinary Meetings

Table 7.2 summarises speakers and subjects at Ordinary meetings during the 1920s. At a *Council* meeting on **15 November 1923**, it was noted that meetings were currently announced in:

- The *Lancet*
- *British Medical Journal*
- *Medical Press and Circular*
- *Nation*
- *Nature, Lond*
- *Times, Lond*
- *Journal of the Royal Society of Arts*
- *Royal Societies Club*

Manson Lecture

On **24 June 1927**, Col Clayton Lane suggested a biennial *Manson Lecture*. This was approved by *Council* later in the year; however, Dr Manson-Bahr felt that this should be postponed until the Society had moved to Manson House (*see* Chapter 8).

Lady members

At a *Council* meeting on **21 February 1929**:

Dr [H S] Stannus suggested that as there were so many lady members of the Society, the name of one of these might be included in the list of nominations for a future Council.

A Charter for the Society?

At a Council meeting on **21 November 1929**, the possibility of a charter for the Society was discussed. It was however decided 'to leave this until

BUCKINGHAM PALACE

15th. December, 1928.

Dear Sir,

I am desired by the Queen to thank

the Council of the Royal Society of Tropical

Medicine and Hygiene for their kind message

of sympathy and good wishes for the King's

speedy recovery, which you sent from their

general meeting.

Yours very truly,

Clive Wigram

The Hon. Secretary,
    Royal Society of Tropical Medicine and
                                Hygiene.
        11 Chandos Street,

Figure 7.8: Letter (dated 15 December 1928) received from Buckingham Palace regarding the illness of King George V (RSTMH archive).

Table 7.2: Communications at *Ordinary* Meetings – 1921–9

Date	Subject	Speaker
1921		
21 January	Humidity and the life-history of mosquitoes	C A Gill
18 February	Pathology of relapsing fever	J C Kennedy (RAMC)
	Fasciolopsis infection	A F Cole
	Chrysops and filaria in West Africa	A Connal
20 May	New treatment of trypanosomiasis*	C H Marshall
3 June	Trachoma	H Kirkpatrick
17 June (14th AGM)	Snakebite in India	R Knowles (IMS)
20 October	Life Insurance in tropics (*presidential address*)	Sir James Cantlie
15 December	Medicine and sanitation in Mauritius	A Balfour
1922		
19 January	Relations between vegetable and human pathology	E J Butler
	Ear disease in tropics	W Salisbury Sharpe
16 February	Relapsing fever in India	F W Cragg
18 May	Medical research in Western Pacific	F W O'Connor
	Malaria in Trinidad	E de Verteuil
22 June (15th AGM)	School latrines in tropics	E P Minett
	House incidence of sprue	A Powell
	Disease in the Gold Coast	J W S Macfie
19 October	Rat-bite spirochaetosis	R Row
21 December	Diagnosis of ankylostome infestation	C T Lane
	Physical sequelae of malaria and dysentery	C F Harford
1923		
18 January	Treatment of trypanosomiasis with 'Bayer 205'	G C Low, P Manson-Bahr
	Tryparsamide in trypanosomiasis	C C Chesterman
15 February	Leprosy and meteorology	L Rogers
17 May	Treatment of refractory dysentery	J G Willmore
21 June (16th AGM)	Plague in East Indies	L F Hirst
18 October	Food and disease causation (*presidential address*)	P W Bassett-Smith
15 November	Yaws in Kenya Colony	J L Gilks
1924		
17 January	Local immunity in Infectious Disease	A Besreaka (Paris)
21 February	'Bayer 205' in African trypanosomiasis	F K Kleine
15 May	Malaria Treatment of GPI	J W S Makfie
19 June (17th AGM)	Kala azar in Assam	T C M Young

Date	Subject	Speaker
23 October	Malaria control in Assam tea-gardens	Sir Malcolm Watson
11 December	Drug addiction in tropics	W E Dixon
1925		
15 January	Cinchona alkaloids in malaria treatment	A T Gage, C Lane
19 February	Goitre and schistosomiasis in Sierra Leone	D B Blacklock
21 May	Serology of relapsing fever in Madras	J Cunningham
18 June (18th AGM)	Malaria during treatment of GPI	Warrington Yorke
15 October	Tropical medicine pioneers (*presidential address*)	A Balfour
17 December	Surgical aspects of amoebiasis	Sir Thomas Carey Evans
1926		
21 January	Diagnosis and vaccine treatment of leprosy	J Hasson
	Plague in Britain	W P MacArthur
18 February	Depopulation of New Hebrides and Melanesia	P A Buxton
20 May	Chemotherapy of *Surra* in India	J T Edwards
17 June (19th AGM)	Malaria in England	S P James
21 October	Chemotherapy and immunity in schistosomiasis	N H Fairley
9 December	Tropical neurasthenia	H S Stannus
1927		
20 January	The haemoglobinurias	J W W Stephens
17 February	Typhus in Britain	W P MacArthur
19 May	Medical research in the tropics	A T Stanton
16 June (20th AGM)	Rat-flea surveys and plague prevention	L F Hirst
20 October	Functions of the spleen (*presidential address*)	J W W Stephens
8 December	Leptospirosis, Tsutsugamushi disease and typhus in Malay States	W Fletcher
1928		
19 January	Health organisation in the Far-east	D H C Given
16 February	Medical and sanitary service for rural African natives	A R Paterson
17 May	Vitamin B deficiency in infants	G W Bray
21 June (21st AGM)	Differentiation of human amoebae	E Brumpt (Paris)
18 October	Surgical aspects of tropical diseases	F P Connor
13 December	Rôle of the spleen in haemorrhage	A K Gordon

Date	Subject	Speaker
1929		
17 January	Experimental Yellow fever	E Hindle
21 February	Malaria control in Italy	L W Hackett
16 May	Pulmonary Tuberculosis in the tropics	V S Hodson
21 June (22nd AGM)	Health problems in British Guiana	J F C Haslam
17 October	Tropical Medicine, 1894–1914 (*presidential address*) (see Chapter 8)	G C Low
12 December	Blackwater fever	Warrington Yorke, F Murgatroyd, D U Owen

*This paper was the basis of the misunderstanding involving the Colonial Office.

the Manson House issue had been concluded', because a charter would be costly – amounting to at least £120.

Advertisements in Transactions

At a meeting on **17 May 1923**, *Council* proposed adoption of the following rules as a guide to advertisements in *Transactions*:

Draft Rules Governing Advertisements

Advertisements, to be admissible to the *Tropical Diseases Bulletin*, must conform to the following rules:-

1. No advertisement will be accepted which, either by intent or inference, would result in deceiving, defrauding or misleading the reader.

2. Extravagantly or vulgarly worded copy is subject either to revision or rejection.

3. Advertisements of proprietary medicines will not be accepted without sufficient documentary evidence as to their efficacy and relative freedom from danger. The Editors reserve the right to refuse advertisements of such products unless the composition is disclosed.

4. Testimonials as to the value of a proprietary medicine or dietetic product will not be accepted unless cited from the text of a reputable medical journal, the reference to which must be attached. Testimonials in the form of letters to the makers or proprietors will in no case be accepted.

5. Except in the case of foods, common disinfectants and household remedies the article must not be also advertised in the lay press.

6. The name of a medical practitioner must not be used in an advertisement without his written permission.

Honorary Fellows

Criteria for election of an *Honorary* Fellow were discussed by *Council* on **15 March 1928**. It was generally agreed that 'they were usually foreigners of such standing that they might have been presidents of the Society'. Owing to the fact that they received *Transactions* gratis it was felt by one member that the number be 'limited to 1 per cent of the total membership'.

At a previous *Council* meeting on **18 March 1921**:

> The following had been proposed, seconded and duly elected:
> Dr Harper
> Dr Flexner (USA),
> Prof Mesnil [France]
> Sir H J Read [Colonial Office].
>
> A proposal of Col [J] Cummins that Dr Richard Strong should be appointed as an Honorary Fellow was rejected on the ground that it was inadvisable to elect more than two of one nation on one occasion.
>
> Sir Ronald Ross raised serious objections [also on 18 March 1921] to the election of Prof Grassi (Rome) [*see* Figure 7.9] as a man who pirated other men's work [*see* Figure 7.10]. He read letters from Lord Lister, Professor Laveran and Professor Koch [*see* Figures 7.11–7.13]. The [proposition] was put that Prof Grassi be *not* elected. 4 votes were recorded for the motion and none against. Professor Grassi was therefore *not* elected.

Council, on **21 June 1923** (preceding the 16th AGM) recommended that Professor E Brumpt of Paris be elected an Honorary Fellow. This was carried unanimously.

Other matters

On **7 October 1920**, a letter was read to *Council* from the Royal Society of Literature requesting books 'to supplement the depleted Medical

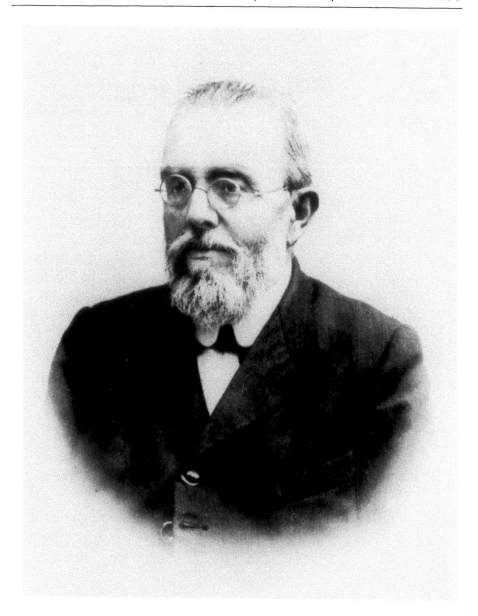

Figure 7.9: Giovanni Battista Grassi (1854–1925), an Italian malariologist who claimed priority in the elucidation of mosquito transmission of human malaria (reproduced courtesy the Wellcome Library, London).

FROM
SIR RONALD ROSS, K.C.B., K.C.MG. F.R.S

TELEPHONE & TELEGRAMS:
PADDINGTON 3100.

36, HARLEY HOUSE,
REGENTS' PARK,
LONDON, N.W.1.

22nd March, 1921.

To the Honorary Secretaries,
  Royal Society of Tropical Medicine.

Dear Sirs,

        At the meeting of the Council held on the 18th inst.,
I lodged a protest against the proposed inclusion of Professor
Grassi's name for the Honorary Fellowship of the Society. In support
of my protest I read letters from Professor Robert Koch, Dr. Laveran
and Lord Lister; and, after my protest had been accepted by the
Council it agreed to file copies of the said letters in connection
with the Minutes. I now send you the required copies; and should
add that the letters have been published, almost complete, in
Science Progress April, 1917, No 44, page 669, and will be reproduced as they stand in my book on malaria which Mr. Murray proposes
to issue during the year.

        I also referred at the meeting to recent publications in
which Professor Grassi's originality with regard to various advances
in science is questioned. These publications are as follows:-

        (1) Professor Claudio Fermi: Si Puo' col Metodo Grassi etc.
        Roma. Tipografia I. Adriani, Via Bonella, 4. 1920

        (2) Prof. Guido Cremonese: La Malaria Fiumicino e il
        Prof. Grassi. Roma. Tipografia C. Lucci. 1921.

                Yours faithfully,

Encls.

Figure 7.10: Letter from Sir Ronald Ross FRS to the Hon Secretaries, RSTMH (22 March 1921).

Libraries in Serbia. Although the Society itself 'had no books that could be spared', it was decided to place a notice in *Transactions* inviting Fellows to send 'spare volumes'.

Copy of a letter dated 1st April, 1901 from Lord Lister to
Major Ronald Ross, I.M.S., Liverpool.

12Park Crescent,

Portland Place,

1st April, 1901

My dear Ross,

Your letter is not too long, considering the
interest of its contents.

It is terribly sad to think of such roguery in men who
call themselves scientific: but you show too serious grounds
for believing that it exists in Grassi and Co.

Laveran's letter, which I return, is also completely
confirmatory of your opinion and Koch's, and its cordial tone
towards yourself is very pleasant.

(The remainder of the letter deals with other matters)

Believe me,

Very truly yours,

(Signed) Lister.

True Copy.

Figure 7.11: Copy of a letter from Lord Lister FRS to Ross dated 1 April 1901.

Relations with other Societies in the 1920s

Representation at meetings and congresses of other societies continued to be deemed important in the 1920s, and *Council* thus chose their representatives with care.

Sir James Cantlie asked at a *Council meeting* on **13 October 1921**, what part the RSTMH should take in the *British Empire Exhibition (BEE)* to be held in 1924? It was suggested that it 'might undertake organisation of

Copy of a letter dated 26th March, 1901 from A Laveran to
Major Ronald Ross, I. M.S., Liverpool.

Paris, 26 Mars.

Mon cher confrère,

Je vous remercie de votre lettre, ainsi que de la copie
de celle de Koch. Je connais trop vos adversaires dans ce
débat pour m'étonner de leur manière d'agir à votre égard. Ceux
qui ont suivi attentivement vos recherches savent à quoi s'en
tenir au sujet des assertions de Grassi, mais c'est le petit
nombre. Vous faites donc bien de vous défendre et de dévoiler les
precédés mesquins et malhonnètes de ceux des auteurs italiens qui
cherchent à diminuer à leur profit l'importance de vos travaux.

Je vous prie d'agréer, mon cher confrère, l'expression
de mes sentiments tout dévoués.

(Signed) A. Laveran.

True Copy.
S. H. Yates.

Figure 7.12: Copy of a letter from Alphonse Laveran to Ross dated 26 March 1901.

the Tropical Exhibit', *ie* assuming various bodies interested in the subject 'agree to co-ordinate under their leadership' (which they subsequently did). A provisional Sub-Committee was set up. This strategy was however, apparently abandoned and Balfour was appointed as the representative of the RSTMH on the Committee of the Tropical Diseases Section of the BEE. The General Manager of the BEE later invited the Society to hold a series of meetings during the 'period of the exhibition'. Although this invitation was declined, it was suggested that individual Fellows of the RSTMH would be prepared to give lectures.

Representation at a Congress of *The Royal Sanitary Institute* was repeatedly discussed by *Council* in 1921–2. There was doubt as to whether the Institute was interested in tropical *hygiene*; however, in March 1922 they were assured that they were! A meeting held at Bournemouth in July 1922 was apparently a success. The RSTMH was invited to send a delegate to the Liverpool Congress (*see CM*, **21 February 1924**); Professor Yorke consented to undertake this. On **18 February 1926**, Col S P James was chosen to represent the Society at the *Imperial Congress* held in July of that year. However, in 1927 no representative was sent because Tropical Medicine and Hygiene did *not* appear on the agenda. At a meeting of *Council* on **15 March 1928**, Balfour was invited to represent the Society at the forthcoming congress. At the *Congress* to be held at Sheffield in July 1929, General Barrow was invited to represent the Society (16 May 1929).

Council resolved on **15 February 1923** to request Stephens to represent the RSTMH at the Congress of the *Royal Institute of Public Health* at Scarborough in May 1924.

Warrington Yorke was invited on **17 February 1927** to represent the RSTMH at the *Royal Microscopical Society*'s Congress at Liverpool in March 1927. The Society also accepted an invitation from the BMA to send representatives to the conference in connection with the *Dogs Protection Bill*.

OTHER ORGANISATIONS, CONGRESSES, ETC

Many other invitations to send a delegate were received; they included the *Entomological* Congress and the 6th Congress of the *Far Eastern Association of Tropical Medicine. Council* decided on **15 February 1923** to ask Bruce to represent the RSTMH at the *Pasteur Centenary celebrations* at Strasburg in May. Unfortunately, he was unable to attend, and on 15 March, Wenyon was chosen in his place. *Council* was informed on **17 March 1927** that an *International Congress of Tropical Medicine* would be held in Amsterdam in 1928. There was limited reference to *Tropical Medicine* at the Dublin Congress of the *Institute of Public Health* in 1928, so the Society did *not* send a delegate. The 7th Congress of the *Far Eastern Association of Tropical Medicine* was held at Calcutta in December 1927 (*see CM*, **19 May 1927**); the Society was represented by the president (Stephens). At a Congress of *Military Medicine and Pharmacy*, the Society was represented by Daukes of the Wellcome Bureau of Scientific Research. A *Congress* was held in Cairo in December 1928, and *Council* unanimously agreed to request the president (Stephens) to attend at the invitation of the Egyptian Minister

Copy of a letter dated 10th February, 1901 from Robert Koch
to Major Ronald Ross I.M.S., Liverpool.

Berlin, W.,
Kurfürstendamm, 25,
10 Feb. 1901.

Hochgeehrter Herr College,
Die Deutung, welche Calandruccio meinem Verhalten
gegenüber Grassi giebt, ist nicht richtig.
Nach meiner Ansicht dürfen wir einem Menschen, auch
wenn er ein Schuft ist, seine moralischen Defekte nicht auf seine
wissenschaftlichen Verdienste, sofern er solche besitzt, anrechnen.
Ich würde deswegen, obwohl ich Grassi für einen Schuft
und einen Räuber auf wissenschaftlichem Gebiete halte, seine
wissenschaftlichen Verdienste, da wo sie erwähnt werden müssen
nicht verschweigen. Aber nach meiner Überzeugung hat er keine
solche Verdienste. Das, was er als solche angiebt, ist gestohlen
oder erlogen und was dann noch übrig bleibt, ist zu unbedeutend,
als dass ich mich für verpflichtet halte, es als werthvolle
Bereicherung der Wissenschaft zu erwähnen. Seine Angaben über
die Entwicklung der Malaria-parasiten im Mückenleib sind, wenn er
sie wirklich so gesehen hat, wie er angiebt (was ich übrigens nicht
glaube nur eine Bestätigung Ihrer Entdeckungen. Seine Abbildungen
sind geradezu Copien derIhrigen. Die ersten Infections-Versuche
welche in Rom von Grassi und seinen Mitarbeitern gemacht wurden
und mit so ausserordentlicher Reclame in alle Welt verkündigt
wurden, halt ich für erfunden; denn sie wurden in einer Jahreszeit
ausgeführt, in welcher es keine frischen Infectionen in Italien
giebt.
Leider ist Grassi nicht der einzige, der in Rom auf
diese Art Wissenschaft macht. Seine unmittelbaren Mitarbeiten
handeln wie ich selbst erfahren habe, nicht besser. Und Marchiafava
hat in früheren Zeiten Golgi und Laveran in ähnlicher Weise zu
berauben versucht, wie Grassi es bei Ihnen gemacht hat. Laveran
hat er in seinem Traité du paludisme 1898, p. 42. Anm. 2
geschildert.
Dieser sogen römischen Schule gegenüber muss man, wie
mir scheint sehr vorsichtig und auch sehr skeptisch sein. Ich
glaube diesen Leuten nichts mehr, als was ganz unwiderleglich und
unter Zuziehung von zuverlässigen Zeugen bewiesen ist.

Mit vorzüglicher Hochachtung,
argebenst,

(Signed) R. Koch.

True Copy.
R.H. Yates

Figure 7.13: (a) Copy of a letter from Robert Koch to Ross dated 10 February 1901.

of Education. However, Stephens could not undertake this, and General
D Harvey was invited in his place.

On **16 May 1929**, Col F A Saunders was invited to represent the Society
at the Centenary celebrations of the *South African College* at Capetown in

Copy of a letter dated 10th February, 1901 from Robert Koch
to Major Ronald Ross I.M.S., Liverpool.

Kurfürstendamm, 25,
Berlin, W.
February, 10th. 1901.

Translation.

Honoured Colleague,
    The interpretation which Calandruccio gives of my
conduct towards Grassi is not correct.

    In my opinion it is not permissible to take account of
the moral defects of a man even if he is a rogue, in considering
his scientific deserts so far as he possesses any.

    For this reason, although I consider Grassi to be a
rogue and a robber in scientific domains, I should not pass over
his scientific deserts where they ought to be mentioned. But it
is my conviction that he has no such merits. What he claims as
his, is either stolen or fabricated, and the remainder is too
small for me to consider myself under any obligation to mention
it as a valuable addition to knowledge. His statements regarding
the development of the malarial parasite in the stomach of the
mosquito, if he really saw them as he states (which, by the way,
I do not believe) are only a confirmation of your discoveries.
His illustrations are nothing more than copies of yours. The
first infection experiments which were made in Rome by Grassi,
and his Colleagues, and so very loudly advertised to all the world,
I consider to be inventions: for they were made in a season
when there are no fresh infections in Italy.

    Unfortunately Grassi is not the only one in Rome to
manufacture science in this manner. His immediate colleagues do
not behave better, as I myself experienced. And in earlier times
Marchiafava tried to rob Golgi and Laveran in a similar way as
Grassi has done with you - Laveran has described it in his
"Traité du paludisme" 1898. p. 42. Ann. 2.

    It seems to me one has to be very careful and also
very sceptical as regards the so-called Roman School. I do not
believe these people further than what is indisputably proved and
is testified to by reliable witnesses.
                        Yours sincerely,
                        (Signed) R. Koch.

True Copy.
  S. H. Yates

Figure 7.13: (b) Translation of the letter from German to English.

October of that year. Although the Society was invited to send a delegate
to the *Tuberculosis Congress* in Newcastle in July 1929, no decision seems
to have been taken (*see CM*, **25 June 1929**). Col W P MacArthur ultimately
represented the Society on 17 October 1929.

An invitation for the president to become a member of the executive of the *Féderation des Sociétés de Médicine d' Hygiène tropicales* was declined by *Council* on **11 December 1930**. *Council* agreed on **19 February 1931** to render assistance at the 'forthcoming *Colonial and International Exhibition* in Paris'; a Sub-Committee consisted of: Stanton, Stannus and Daukes, together with the Society's officers. The *French Colonial Exhibition* was to be held in Paris from 22–31 July 1931, and the Society's delegates were to be: Stannus, Gordon Thomson and Wenyon.

The fourteenth to twenty-second annual reports

The number of Fellows 'on the books' increased during this decade from 724 in 1921 to 1,393 in 1929.

In the financial year 1920–21, receipts amounted to £627 9s 11d (plus Mrs A J Chalmers' gift of £500). However, this rose to £1,189 2s 1d the following year. A separate 'House Fund' is recorded in the report for 1922–3, when a further £500 from the Society's assets was transferred to this new initiative. The Treasurer's Report for the year ended 31 March 1929 indicated that the Society's finances continued to be in a sound state; a balance of £339 3s 11d was carried forward, and the *Manson House Fund* then stood at £4,352 6s 6d. Furthermore, the total value of investments stood at £5,139 1s 1d.

References and Notes

1   **James Cantlie** was born in Banffshire and educated at Aberdeen University and Charing Cross Hospital. After a spell as instructor in Anatomy in London, he accepted Manson's invitation to join him in Hong Kong. Returning to London in 1896, he was appointed to the LSTM in 1899 and became the major figure in the founding of the (R)STMH. Another major interest was emergency medical aid; he joined the St John's Ambulance and Red Cross. *See*: M Harrison. Cantlie, Sir James (1851–1926). In: H C G Matthew, B Harrison (eds). *Oxford Dictionary of National Biography.* Oxford: Oxford University Press 2004: 9: 962–4; Anonymous. Cantlie, Sir James. *Who Was Who, 1916–1928* 5th ed. London: A & C Black 1992: 132.
2   J Cantlie. The extra premium charged to tropical residents by life insurance companies. *Br med J* 1897; i: 1487–8. [*See also*: Anonymous. Extra insurance premiums for tropical medicine. *Br med J* 1897; i: 1494].
3   J Cantlie. Presidential address: Life Insurance in the tropics. *Trans R Soc trop Med Hyg* 1921–22; 15: 109–16.

4   **Percy Bassett-Smith** was educated at St John's College, Hurstpierpoint and the Middlesex Hospital. He had a distinguished career in the Royal Navy and afterwards served at the London School of Tropical Medicine. He became Professor of Pathology and Lecturer in Tropical Medicine at the RN College, Greenwich. He wrote extensively on tropical medicine. *See:* Anonymous. Bassett-Smith, Surgeon-Rear Admiral Sir Percy William. *Who Was Who, 1916–1928* 5th ed. London: A & C Black 1992: 49–50.

5   K J Carpenter. *Beriberi, white rice, and vitamin B.* London: University of California Press 2000: 282.

6   P Bassett-Smith. Presidential address: The relation of food to the causation of disease in the tropics. *Trans R Soc trop Med Hyg* 1923–24; 17: 223–44.

7   **Andrew Balfour** was born in Edinburgh and educated at the University of Edinburgh. He became Director of the Wellcome Research Laboratories at Khartoum, Sudan, and during the Great War served in the Middle-East. After the war, he was appointed Director of the LSHTM in 1923 but, suffering from a bi-polar disorder (a manic-depressive psychosis), committed suicide in 1931. *See*: A S MacNalty, M E Gibson. In: H C G Matthew, B Harrison (eds). *Oxford Dictionary of National Biography.* Oxford: Oxford University Press 2004: 3: 493–4; Anonymous. Balfour, Sir Andrew. *Who Was Who, 1929–1940* 2nd ed. London: A & C Black 1967: 57.

8   G C Cook. Management of cholera: the vital role of rehydration. In: B S Drasar, B D Forrest (eds) *Cholera and the ecology* Vibrio cholerae. London: Chapman and Hall 1996: 54–94.

9   A Castellani. A J Chalmers. *Manual of tropical medicine.* London: Baillière, Tindall and Cox 1919: 2436.

10 Anonymous. One hundred years ago: the knowledge of Tropical Diseases in 1813. *Br med J* 1913; i: 455–6.

11 A Balfour. Presidential address: Some British and American pioneers in tropical medicine and hygiene. *Trans R Soc trop Med Hyg* 1925–26; 19: 189–230.

12 **John Stephens** was born in Carmarthenshire and educated at Cambridge and St Bartholomew's Medical School. He subsequently became a bacteriologist to the Government of India. Stephens later worked on malaria control in Africa and in Lahore. On return to England, he was appointed to the Liverpool School of Tropical Medicine which he served until retirement. See: W F Bynum. Stephens, John William Watson (1865–1946). In: H C G Matthew, B Harrison (eds). *Oxford Dictionary of National Biography.* Oxford: Oxford University Press 2004: 52: 476–7; Anonymous. Stephens, John William Watson. *Who Was Who, 1941–1950* 5th ed. London: A & C Black 1980: 1099.

13 J W W Stephens: Presidential address: The functions of the spleen. *Trans R Soc trop Med Hyg* 1927–28; 21: 161–84.

14 C H Marshall. A new method of treatment of trypanosomiasis. *Trans R Soc trop Med Hyg* 1921–2; 15: 10–20.

Chapter 8

George Carmichael Low's presidency and removal to Manson House – 1929–33

Problems with accommodation regarding (i) a suitable room for the running of the Society, and (ii) a venue for *Ordinary* meetings had begun shortly after foundation of the Society (*see* Chapter 2). However, they were to reach a crescendo in the early 1920s, *ie* the decade leading to the acquisition of a *permanent* home (Manson House).

Initial accommodation at the Royal Medico-Chirurgical Society and RSM (*see* Chapter 1), and later use of a room at the Medical Society of London (MSL) in Chandos Street, W1 (*see* Chapter 2) had proved only partially satisfactory. At a meeting of *Council* on **11 June 1920**:

> The Secretaries reported that owing to Miss Hooper's resignation [*see* Chapter 5], they thought the time opportune to raise the question of removal of the Society to 23 Endsleigh Gardens [where both the HTD and LSTM were then accommodated – *see* Chapter 7]. There were obvious advantages in the Society being under the same roof as other Institutes in London concerned with *tropical medicine*. Objections … were (1) that removal to the same building as the [LSTM] would be displeasing to the other Schools, owing to the advantage that would accrue to the London School, and (2) that the position was less convenient than Chandos Street [to those with private practice in the 'medical quarter']. It was pointed out that the Society would be the tenant of the Seamen's Hospital Society [SHS] and not of the School. Other aspects of the suggested move were discussed. The President [at that time, Simpson] considered that the Society should have the exclusive use of a room for their paid Secretary and … Balfour said that if the [SHS] were unable to find a room he would provide one at the Wellcome Bureau [of which he was Director]. Finally, the Secretaries were directed to write to the Secretary of the [SHS], stating the requirements of the Society, offering a sum not

exceeding £70 [per annum] for accommodation including rates, heating and lighting, and bearing stress on the need for security of tenure.

One week later:

A letter sent by the [Hon] Secretaries to the Secretary of the [SHS] was read, enquiring if [they] could accommodate the Society @ 23 Endsleigh Gardens, and [also] the Secretary's reply thereto which stated that the proposal was received favourably by the [SHS] Committee of Management. A general discussion took place. Dr [W T] Prout suggested that there had not yet been time to give the matter such consideration as it merited. Major [E E] Austen asked if quarters could be obtained in Burlington House. Dr [C F] Harford thought that the possible disadvantages of the proposed removal should be very carefully weighed. Dr [G C] Low [an Hon Secretary at the time] suggested that ... proximity to a large library would be a great advantage, and said that comparatively few Fellows visited the room at 11 Chandos Street. The President doubted whether there was room enough at 23 Endsleigh Gardens, having regard to probable expansion of the [LSTM]. Other speakers dwelt on the obvious advantages of the Endsleigh Gardens proposal. The Secretary said that, according to Mr Bethell, the [MSL] would not insist on ... six months notice being given on June 24th, so that there was no necessity for an immediate decision. Finally, on the motion of Dr Prout, it was resolved that a *Council* meeting should be convened on June 28th for the special purpose of discussing the proposed removal.

At the meeting on **28 June**:

A letter was read from Professor [J W W] Stephens in which he expressed the opinion that the Liverpool School of Tropical Medicine had no ground of complaint if the Society moved to 23 Endsleigh Gardens, but that this course would inevitably result in loss of independence by the Society. The discussion of June 18th was renewed, each of the members present expressing his opinion. The President and Messrs Prout, Austen, Harford and King spoke *against* [author's italics] the proposed removal to 23 Endsleigh Gardens on the grounds that the Society's independence would be lost, or that the Society would become identified with the London School. Removal was *supported* [author's italics] by Messrs Balfour, Dobell, Low, Hartigan, James, Bassett-Smith, Wenyon, Cummins and Bagshawe. Dr Balfour suggested that such an increased membership would result that the Society would eventually have the funds to get its own premises. Dr Hartigan [Treasurer] thought that if the Society remained at Chandos St it would eventually have to pay a much larger rent, probably £140. Colonel Cummins thought that loss of identity in the eyes of the public was immaterial, and that as the policy was settled by the Fellows there was little fear of loss of independence.

It was generally agreed [in conclusion] that it would be better to remain at Chandos Street than to have dissention in the Society. The President [Simpson] said that the room suggested for the Secretarial work at 23 Endsleigh Gardens was [in any case] unsuitable, and Dr Balfour renewed his offer of a room at 25 Endsleigh Gardens [the Wellcome Bureau of Scientific Research]. A proposal by Dr Harford to postpone the decision for 6 months for the purpose of consultation with the Fellows was negatived. Finally, on the motion of Surgeon Rear Admiral [P W] Bassett-Smith, seconded by Colonel [W G] King, it was resolved that the Society remain at Chandos Street till a suitable house [could] be found and that the Secretaries be asked to look for accommodation in the neighbourhood of Endsleigh Gardens other than the [SHS] building. Dr Balfour suggested that accommodation might be available in University College.

George Carmichael Low (1872–1952)

Low (the twelfth president), as well as being a joint founder of the Society, was in many respects the greatest figure in its history. In 1994, HRH the Princess Royal officially opened the refurbished lecture-theatre at Manson House – which she named the *George Carmichael Low* auditorium. In his presidential address in 1929 (*see* below), Low outlined the development of the formal discipline of *tropical medicine* (*see* below). Furthermore it was he who in many ways did more than any other Fellow to create a *permanent* home for the Society at 26 Portland Place

(Manson House). It was during his presidency that the removal from the MSL's premises in Chandos Street, took place, and Manson House was officially opened by the Prince of Wales (*see* below).

Only two Fellows to date have been elected to the Presidency for *two* terms; the first of these was George Low MA MD FRCP (1872–1952)[1] (Figure 8.1) who held office from 1929 to 1933. The title of his Address was: **A retrospect of tropical medicine from 1894 to 1914**. He apparently chose this period, he claimed, for three reasons:

> ... first, because [these years] form a period wherein all the isolated efforts of that wonderful body of pioneers, who worked in the tropics in the past, became welded together; second, because some of the most remarkable discoveries ever made in medicine, both in the etiology and treatment of disease have been recorded during that time; and, third, because *Tropical Medicine* then became definitely defined as a special branch which involved the study of subjects *not* included in the ordinary medical curriculum.
>
> To one man [he claimed], we owe much of this. I refer ... to Sir Patrick Manson, our first President, my teacher and my friend. ... his biography [had been written] by ... Manson-Bahr and ... Alcock.[2]
>
> ... I must point out emphatically [Low continued] that medicine as practised in hot climates [is] *not* a new thing, while the diseases met with there were not then discovered for the first time. To prove this it will suffice if I again call attention to ... Balfour's presidential address [*see* Chapter 7], wherein he clearly showed the work of the pioneers, unaided and untaught. In this connection he mentioned the Indian work of Martin, Annesley, Morehead, Chevers, Lewis, Cunningham, Fayrer, the African work of David Livingstone, and the work of Finlay in Havana – to quote only a few.
>
> The term 'Father of *Tropical Medicine*' has, however, been applied to ... [Patrick] Manson because it was his genius that first established the ... fact that insects transmit disease, and it was his discoveries on filariasis and malaria that drew special attention to *Tropical Medicine* ... Sir Patrick, in his conversations with me, always gave the greatest credit to Chevers and the other men of the Indian Medical Service who did such pioneer service

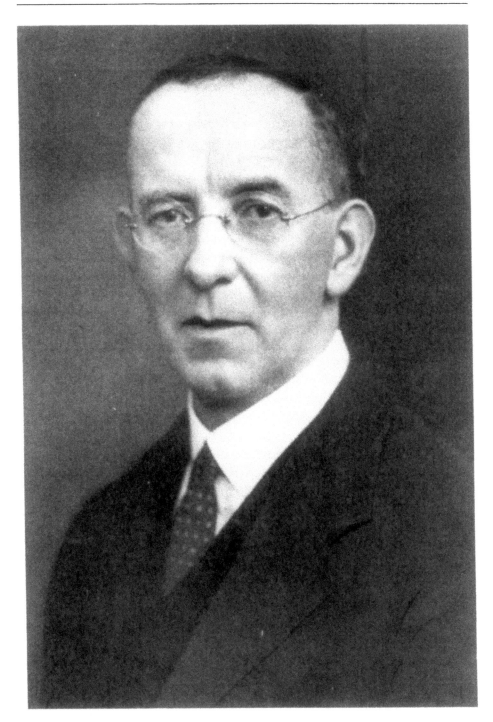

Figure 8.1: Dr George Carmichael Low – the twelfth president of the Society (who served two terms, and presided over the removal to Manson House) (RSTMH archive).

in India; the point he emphasised was, not that there were no workers on *Tropical Medicine*, but that there was no adequate teaching of the subject in England apart from the lectures to the Army and Indian Medical Service doctors at Netley ...

This was, in retrospect, an opportune moment to emphasise the past and to build on the lecture by Balfour (*see* Chapter 7) on the earlier history of *tropical medicine* (the diseases of warm climates). Low proceeded to give succinct accounts of the more important milestones in elucidation of the aetiology and pathogenesis of several major tropical diseases: *malaria, filariasis, yellow fever, trypanosomiasis, ankylostomiasis, kala-azar, undulant fever* [brucellosis], *schistosomiasis, plague* and *beri-beri*. He also included sections on 'The use of intravenous antimony', and 'The use of emetine'. But two sections of the address warrant special attention, *ie* those devoted to '*The Foundation of the schools of tropical medicine (1899)*', and '*The foundation of the Society of Tropical Medicine and Hygiene (1907)*' (*see* Chapter 1). In the first of these, Low described the early days:

> ... Manson had begun lecturing and giving instruction in tropical diseases in 1894, and as time went on he realized more and more the necessity that men outside the Army and Indian Medical Service should have special teaching before proceeding abroad. His fortunate appointment as Medical Adviser to the Colonial Office, in July, 1897, gave him the chance he desired. By it he was brought into intimate touch with Mr Joseph Chamberlain [1836–1914], one of the most brilliant and far-seeing statesmen in England at that time, and this association soon bore fruit. On 11th March, 1898, ... Chamberlain addressed a circular letter to the *General Medical Council* and the leading medical schools of the United Kingdom, pointing out 'the importance of ensuring that all medical officers selected for appointments in the tropics should enter on their careers with the expert knowledge requisite for dealing with such diseases as are prevalent in tropical climates, and that it was very desirable that, before undergoing such special training, the future medical officers of the Colonies should be given facilities in the various medical schools for obtaining some preliminary knowledge of the subject'.
>
> The *General Medical Council* replied in favourable terms to this letter, and considered it highly advisable that the Government

should arrange for special instruction in *tropical medicine*, hygiene and climatology for doctors selected for the *Colonial Medical Service* or for those who proposed to practise in tropical countries.

Following this up ... [Joseph] Chamberlain, on 28th May, 1898, addressed a circular to the governors of all Colonies. In this he stated that largely through the interest taken in the matter by ... Manson, who had succeeded Sir Charles Gage Brown [1826–1908] as Medical Adviser of the Colonial Office, his attention was more definitely directed to the importance of scientific inquiry into the causes of *malaria*, and of special education in *tropical medicine* for the medical officers of the Crown Colonies. He then advised that a special training school in *tropical medicine* should be established, where officers, newly appointed to the medical services of the Colonies and Protectorates, might be given systematic instruction, with special facilities for clinical study, before leaving England to take up their appointments; and where doctors already in the service might, when on leave, have opportunities of bringing their professional knowledge up to date.

The result of this circular was the formation of the Liverpool and London [LSTM] Schools of *Tropical Medicine* in England. ... the Liverpool school ... came into being first and was entirely due to the energy and public spirit of two men [both subsequently knighted], Alfred Jones [1846–1909] and Rubert Boyce [1863–1911]. ... The Staff of the [LSTM] was appointed in May, 1899; teaching commenced on 2nd October, 1899 [and it] officially opened on 3rd October, 1899. Previous to this, Manson had been actively instituting inquiries as to where the [LSTM] should be located, and as early as May, 1897, had tabulated a scheme with the Secretary of the Seamen's Hospital Society [SHS] (Mr [later Sir James] Michelli [1853–1935]) to have the school established at the Albert Dock Hospital.[3] ... Chamberlain wrote to the Board of Management of the [SHS] about the matter, and the latter acceded to his request, and decided to throw the course open to all medical graduates who desired to come. On 14th October, 1898, a minute was passed 'That a Sub-Committee be appointed, consisting of Mr H J [later Sir Herbert] Read [1863–1949], of the Colonial Office, and others, to formulate a scheme for the organization and management of the new School of *Tropical Medicine*, with powers to co-opt members of the medical profession interested in tropical diseases and bacteriology'. The Sub-Committee met several times, and on 10th March, 1899, drew up the rules and arranged for advertising for members for the teaching staff. ...

... Success has attended both schools. Manson suggested Ross's name for the Liverpool School [of Tropical Medicine] ... A larger staff was appointed in London [than in Liverpool]; in addition to Manson, there were Cantlie, Simpson, Duncan, Baker, Hewlett and Sambon, and systematic lectures were given as well as clinical instruction and the laboratory course. Dr [D C] Rees was the first Medical Tutor. ... Dr [R T] Leiper came in January, 1905, and Dr [C M] Wenyon in May of the same year when special departments of helminthology and protozoology were started, these being followed by one of entomology with Colonel [A W] Alcock in charge.[4] ...

In Liverpool ... J W W Stephens followed [H E] Annett as Demonstrator of Tropical Pathology in 1902, and ... Warrington Yorke was appointed Research Assistant at the Runcorn Laboratory in 1909, becoming Director in the following year. ... [John] Stephens became Professor of *Tropical Medicine* (Alfred Jones Chair of *Tropical Medicine*) in 1913, and in the same year ... Yorke was appointed to the Walter Myers Chair of Parasitology.[5] ...

... By the end of 1913 the Liverpool School had sent out to the tropics no fewer than thirty-one expeditions for the study of disease, and at that same time the London School had also sent out several, while an average of sixty students a session, 180 in the year, were now attending the courses. This had necessitated enlargements of the schools several times, and also of the hospital to meet these requirements. The University of Cambridge instituted a Diploma in *Tropical Medicine* in 1903, and Liverpool University some little time later. In 1911 the Royal College of Physicians and the Royal College of Surgeons started a *Diploma in Tropical Medicine and Hygiene* in London. Other nations soon followed the lead of England by establishing Schools of Tropical Medicine – Paris, Germany (Hamburg) in 1900, Belgium and, later, the United States of America and other places. The seed sown by Manson had thus borne abundant fruit.[6]

Low then concentrated on the early days of the Society[7]; he continued:

> ... [by 1907] *tropical medicine* had advanced [and] with such
> enormous leaps and bounds that it was fitting it should have
> further recognition than that given to it by the tropical schools
> [*see* Chapter 1]. ... The necessity that this Society should have its
> own home [had] been realized for several years [he continued],
> and the appeal for money for the Manson House, as the home is
> to be called, is doing well, and we hope soon to be able to secure
> a suitable building [*see* below].

Low also embarked on an account of *research* into tropical diseases
between 1894 and the date of this lecture (1929). He began with an
account of the role of the mosquito in malaria transmission, and outlined
the various contributions of Ross and Manson to the saga.[8] Next, came
the history of filariasis research – beginning with Demarquay's work in
1863, and ending with his own work on the mosquito-man dimension
of the filaria life-cycle in 1900.[9] Of course Manson's seminal discovery in
Amoy, China in 1877 revealing the man-mosquito component received
in-depth coverage. This was followed by discovery of *Aëdes* sp in the
transmission of a viral infection – yellow fever – by the American Yellow
Fever Commission in Cuba in 1900.[10] The history of a solution to the
'negro lethargy' or Sleeping Sickness problem in Uganda – in which Low
himself was involved – received detailed coverage, ending with Bruce's
work in 1903.[11] Next, came Looss's work on ankylostomiasis in 1897; he
had demonstrated invasion via intact skin, and this of course led to the
Rockefeller *Sanitary Commission* and *International Health Board*'s efforts at
world-wide eradication of this infection.[12] Kala azar, formerly considered
a form of chronic malaria or ankylostomiasis and confined to Assam,
received detailed attention. Research on brucellosis, schistosomiasis and
plague was also summarised.[13] Low then turned his attention to beri-
beri which before it was known to be a deficiency disease (*see* Chapter
7), posed a significant dilemma and was originally felt to be due to an
environmental factor.

Low included in his 20-year history of *tropical medicine* some remarks
on chemotherapy of these 'exotic' infections, beginning with the use of
intravenous antimony:

> Nicolle and Mesnil first proposed the use of antimony salts
> ... namely, for *trypanosomiasis* [in 1906]. These authors, not
> satisfied with the results obtained by atoxyl and other arsenicals,

suggested that antimony might be given a trial. Plimmer and Thomson followed up this suggestion and gave subcutaneous injections of both the sodium and potassium tartrate of antimony to experimental rats heavily infected with *trypanosomes*, and were astonished with the sterilizing effect the drug had upon these infections. ... [Patrick] Manson, considering these results [to be] very promising, then gave two human cases of *trypanosomiasis* similar subcutaneous injections, but the local reaction produced was so severe and such extensive sloughing of the tissues followed that they had to be abandoned. He then tried giving the drug by ... mouth, but its emetic action stopped this route effectively.

About the same time Broden and Rodhain, working in the Congo with cases of sleeping sickness, found the same difficulties in administering antimony, and as an experimental trial gave some natives who were *in extremis* [a small dose] ... into the veins. The result was extraordinary, the drug, instead of sloughing the walls of the veins, disappeared into the circulation without producing any ill effects, and ameliorated the condition of the patient in a most remarkable manner. Larger doses were then tried, and the intravenous route was established. [it can] without exaggeration [be said that] this discovery ... is one of the greatest that medicine has ever seen. It has enabled us to control *trypanosomiasis* (partly), kala-azar, ulcerating granuloma and bilharziasis, and to rob these horrible diseases of their terrors. ... Before its introduction, for example, 95 per cent of kala-azar cases died, now the conditions are entirely reversed, 90 percent or so recovering. Yet if one were to ask the man in the street [whether] ... he had ever heard of [these investigators] and their work, he would probably invariable reply in the negative. It is strange that when any really big or important discovery is made a second person almost always claims to have made it independently ... Leboeuf says he also discovered it, but as regards publication Broden and Rodhain have undoubted priority.

The new treatment was soon applied to white people suffering from *trypanosomiasis*. Martin and Darré tried a combined treatment of atoxyl subcutaneously and antimony intravenously in a series of cases; very good results were again obtained. Still later, Kerandel, a French doctor, who had unfortunately acquired *trypanosomiasis*, published his own case. At first treated by atoxyl, he did not improve, so he tried antimony by [the oral route], having heard of the cases that [Patrick] Manson had tried to treat in this way. The drug caused sickness, and could not be tolerated, so nothing remained but to try ... intravenous administration. Martin and Darré carried this out at the *Hospital of the Pasteur Institute* with complete success, a cure resulting. Intravenous antimony was thus established as a treatment for human *trypanosomiasis*.

The first records of the use of tartar emetic injections in *leishmaniasis* were made at the *Brazilian Society of Dermatology* in 1913, when Machado and Vianna showed cases of cutaneous leishmaniasis successfully treated in this manner. In the same year (1913) Arãgao and Vianna treated cases of *ulcerating granuloma* by the same method with excellent results. ... Terra and Rabello confirmed this work, and the treatment then became generally adopted for this loathsome disease. During 1914, further papers on the treatment of cutaneous leishmaniasis by intravenous injections of tartar emetic were published by Da Silva and Carini in Brazil. In the latter part of the same year (1914) Castellani treated a case of kala-azar in Ceylon in this way. Subsequent work on the treatment of kala-azar with antimony falls out of my period, as does also Christopherson's discovery of its efficacy in bilharzial disease.[14] ...

Low also had something to say on the use of *emetine*:

... Ipecacuanha was long known to possess a therapeutic action on cases of *amoebic dysentery*, but its action was not clearly understood. On 6th February, 1911, Captain Edward B Vedder, Medical Corps, US Army, read a paper before the *Manila Medical Society*, entitled, 'A Preliminary Account of some Experiments Undertaken to Test the Efficacy of the Ipecacuanha Treatment of Dysentery'. He had found that one of the alkaloids of ipecacuanha, namely emetine, was very toxic to amoebae *in vitro*. Sir Leonard Rogers [*see* Chapter 9] in Calcutta put Vedder's experimental work to the clinical test, and devised the method of giving the alkaloid hypodermically. This allowed of greater control in giving the drug, and led to a revolution in the treatment of *amoebic dysentery* and the disappearance to a large extent of its serious complication – liver abscess.

In conclusion, he acknowledged the fact that during the period under review (1894–1914) much more had been accomplished than his time allowed:

> ... I need only mention the work that has emanated from the different Tropical Schools, associating the names of Boyce, Stephens, Dutton, Todd, Yorke, the Thomsons and Sinton with the Liverpool School; Rees, Daniels, Leiper, Wenyon, Alcock, Newham and Manson-Bahr with the London School; Laveran, Blanchard, Mesnil and Brumpt with Paris; Nocht, Giemsa and Fülleborn with the Hamburg School; Ziemann with Berlin; and Marchiafava, Grassi, Bignami, Bastianelli and others in Italy. Then there [was] the work of Balfour in the Sudan; of Ross, Rogers, James, Christophers and Giles in India; of Gorgas, Darling and Strong in America; of Sergent and Nicolle in North Africa; of Schüffner, Van Loghem, Swellingrebel and others in the Dutch East Indies; of Kitasato and Shiga in Japan; and a host of others throughout different parts of the world. ...
>
> The textbooks of [Patrick] Manson, published in 1899 [sic], of Daniels in 1909, and that of Castellani and Chalmers in 1910, with the practical works of Stephens and Christophers (1903) and Daniels (1903), etc, have crystallised the knowledge gained during my period, and the names of all the workers will be found in them.

Low ended his address by stressing that there was still much to be discovered, including: 'the etiology of *blackwater fever*, *sprue*, and other diseases ... and the whole field of *prevention* is [still] an open one'.

> It is not sufficient to discover the cause of a disease alone; this is only a means to an end, the grand finality being the complete eradication and removal of that disease from the surface of the globe ...

Low's last theme is almost as pertinent today as it was in 1929; only limited progress has in fact been made in disease (both cause and prevention) in warm climates since then![15]

The Society during Low's presidency

The Society's accommodation

By the early 1920s the Society was still installed in a room at the MSL's house at 11 Chandos Street, W1 (*see* Chapter 7). However, on 11 June 1925, Dr Des Voeux, Treasurer of the MSL, proposed that the new Secretary/Registrar (Bethell was retiring) should control the secretarial work of all those Societies which were tenants of the MSL and that they should all contribute to the salary of the MSL's Secretary. *Council* of the RSTMH felt unanimously however, that the [RSTMH] could '*not* sacrifice its independence in this way'; and their Assistant Secretary would thus continue as before!

Council agreed incidentally, on **15 October 1925** that the Society's office (at the MSL) would be closed in August and September of each year, and on 19 May 1927, they reluctantly agreed to a rent increase of £188 per annum to the MSL; however, this was subsequently reduced to £175 because the MSL proved to be exempt from 'certain rates' under the 'Scientific and Learned Societies Acts'. In view of these problems with accommodation over the years, it was in fact considered imperative that the Society possessed its own property.

When the Society removed to Manson House on 24 June 1931 (*see* below) they were requested to pay for redecorating the 'room at the MSL which they were vacating'; *Council* 'did not [however] see its way to authorising this payment'.

The permanent Headquarters

G C Low (then Treasurer) pointed out to *Council* as early as **4 July 1923** (*ie* during Bassett-Smith's presidency – *see* Chapter 7): 'the advantages to be gained by starting a special fund for [the] purpose' of obtaining a *permanent* home. He duly proposed that 'a *House Fund* should be instituted', and '£500 of the accumulated funds of the Society [were immediately] transferred to [this] Fund'. The news was conveyed by Bassett-Smith to an *Ordinary* meeting of the Society on **18 October** of that year; he also alluded to the 'House Fund' at the 18th AGM.

By **15 November**, the *House Fund* amounted to £533 5s 0d, and *Council* suggested that a public appeal be initiated. Since this was now a '*Royal*' Society it might be possible, it was suggested, to seek the patronage of the King (George V); the Prince of Wales might also be approached.

A draft letter to Fellows regarding the *House Fund* was finalised by

Council on **21 February 1924**, and the Secretaries were duly authorised to send a copy to all Fellows. On **15 May**, *Council* agreed to transfer a further £50 to the *House Fund*, which now amounted to £647 0s 1d. By October of that year, the fund stood at £737 12s 7d, and it was suggested by *Council* that a page in *Transactions* should be devoted to the Fund. By January of the following year, £761 had been received (£261 of it from Fellows). At a *Council* meeting on **15 October 1925** it was however, reported that only 68 Fellows had contributed to the Fund which had then been in existence for two years; a Sub-Committee to deal with the matter was set up. On **21 January 1926**, Balfour (president) undertook to write to every Fellow, in a further appeal for contributions; the total was then £904 2s 4d, and at the following *Council* meeting he also agreed to write to surviving past-presidents of the Society. On 20 May 1926, a further £200 was transferred from the Accumulated Fund, and further donations were announced on **21 October** and **18 November 1926**, and **20 January 1927**.

Manson House

To name the *permanent* home *Manson House* as a memorial to Sir Patrick Manson, who had died in 1922, was suggested to *Council* on **20 January 1927** and this was ratified in May of that year. At a *Council* meeting in March, Manson-Bahr promised to donate to the Fund 50% of profits on his 'The Life of Sir Patrick Manson'[16] just published.

On **19 May**, *Council* agreed to transfer a further £361 4s 2d from the Accumulated Fund, bringing the total to £1,577 3s 3d. That meeting also agreed that a letter should be sent to all former students of the LSTM requesting donations; it was suggested that they contribute to this 'Imperial and international memorial' to Manson. In June, Sir Harry Waters told *Council* that he would invite donations to the fund from 'various business firms' with branches in the tropics.

By **21 June 1928** the total had risen to £3,326 3s 5d, and on reaching £3000, a *Public* appeal had been launched. *Council* discussions (*see* for example *CM*, **17 May**) referred to whether 'Patrick Manson House' might be a preferable name! Dr H S Stannus, it seems, was concerned that *Manson House* might be confused with Mansion House!

SEARCH FOR A SUITABLE PROPERTY

At the *Council* meeting on **18 October 1928**, it was announced that the fund had reached £3,420 18s 11d. It was considered time to consult a local house agent; Manson-Bahr and the Secretaries (Wenyon and Clayton Lane) duly met Mr Bedford who had actually known Manson. This Sub-Committee which reported to the next meeting in November indicated that every Fellow should be personally invited to contribute to the fund, and a property which by then had been inspected by the Sub-Committee was in many ways suitable. Twenty-nine Portland Place had been inspected, and provided the Superior landlords (Howard de Walden Estate) agreed to grant a 999-year lease on reasonable terms to the Society, it was decided to recommend its 'adoption by the *Council'*. In the event the Superior landlord would only grant a 45-year lease – which was deemed totally 'unsuitable to purchase' as a *'permanent* memorial to Sir Patrick Manson'.

Manson-Bahr, Low and Sir Leonard Rogers had meanwhile promised loans ranging from £500 to £2000 *without interest*. At the next meeting (in December) it was announced that Dr H S (later Sir Henry) Wellcome had donated two hundred guineas.

By **21 February 1929** the Fund stood at £4,240 3s 10d, and Low was unanimously nominated by *Council* to be the next president; he declared that 'he hoped to see Manson House actually established during his term of office'. This sentiment was also expressed at the 1929 AGM, when he took office as president. Table 8.1 gives an impression of the widespread interest throughout the British Empire in the establishment of a *permanent* memorial to Manson.

On **16 May** it was reported that several other houses had been inspected by the Sub-Committee; one considered 'quite suitable' had however been disposed of *before* authority from *Council* to make a definite offer could be obtained. That meeting decided therefore, that in future the Sub-Committee should be given 'full power' to go ahead.

Several substantial donations were recorded on **17 October**, when it was unanimously agreed that a suitable appeal letter should be drafted and sent to *The Times*; it was hoped that the Editor would also arrange for a *leader* to appear on the subject. At their meeting on **21 November** *Council* approved a draft of the letter to *The Times* – signed by Low, Ross, Balfour, Stephens, Bagshawe and Wenyon. It was hoped that it would be followed by letters from Sir John Rose Bradford, Lord Inchcape, J L Maxwell, Lord Reading and Neville Chamberlain. Sir Austen Chamberlain had signed a covering note to be sent out with the *Times* letter and leader – as part of a *Public Appeal*. The Secretary of State for the Colonies (Lord Passfield) was also asked for his help. The total at **20 February 1930** was £7,534 15s 1d

Table 8.1: Some references to newspaper/journal articles referring to the Manson House Fund, to institute a *permanent* memorial to the first president – purchase of 26 Portland Place

Country/ continent	Newspaper/journal	Date
1928		
Ceylon	*Times*, Ceylon	24 December
1929		
UK	*Times, Lond* (+ leading article)	18 "
	Times, Lond	21 "
	Observer	22 "
	Med Press Circ.	25 "
	Times (Weekly Ed)	26 "
	Yorkshire Herald	27 "
	Country Life	28 "
	Aberdeen Press	30 "
	Times, Lond	28/30 "
Africa	*Star*, Johannesburg	13 March
	Lourenço Marques	19 "
	West Africa	28 December
1930		
UK	*Times*, Lond	11 January
	Lancet	18 "
	Br med J	18 "
	Children's newspaper	18 "
	Wakefield Express	25 "
	Med Press Circ	31 "
	Times, Lond	13 February
	Med Press Circ (Times reprint)	19 "
	Answers	8 March
	Lloyd's List	10 April
	Farmer's Weekly	11 "
	Co-operative News	19 "
	Cancer	[?] July
	Br med J	12 "
	Med Press Circ	[?] "
	Sub-tropical gardener	[? Date]
Australia	*Med J Aust*	1 March
India	*The Pioneer*, Allahabad	19 January
	Daily Chronicle, Delhi	28 March/9 April
	Indian Textile Journal	[?] May
Hong Kong	*Hong Kong Telegraph*	4 April

Country/ continent	Newspaper/journal	Date
Africa	*African World*	5 February
	Tanganyika Opinion	4 March
	Tanganyika Standard	8 "
	Mombasa Times	12 "
	Tanganyika Times	15 "
	Natal Mercury	16 December
1931		
UK	*Times, Lond*	28 March
	Times, Lond	[?] June
	Evening News, Lond	24 "
	Nature, Lond	4 July
	Med Press Circ	22 "
	Medical Officer	August
Africa	*West Africa*	11 July
South Africa	*Natal Mercury*	6 November

(of which £1,153 had come from the Public Appeal). And a month later, Wenyon had written to Wellcome (*see above*) suggesting that an appeal be also launched in the USA. *Council* was told in May that Passfield (*see above*) was very enthusiastic for a *permanent* memorial to Manson, and had 'sent a dispatch to the Governors of various colonies urging their support …'.

On **11 December** of that year, Low, now the president, 'informed *Council* that 26 Portland Place (*see* Figures 8.2 and 8.3) was again in the market at a price of £22,000'. The House Sub-Committee was unanimous in recommending purchase of this property.

HISTORY OF 26 PORTLAND PLACE

The developers of the impressive thoroughfare, Portland Place (where Manson House stood), on land owned by the Duke of Portland, were the Adam brothers – Robert and James. The project had first been conceived in 1773, the initial idea being to build a series of detached private palaces flanking a wide avenue which ran northwards from Foley House, the Duke's mansion (situated on the site now occupied by the Langham Hotel). However, this initial plan was abandoned (due apparently to unforeseen economic factors) and in 1776 a series of large terraced

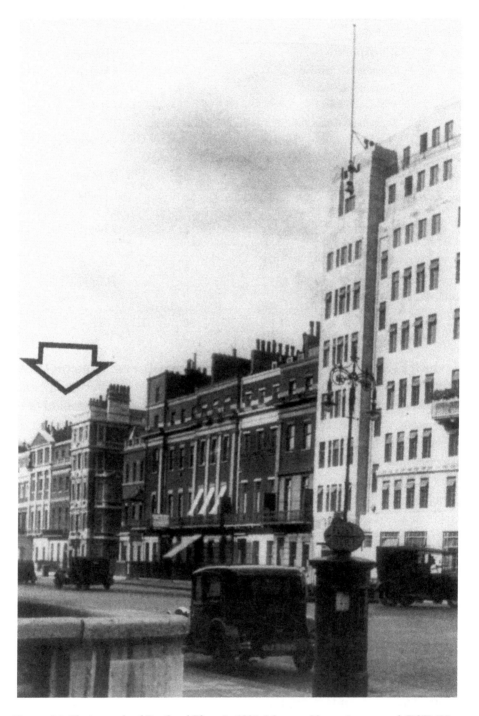

Figure 8.2: Photograph of Portland Place in 1931; Manson House is arrowed (RSTMH archive).

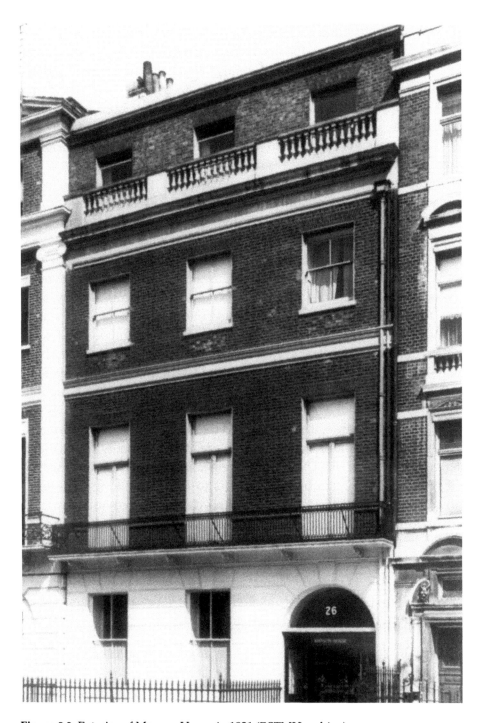

Figure 8.3: Exterior of Manson House in 1931 (RSTMH archive).

houses were built on each side of the new street (Portland Place). These were of high quality, and each encompassed 'Adam style' features.

No 26 (which became Manson House) is arguably one of the finest of these terraced houses – which retains much of the original Adam decoration; it was probably completed in 1778.

In 1781, the house was occupied by the diplomat, Lord Stormont[17] at which time it had been the site of an interesting historical event: on 26 November of that year Lord Germain (1716–1785), Commissioner of Trade and Plantations and Secretary of State for the Colonies (1775–1782), accompanied by his Secretary, Lord Walsingham, arrived with 'stop press' news of General Cornwallis's [1738–1805] surrender, on 19 October, at Yorktown, Virginia. After France and Spain, both with powerful fleets, entered the 'War of American Independence' (1775–1783) against Britain, the Royal Navy (RN) briefly lost control of the seas. Cornwallis had retreated with his army to Yorktown, where he was relatively secure provided he could receive supplies by sea. On 17 October, a British rescue fleet had set out from New York – but too late; Cornwallis was already outnumbered, outgunned, and was rapidly running out of food. When the RN failed to come to his aid he was therefore forced to surrender his army to the colonialists, a defeat which heralded the British Government's abandonment of the struggle, independence of the colonies being recognised at the 'Peace of Paris' in 1783. Shortly afterwards, they developed their own form of government, eventually uniting under the presidency of George Washington in 1787. After collecting the Lord Chancellor, they called on the Prime Minister, Lord North (1732–92), to break the news to him. Following this, they proceeded to inform King George III of this disastrous episode.

Lord North and George III (1738–1820) (who possibly suffered from porphyria) were subsequently blamed for the loss of the American colonies![18]

26 Portland Place receives Council's backing

At the *Council* meeting on **11 December 1930**, the following was minuted:

> After a discussion it was decided that an effort should be made to secure the property [26 Portland Place] for the Society. The Treasurer [Bagshawe] proposed that the *Council* authorise the Hon Secretaries to proceed with the negotiations for the purchase at a maximum price of £22,000 provided that a satisfactory

surveyor's report [was] obtained, and that an examination of the terms of the lease [showed that] there were no restrictions which might hamper the development of the Society. The Resolution was seconded by Dr [A T] Stanton and after some further discussion was carried unanimously.

It was agreed that Messrs Pothecary and Barratt should be appointed to act as the Society's solicitors for the negotiations and that Messrs Daniel Smith, Oakley and Garrard ... make a survey of 26 Portland Place and report thereon as soon as possible.

And at the following meeting of *Council*:

The Secretary read the Report which had been sent in by the Surveyors ... and also a letter from the solicitors ... saying that Mr [G P] Joseph the present holder of the lease was willing to accept £22,000 on condition that the Society would purchase certain fittings at a sum of approximately £500. A discussion took place ... in the course of which Dr H H [later Sir Harold] Scott drew attention to the fact that the building was an old one, that the Report mentioned various structural defects and that the cost of the proposed improvements would be heavy. Dr Bagshawe pointed out that in the previous report by Mr Skues the site alone was described as very valuable.

It was finally agreed as proposed by Dr Manson-Bahr and seconded by Dr Bagshawe that an offer of £22,500 or less be made for 26 Portland Place provided that the fixtures, as they stand in the inventory, are included [and a] detailed Surveyor's Report on the structure and drains be obtained. It was also agreed that the price to be paid for the fixtures was to be determined by a valuation. Dr Stanton and Dr Horn [sic] both emphasized the desirability of having at least one room available for the use of Fellows as a reading or writing room.

In order to empower the Society to borrow money with a view to the purchase of a house or other similar object the President [Low] proposed that the Laws of the Society be altered by adding the following paragraph to Law 22:

The *Council* may, from time to time raise and borrow on mortgage or charge of any of the property of the Society or otherwise any sum or sums of money for the purchase of land

and buildings, the erection of buildings or provision of plant and equipment or for such other purposes tending to promote the objects of the Society as the *Council* may determine.

The resolution was duly seconded by Dr Hamilton Fairley [Hon Secretary] and the *Council* agreed.

The Secretaries were instructed to take the usual steps to inform the Fellows of the proposed alteration in the Laws by posting a note in the Society's rooms; and to call a *Special General meeting* in accordance with Law 42 to which the proposal should be submitted.

Low continues as president and a bridging loan is obtained

On **15 January 1931**, Dr A T Stanton indicated to *Council* that 'it would be a very great advantage to the Society if Dr Low could continue to hold office as president for a further period [in order to oversee the removal to 26 Portland Place and the financial efforts involved]'. This meant an amendment to Law 12 (originally 14), which was accomplished at a *Special General Meeting* on 26 March.

On 19 February a letter from the Westminster Bank was read to *Council* agreeing a loan of £15,000 to the Society, at a rate of 1% above Bank Rate with a minimum of 4½% (the current rate being 3%). The Fund then stood at £11,074 10s 8d.

At a crucial *Council* meeting on **19 March**:

It was announced that the negotiations with regard to 26 Portland Place were now almost complete with the exception of the price to be paid for the fixtures which the *Council* had agreed to purchase on valuation and for a sum not exceeding £500. Valuations had been made by the Society's representative and also by Mr [G P] Joseph's (the present owner). These showed a difference of nearly £200 and the alternative was to accept the price of £500 asked by Mr Joseph, or appoint an umpire and accept his decision.

After some discussion the following resolution was proposed by Dr Stanton, seconded by Dr Fletcher and carried unanimously:

With regard to the purchase of fixtures at 26 Portland Place it is agreed to accept the umpire's decision, even should the sum of £500 fixed by previous resolution of the *Council* be exceeded.

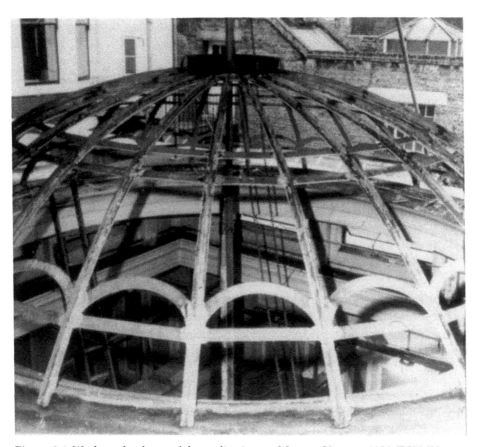

Figure 8.4: Work on the dome of the auditorium at Manson House – 1931 (RSTMH archive).

[Also] the following Resolutions were put by the Chairman and carried unanimously:

(i) … that the leasehold property 26 Portland Place be transferred into the names of the Trustees of the Society.

(ii) … that the Society's Bankers the Westminster Bank Limited, be requested to advance to the Society from time to time sums not exceeding £15,000 against the deposit of the title deeds or other documents of title of 26 Portland Place which title deeds or documents of title are or will be in the names of the Trustees of the Society …

It was unanimously decided by *Council* on **21 May** to build a hall at 26 Portland Place; plans prepared by the architect also showed a 'new staircase with cloakrooms and other accommodation'. This meeting appointed Mr J N Randall Vining FRIBA as architect. Figure 8.4 shows the dome of the auditorium during construction.

Low reminded the 24th AGM that that was the last meeting at 11 Chandos Street; after 24 June 1931 the Society's address would be Manson House, Portland Place. Removal was in fact announced in the lay and medical press (*see Times, Lond* 1931: 25 June; *Med Press* 1931: 1 July; *Nature, Lond* 1931: 4 July; *Med Press* 1931: 22 July; *Med Officer* 1931: 29 August). The first *Council* meeting was held at 26 Portland Place (Manson House) on **16 July**, the local Secretary for Sarawak – Mrs [E J O] Le Sueur being in attendance; this was the first time that a lady had attended a meeting of *Council*!

At that first (*Council*) meeting at Manson House the meeting had considered:

> The financial position in relation to [26 Portland Place] and the proposed alterations and building a hall. A loan of £15,000 had been arranged with the Westminster Bank at ½ per cent above Bank Rate and it was hoped that an additional £1,400, if required, could be raised by a further appeal to the Fellows.
>
> Specifications and drawings had been prepared by the Society's architect [*see above*] ... and sent out to three firms of contractors. The estimate received from Messrs Minter and Co was the lowest (£3850) [of these] which with the estimates for the other necessary work and architect's fees and expenses made up a total of £4,576.
>
> After some discussion it was agreed that the contract should be signed with Messrs Minter & Co and the work put in hand at once. The following were elected as members of the House Committee with power to co-opt others if considered advisable: Dr Stanton, Dr Stannus, Dr Daukes and Dr William Fletcher. ...
>
> Dr Wenyon called the attention of the *Council* to the beautiful ivory Chairman's hammer which the President [Low] had presented on the day the Society entered into occupation of its own home. Members of the *Council* expressed their appreciation of the useful gift. Other gifts had been made to the library by the President of various early volumes of the *Transactions* and of the *Journal of the School of Tropical Medicine*. Dr Oswald Marriott was also thanked for presenting the three volumes of Byam and Archibald's *Practice of Medicine in the Tropics*.[19]

At the *Council* meeting on **15 October**, the Treasurer (Bagshawe) indicated that as well as the £15,000 loan, a further £950 would be required 'to meet the cost of building and furnishing'. Meanwhile, the president's Appeal had so far raised £188 5s, which had risen to £531 7s 11d by January 1932. The Marylebone Borough Council confirmed that the Society was exempt from local rates – an annual saving of £163.

Figures 8.5a–8.5d show the interior of rooms (including the auditorium) after renovation of Manson House as they appeared in 1931.

Tenants of Manson House and associated property

The first tenant was Mr G P Joseph who rented the maisonette and garage for twelve months from September 1931. The *British Society for the Study of Orthodontics* requested accommodation (the hall and council room) seven times a year; *Council* suggested on **21 January 1932** that an annual rent of £50 should be charged, and this was subsequently accepted.

First Ordinary Meeting at Manson House

It was suggested to *Council* on **19 November 1931** that the Prince of Wales might be invited to open Manson House the following spring. This matter was again aired on 10 December; if the Prince was unable to perform the ceremony, the Duke of York would be invited instead. The president (Low) told a meeting of *Council* on **10 December** that the new hall would be ready for the *Ordinary* meeting in January 1932. This meeting duly took place on **21 January 1932**, and Low gave a short account of the Society's history, since 1907, paid tribute to the architect (Vining), the Society's Secretary (Miss Wenyon), and thanked four donors for gifts to Manson House (*see* below). Before he read his paper (*see* Table 8.2), Dr C M Wenyon (Hon Secretary) referred to the carved oak rostrum, chairs, lectern and clock which had been presented by the president. Wenyon's paper was entitled 'Leishmaniasis and the problem of its transmission'; Col J A Sinton VC, Dr E Hindle, Dr N J Smyly, Prof J G Thomson, Wing Commander Whittingham and Prof Warrington Yorke took part in the subsequent discussion.

The official opening

At the *Council* meeting on **18 February 1932** it was announced that HRH The Prince of Wales had agreed to formally open Manson House on 17 March 1932. Low expressed appreciation of the help rendered by Sir

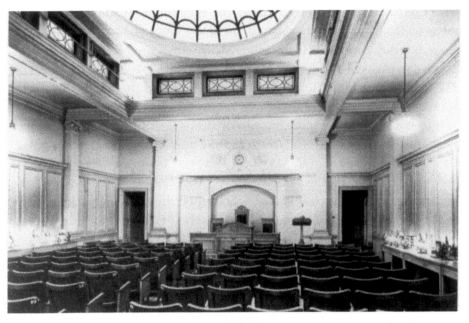

Figure 8.5a: The auditorium (or Hall), Manson House in 1931 (RSTMH archive).

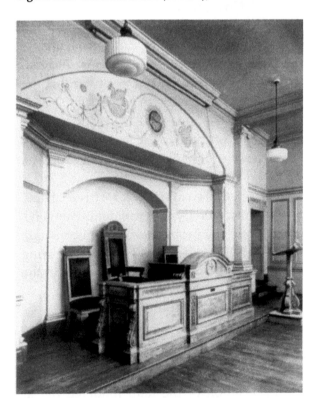

Figure 8.5b: The presidential rostrum and lectern at Manson House – 1931 (RSTMH archive).

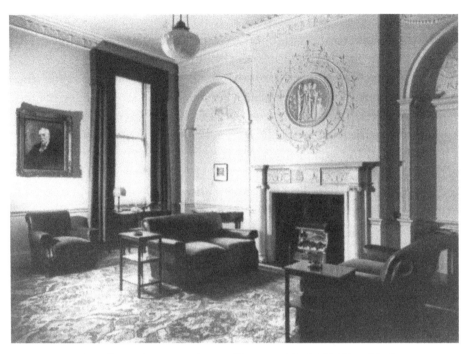

Figure 8.5c: The Fellows' Room at Manson House c.1931 (RSTMH archive).

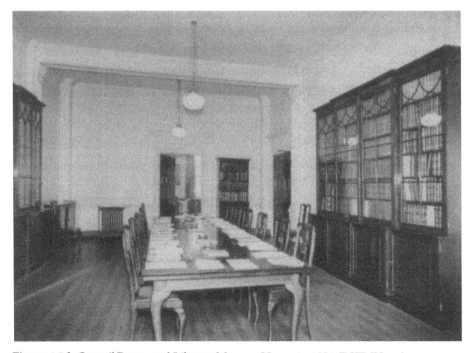

Figure 8.5d: *Council* Room and Library, Manson House in 1931 (RSTMH archive).

Austen Chamberlain and Sir Herbert Read in approaching the Prince. Thanks were again expressed to the architect for helping in the design of the Hall, and in carrying out various structural alterations.

The next meeting of *Council* took place on **22 March** (*ie after* the opening ceremony had taken place) when the 'successful function' of the previous week (the official opening – *see* below) was referred to; messages of good wishes from several Fellows (including Ross) who were unable to be present at the ceremony were read out. At that meeting, it was agreed that The Prince of Wales be invited to become a Vice-Patron, and Sir Austen Chamberlain, an Honorary Fellow of the Society; both sent written acceptance.

Figures 8.6a and 8.6b show the order of proceedings at the formal opening of Manson House on 17 March 1932. The following is an account of the opening ceremony published in the London *Times* of Friday 18 March 1932:

> The Prince of Wales [later King Edward VIII] yesterday opened Manson House [*see* Figure 8.7], the new headquarters of the [RSTMH] in Portland-place, W. The premises will perpetuate the memory of Sir Patrick Manson, the father of tropical medicine.
>
> The Prince was received by Sir Austen Chamberlain, MP KG, and Dr Carmichael Low, the president of the society, and was conducted to the Fellows' Room, where presentations were made. He afterwards went to the hall, where the opening ceremony took place in the presence of a large gathering, which included Lady Manson.
>
> **Dr Carmichael Low** spoke of the Prince's appreciation of the importance of *tropical medicine* and the fact that his Royal Highness had acquired through personal experience an intimate knowledge of one of the chief tropical maladies – *malaria*. The society had on its roll over 1,700 Fellows. Every institute of note dealing with *tropical medicine* and nearly every country was represented. Contributions to the fund for establishing the new headquarters had been received from all parts of the world [*see* Table 8.1], testifying to the increasing appreciation of the pioneer work inaugurated by Sir Patrick Manson. To meet their obligations a further sum of £15,000 was required.
>
> *Malaria in Kenya.* **The Prince of Wales** said: From my fairly extensive travels I have always been very interested in tropical

research, and, knowing its great value, I was very pleased to have been asked to perform this ceremony. It is not the first function that I have done for the [RSTMH], but I feel more fitted to speak on this subject than I did on the last occasion. I am not going to claim that I have devoted any time to research, but as your president has mentioned my having been stricken with one of those tropical diseases, from which at times I still suffer, I can claim, at any rate, some experience and some knowledge of the nature, at least, of one of those diseases, and I hope more than most of you here this evening. (Laughter.) It may even interest you to know that when I was convalescent after my first attack of *malaria* in Kenya Colony some of my friends were pleased that I was so quickly convalescent because they thought it was a good advertisement for the Colony. *Malaria* is looked on there as not very much more than a bad go of 'flu, and when they knew I was convalescent they were really quite pleased.

One of the great obstacles to the development of tropical countries is not so much the climatic conditions but the diseases which are prevalent in them. As so many of our Possessions and many of the countries which provide an outlet for our people are in the tropical regions, this has, therefore, become a vital problem in this country and throughout the British Empire, and it is not surprising that, although these diseases are still prevalent in those tropical countries, yet a very great deal of progress and improvement has been made in the last 30 years. This improvement is due to the discoveries made by our pioneer investigators who devoted their lives to the study of tropical diseases and medicine on the spot, revealing the cause of many unknown diseases, and, what is still more important, the way in which they are spread, and the remedies for their successful treatment. It is impossible to over-estimate the importance of these discoveries which have saved the lives of hundreds of thousands of those whose lot it has been to live in tropical lands, not only Europeans, but also the native population.

Manson's great work. When we think of our great pioneer investigators – those fine men who devoted their lives, very often at the expense of health, in order to gain this end – the name that naturally comes to our minds this evening is Patrick Manson, after whom this house has been so fittingly named. We are privileged

The Royal Society
OF
Tropical Medicine and Hygiene

MANSON HOUSE, 26 PORTLAND PLACE,
LONDON W.1

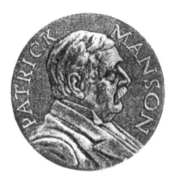

Order of Proceedings

AT THE

Opening of Manson House

Headquarters of the

Royal Society of Tropical Medicine & Hygiene

by

H.R.H. The Prince of Wales, K.G.

ON

THURSDAY, 17th MARCH, 1932

at 5.30 p.m.

Figure 8.6a: Front cover of 'Order of Proceedings' of the opening of Manson House on 17 March 1932.

The Opening of Manson House

Order of Proceedings

5.30 H.R.H. THE PRINCE OF WALES arrives at Manson House and will be received by The Rt. Hon. Sir Austen Chamberlain, K.G. and Dr. G. Carmichael Low, F.R.C.P., President of the Royal Society of Tropical Medicine and Hygiene.

His Royal Highness will be conducted to the Fellows' Room, where Presentations will be made.

The Prince of Wales will be escorted to the new Hall by Sir Austen Chamberlain, the President and the Honorary Secretaries.

An Address of Welcome to His Royal Highness will be delivered by the President.

HIS ROYAL HIGHNESS THE PRINCE OF WALES will reply to the Address and will declare open Manson House.

A Vote of Thanks to His Royal Highness will be proposed by The Rt. Hon. Sir Austen Chamberlain, K.G.

Colonel W. P. Mac Arthur, D.S.O., K.H.P., R.A.M.C., will second Sir Austen Chamberlain's proposal.

Before leaving Manson House, His Royal Highness will proceed to the Library, where there will be a Demonstration of Microscope slides illustrating the stages of the malaria parasite in man and in the mosquito.

Figure 8.6b: Order of Proceedings of the formal opening of Manson House, 26 Portland Place, W1.

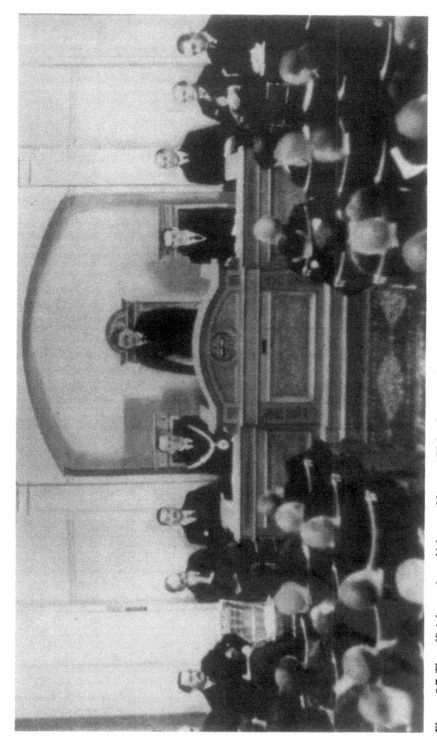

Figure 8.7: The official opening of Manson House, 17 March 1932: The Prince of Wales is in the centre, with Low to his right and Sir Austen Chamberlain to his left (RSTMH archive).

Table 8.2: Communications at *Ordinary* Meetings 1930–33

Date	Subject	Speaker
1930		
16 January	Aetiology of yellow fever	M H Kuczynski
20 February	Physiology of disease-carrying insects	V B Wigglesworth
15 May	Pellagra in Nyasaland	H M Shelley
	Anatomy and histology of pellagra	W Susman
19 June (23rd AGM)	Pathology, biochemistry and treatment of sprue	N H Fairley
16 October	Heatstroke and sun traumatism	F Marsh
11 December	Epidemic dropsy in Bengal	G Shanks
	Minor tropical diseases	A Castellani
1931		
15 January	Induced malaria in England	S P James
19 February	Leprosy: experimental and treatment	H C de Souza-Araujo
21 May	Epidemic catarrhal jaundice	G M Findlay, J L Dunlop, H C Brown
18 June (24th AGM)	Treatment of leprosy	E Muir
15 October	Antimony compounds in treatment of bilharzia and kala-azar	W H Gray, J W Trevan
10 December	Rift-valley fever	G M Findlay
1932		
21 January*	Transmission of leishmaniasis	C M Wenyon
18 February	Tryparsamide in Gambian trypanosomiasis	C C Chesterman
21 May	*Wuchereria bancrofti* infection	F W O'Connor
16 June (25th AGM)	Synthetic anti-malarials and quinine	S P James
20 October	Blackwater fever in British Guiana	G Giglioli
	Blackwater fever in England	P Manson-Bahr, N H Fairley
8 December	Climatic conditions and insects	P A Buxton
1933		
19 January	Bacteriological nature of bacteriophages	F M Burnet
	Bacteriophage work in India	F P Mackie
16 February	Immunity in malaria	J G Thomson
18 May	Australian snake venoms	C H Kellaway
15 June (26th AGM)	*Entamoeba histolytica* carriers	H W Acton
19 October	Disease forecasting in India (presidential address) (see Chapter 9)	Sir Leonard Rogers
14 December	Cysticercosis in the British Army	W P MacArthur

*The first *Ordinary* Meeting at Manson House.

to-day by the presence here of Lady Manson. (Cheers.) A certain amount had been accomplished before Manson's day, but he was the first to associate experimentally a blood-sucking insect with the transmission of human disease. It was he who asked Ross to carry out the epoch-making investigations which led to the detection of the *anopheles* mosquito as the carrier of *malaria*, and it was he who first realized the want of schools where medical men destined for work in the tropics could be taught the latest knowledge on the subject. He was, in fact, the father of modern *tropical medicine*, and the practical effects of his genius were especially exemplified by the success which enabled the Panama Canal to be constructed through one of the unhealthiest regions of the world. Patrick Manson was not only a brilliant scientific investigator, but it was he who, with the help of Mr Joseph Chamberlain [1836–1914], that far-sighted statesman, founded the *School of Tropical Medicine in London*. But he also realized that there was [a] need for something more than just a school of *tropical medicine*; he realized there was [a] need for a clearing-house of knowledge, and so he it was who was the first president of this society, which was founded in 1907.

The Prince observed [how] conditions in ... tropical countries were changed, and one of the most striking changes during the last 10 years had been the improvement in communications. Improved communications, unless precautions were taken, would tend to increase the spread of disease in the tropics, but those same communications on the other hand would increase the facilities for the control of disease. How could that be done? First of all, he thought, by making possible the rapid collection of pathological material for investigation, and secondly, by allowing a centralized research and dispatch to help other centres in the investigation and control of epidemics. In that house those who had made discoveries and those who had gained great experience in tropical lands would be able to pool their opinions for the help of those who would have to face those problems in the future. He hoped that the fine house would receive the support it deserved. (Cheers.)

Sir Austen Chamberlain, expressing the society's thanks to his Royal Highness, recalled the horror with which his father [Joseph Chamberlain] in his early days at the Colonial Office learned how heavy was the toll of life taken by tropical diseases among the young men whom it was his duty to appoint to the Colonial Service. When, two years after his father had received the seals of office, the appointment of the medical adviser to the Colonial Office fell vacant, he set himself to discover who in London knew most about tropical disease, and that inquiry rapidly got him acquainted with Sir Patrick Manson. The immediate result of that first cooperation was the establishment of the School of Tropical Medicine in London and of a similar school in Liverpool, for, although the Liverpool school was independently funded, its inspiration came from Sir Patrick Manson. In 1896 the average death-rate was 100 per 1,000 a year in our tropical possessions. To-day it was only between eight and nine per 1,000.

Colonel W P MacArthur said that among the letters received in response to their appeal was one from a cricket club in Rhodesia [now Zimbabwe], in which it was explained that the members realized that had it not been for the work of Sir Patrick Manson they would not have been able to play cricket in Rhodesia to-day.[20]

At a meeting of *Council* on **21 May**, a letter was read from the vice-Chancellor of Hong Kong University (Sir William Hornell – 1878–1950), both congratulating the Society on the formal opening of Manson House, and referring to 'the early association of Manson with the Hong Kong College of Medicine for Chinese'.

Other Society matters during Low's presidency

Financial concerns continue

There were continuing financial concerns however, as this *Council* minute in May indicates:

> Reference was made to the letter from the Westminster Bank asking that the loan of £15,000 should be repaid before August 25th 1932. The Treasurer [Bagshawe] pointed out that there was as shown on the Balance Sheet a net deficit of £475 in addition to the loan and that the builders' final account had not yet been received; this it was hoped would not exceed £550. There was thus needed, beyond the £15,000 loan, approximately £1,000 to meet the Society's obligations in full.

At the following *Council* meeting one month later:

> It was announced that … Manson-Bahr had very generously lent to the Society £1,000 at a nominal interest of one per cent per annum. This enabled the Treasurer to repay £1,000 to the Bank; an arrangement had also been made by which £1,000 received in April by bankers order payments had been, for a few months until needed for current expenses, used to repay temporarily a further £1,000 thereby effecting a saving of over £3 a month.
>
> The Treasurer [indicated] that the Bank would not be willing to continue the loan permanently and that one of the following alternatives would have to be considered before long:
> 1.   To issue debentures
> 2.   To effect a mortgage with a building society, insurance company or a private lender
> 3.   To borrow from the Fellows at some fixed rate of interest.

On **20 October**, Bagshawe again reminded *Council* that the Builders' final account – which would probably be 'not far short of £700' – had not yet been received. He hoped however that it would be possible to settle this … before the end of the financial year. He referred to the three options set out at the last meeting; the rate of interest paid to the Westminster Bank was only 4½ per cent, but should the Bank Rate [rise], the Society's rate would increase to 5 per cent. It was decided to make a concrete proposal to the next meeting of *Council*.

The £15,000 loan was further discussed at [the next] *Council* meeting …, when it was agreed that they should arrange 'an ordinary mortgage if this could be obtained on easy terms', *ie* assuming a 'definite term of five years could be guaranteed'.

On **16 March 1933**, *Council* was provided with a further update on the finances:

> … Bagshawe made a brief financial statement and explained that the Charity Commissioners in authorising the Society to borrow £13,000 stipulated that a sum of not less than £297 should be invested yearly until the whole [was] repaid. This £297 would be invested by the Trustees of the Charity Commissioners (GCL) in the name of the Society.
>
> The Treasurer informed the Council that in accordance with the Resolution of the *Council* passed at the meeting held on 17th

November 1932 [*see* above], arrangements had now been made to borrow from Lt Col James Archibald Innes DSO and Humphrey Smith Esq, the sum of £13,000 at interest at the rate of 4¼ per cent per annum to be secured on permanent mortgage of Manson House.

The following Resolution was then proposed by Dr A T Stanton, seconded by Dr Manson-Bahr and carried unanimously:

> That the Trustees of the [RSTMH] be and they are hereby authorized to execute the necessary Instrument of Charge of the property known as Manson House, 26 Portland Place and 4a Cavendish Mews South in favour of Lt Col James Archibald Innes, DSO and Humphrey Smith Esq, to secure the re-payment of the said advance and interest.

The following Resolution was [then] proposed by Colonel W P MacArthur and seconded by Professor Warrington Yorke:

> That the Treasurer and Honorary Secretary of the [RSTMH] be authorized to instruct the Manager of the Westminster Bank Ltd, Cavendish Square to hand over to Messrs Pothecary and Barratt, Solicitors, of 73/76 King William Street, the Documents and Title relating to Manson House on payment to the Bank of £13,000.

On being put to the meeting the Resolution was carried unanimously.

The Treasurer explained that a further £1,000 was to be borrowed from the Westminster Bank to meet payments due during the latter part of the financial year. This would be repaid early in April when a considerable sum was received in annual subscriptions paid by Bankers Order.

In connection with this loan the following Resolution was proposed by Dr William Fletcher and seconded by Group-Capt H E Whittingham:

> That the Executive of the Society be at liberty to borrow from the Westminster Bank Ltd, any sums that may be required from time to time, but the total amount outstanding shall not at any time exceed the sum of £1,000 after repayment of £13,000 from the existing loan. Further that the President be

authorized to sign the Bank's form of charge covering £425.4.2. 3½ per cent *War Loan*: and £820, 2½ per cent *Consols* which [were] now inscribed in the books of [the] Bank of England in the names of William Hartigan MD, 10 Bond Court, Walbrook, EC4; Ernest Edward Austen DSO, British Museum (Natural History), South Kensington, SW7; George Carmichael Low MD, 86 Brook Street, W1. Trustees of this Society.

The Resolution on being put to the meeting was carried unanimously.

On **18 May**, *Council* was brought up to date with the state of the finances:

The Treasurer referred to the arrangements which had now been completed in regard to the £15,000 on loan. He stated that this was made up of three items:
1.   £1,000 very generously lent by Dr Manson-Bahr without interest
2.   £13,000 borrowed at 4¼ per cent on mortgage from Colonel Innes and Humphrey Smith Esq
3.   [The sum of £1,132 which had] been borrowed from the Westminster Bank.

This last £1,000 the Society had been able, early in April, to repay to the Westminster Bank and in view of this the following Resolution was proposed by Dr H S Stannus:

That the *Council* hereby cancels the instructions, relating to loans from the Westminster Bank passed at the last meeting of the *Council* ...

This Resolution was seconded by Dr Manson-Bahr and carried unanimously ....

The Treasurer stated that following the [by then] usual custom £660.5.6 available balance of the Accumulated Fund had been transferred to the Manson House Fund – the *Council* expressed its approval of this.

The following Resolution was then proposed by Dr Stanton:

That the balance of £92.8.9 being the excess of income over expenditure for the year ended 31st March 1933 be transferred to the Manson House Fund.

This Resolution was seconded by Professor Gordon Thomson and carried unanimously.

Gifts to the Society at the time of removal

On **21 June 1929** it had been recorded at a meeting of *Council* that Dr Manson-Bahr had donated some of Manson's early publications and photographs. Dr C M Wenyon had [also] written to the Chinese Maritime Custom's London Office regarding Manson's early papers. The president (Stephens) referred to the famous dispatch of Mr Joseph Chamberlain and asked if it was possible to secure a copy. A set of reports by Manson was received by the Society in December 1929. Ross and Bruce had also donated various papers and drawings.

Before the first *Ordinary* meeting at Manson House [*see above*], the following gifts were announced:

- A portrait of Sir Patrick Manson by Young Hunter from Mrs Manson-Bahr [*see* Figure 8.8].
- A library bookcase in memory of Sir Andrew Balfour [*see* below] from an anonymous donor.
- A lantern for the meetings from Dr Manson-Bahr.
- Chair, and various fittings for the Fellows room and cloakrooms from Mrs Hamilton Fairley.

At a *Council* meeting on **22 March 1932** attention was drawn to a gift from an artist – Mr Turnbull – of an etching of Manson, by himself. At the same meeting, the loan of carpets, etc by Mrs Fairley for the opening ceremony [*see above*] was also acknowledged.

Representation at other Society meetings

Dr Andrews consented to represent the Society at a *Veterinary* Congress (*see CM*, **20 February 1930**).

An *International Congress of Tropical Medicine* was to be held at Amsterdam in May 1932 and it was agreed by *Council* on **19 June** that the RSTMH should take part. Suitable subjects were considered to be:

- Sprue.
- Leptospirosis and typhus-like diseases.
- Diet deficiency and disease.

However, this meeting was later cancelled owing to the 'present financial situation'.

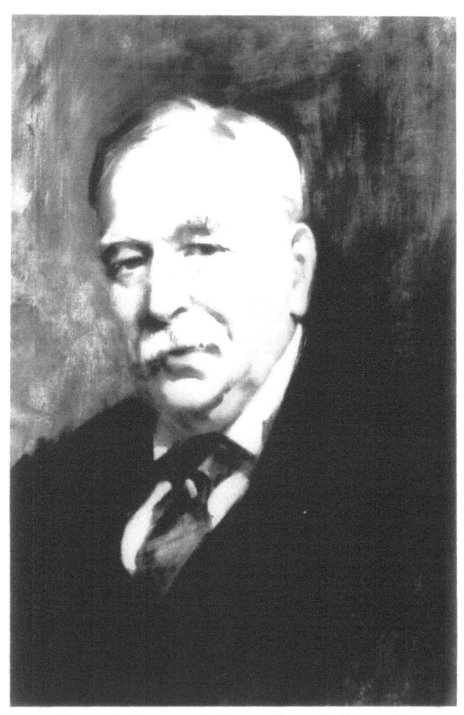

Figure 8.8: Portrait of Sir Patrick Manson (first president – in the Fellows' Room (*see* also: Figure 8.5c) of Manson House) (RSTMH archive).

At the *Annual Conference of the National Association for the prevention of Tuberculosis* in July 1930, Sir Harry Waters represented the Society (*see CM*, **19 June 1930**).

A delegate from the RSTMH was invited to attend the *British Association for the Advancement of Science* Annual Meeting in London in September 1931; at a meeting on **18 June 1931** it was agreed that it should be the president (Low).

Council on **21 May 1932** appointed Dr C A Hoare to represent the Society on a *Royal Microscopical Society* Committee to enquire into the 'standardization of biological stains and staining materials in England'.

Obituaries

The death of Sir Ronald Ross (the second president) was referred to by Low at a *Council* meeting on **20 October 1932**; the president reminded them that a mere few months previously (January), Ross had attended a *Council* meeting at Manson House. He also announced this to the *Ordinary* meeting in October.

Sir Andrew Balfour's death (he had committed suicide) was reported to *Council* at the *Ordinary* meeting on **19 February 1931**; a letter was sent to Lady Balfour referring to this 'tragedy which had overtaken tropical medicine and medical science generally'. The death of Prof W J R Simpson (the seventh president) was reported to *Council* on **15 October**. An original Honorary Fellow, Prof Kitasako, had also died. And at a meeting on **10 December**, the death of Sir David Bruce (the sixth president) was also announced. Dr Fülleborn (an Honorary Fellow) of Hamburg's death was reported to *Council* on **19 October 1933**.

The twenty-third to twenty-sixth annual reports

The number of Fellows increased significantly during Low's presidency – from 1,498 to 1,610 in March 1933.

The balance carried forward was £396 18s 1d and the Society's investments on 31 March 1930 stood at £5,257 12s 2d. However, finances during this period were overshadowed by the 'Manson House Fund', and the debt of £15,000 was emphasised in the 26th annual report.

References and Notes

1   **George Low** was born at Monifieth, Forfarshire and educated at St Andrew's and Edinburgh Universities. He joined Manson at the London School of Tropical Medicine (LSTM) in 1899. His first research project was demonstration of the mosquito-man component of the lymphatic filariasis life-cycle. In 1900, he took part in an expedition to the Roman Campagna which established beyond doubt, the mosquito transmission of *human* malaria. He subsequently undertook research in the West Indies (1901–1902) and headed the first Royal Society Sleeping Sickness expedition to Uganda (1902–3). Most of his subsequent career was spent in London, where he was a 'tower of strength' at the LSTM and later the Hospital for Tropical Diseases, Endsleigh Gardens. He was a joint founder and extremely valuable Fellow of the (Royal) Society of Tropical Medicine and Hygiene. *See*: Anonymous. Low, George Carmichael. *Munk's Roll* 4: 594–5; M Worboys. Low, George Carmichael (1872–1952) In: H C G Matthew, B Harrison (eds). *Oxford Dictionary of National Biography*. Oxford: Oxford University Press 2004: 34: 550–1; G C Cook. George Carmichael Low (1872–1952): an underrated pioneer, and contributor to the (Royal) Society of Tropical Medicine and Hygiene. *Tropical Medicine: an illustrated history of the pioneers*. London: Academic Press 2007: 127–43; G C Cook. *Caribbean Diseases: Doctor George Low's expedition in 1901–02*. Oxford: Radcliffe Publishing 2009: 229.

2   P H Manson-Bahr, A Alcock. *The Life and Work of Sir Patrick Manson*. London: Cassell and Co 1927: 273.

3   G C Cook. *Disease in the Merchant Navy: a history of the Seamen's Hospital Society*. Oxford: Radcliffe Publishing 2007: 630.

4   P Manson-Bahr. *History of the School of Tropical Medicine in London (1899–1949)*. London: H K Lewis 1956: 328.

5   P J Miller. 'Malaria Liverpool': an illustrated history of the Liverpool School of Tropical Medicine 1898–1998. Liverpool: Liverpool School of Tropical Medicine. 1998: 78.

6   G C Cook. *From the Greenwich Hulks to Old St Pancras: a history of tropical disease in London*. London: Athlone Press 1992: 338.

7   G C Low. The history of the foundation of the Society of Tropical Medicine and Hygiene. *Trans R Soc trop Med Hyg* 1928; 22: 197–202.

8   G C Cook. *Tropical Medicine: an illustrated history of the pioneers*. London: Academic Press 2007; 51–60, 81–102.

9   *Ibid*: 127–43.

10 *Ibid*: 103–13.

11 *Ibid*: 145–56.

12 *Ibid*: 163.

13 *Ibid*: 145–9, 157–65, 219–23.

14 A Crichton-Harris. Undercurrents on the Nile: the life of Dr John B Christopherson (1868–1955). *J med Biog* 2006; 14: 8–16.

15 G C Low. Presidential address. A retrospect of tropical medicine from 1894–1914. *Trans R Soc Trop Med Hyg* 1929–30; 23: 213–32.

16 *Op cit. See* Note 2 above.

17 H M Scott. Murray, David, seventh Viscount Stormont and second Earl of Mansfield (1727–1796). In: H C G Matthew, B Harrison (eds). *Oxford Dictionary of National Biography.* Oxford: Oxford University Press 2004; 39: 884–7.

18 G C Cook. Evolution: the art of survival. *Trans R Soc trop Med Hyg* 1994; 88: 4–18. [*See also:* Anonymous. *Royal Society of Tropical Medicine and Hygiene 1907–1957:* RSTMH archive].

19 W Byam, R G Archibald. *The practice of medicine in the tropics.* London: Henry Frowde & Hodder and Stoughton 1921–23 (3 vols): 2550.

20 Anonymous. Royal Society of Tropical Medicine and Hygiene: Opening of Manson House: The Prince of Wales on a vital Empire problem. *Times, Lond* 1932; 18 March.

Chapter 9

The mid 1930s: the Society safely installed in its own house

Presidential addresses – 1933–1937

The Society was now well installed at Manson House, although it would still be some years before the debt was paid off. There were, in the mid-1930s, two presidential addresses.

Rogers' address

The presidential address for 1933 (the first to take place at Manson House) was delivered on 19 October. Major-General Sir Leonard Rogers KCSI MD FRCP FRCS FRS IMS (Retd) (1868–1962)[1] (*see* Figure 9.1) spoke on **The methods and results of forecasting the incidence of cholera, smallpox and plague in India**:

> It was in 1895, nearly forty years ago [he began] that I commenced investigating the *relationship of climatic conditions to the seasonal incidence of disease in India* [author's italics]. I was then in charge of an Indian regiment on the plateau of Chota Nagpur and examined unstained blood films, as then recommended, of all my fever cases for malarial parasites and kept records of the rainfall and of the fluctuations in the ground-water levels, which varied over 30-ft in the different seasons, and I found a close relationship between the rise of the ground-water and the fever incidence[2] which was in accordance with the air-borne theory of infection then generally accepted [Ross's discoveries were not made until 1897–8]. Indeed I planned in the next rainy season to try to trap the organisms in the air during monsoon months, but fortunately was saved from what would doubtless have produced negative results by a transfer to Assam. I also plotted out the monthly fever cases in the regiments at Ranchi for twelve years with the rainfalls[3] and found that high monsoon rains were always

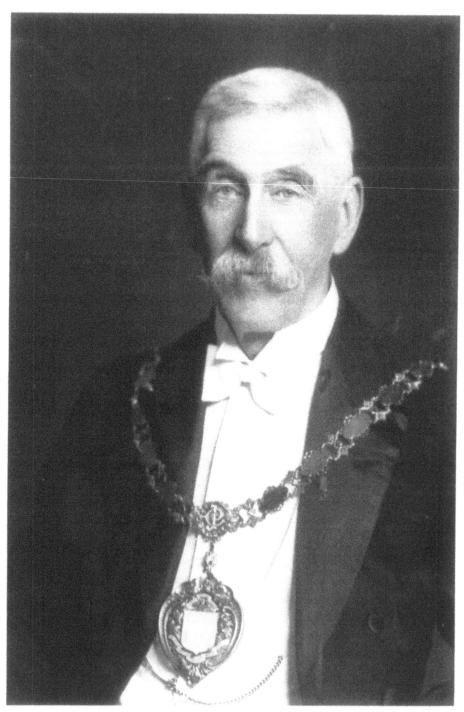

Figure 9.1: Sir Leonard Rogers FRCP FRCS FRS – the thirteenth president 1933–5 (reproduced courtesy the Wellcome Library, London).

followed by high *malaria* incidence. I also observed that the cases in the first five dry months of the year, which I had found to be all benign tertians [*Plasmodium vivax* infections], were in proportion to the incidence in the last six mainly wet months of the previous year, and in the four years in which the regiment was changed about January the cases were in proportion to those the incoming regiment had suffered from in their previous station, proving that they were at least mainly relapses and not new infections.

When studying in the following year the origin of the Assam *kala-azar* epidemic[4] I found that in the monsoon flooded deltaic region of Eastern Bengal bordering on Assam most *malaria* occurred in years of low rainfall, because there was a longer dangerous drying-up period before the minimum temperature fell to 60° C., which I noted was immediately followed by a rapid decrease in new malarial cases owing, as we now know, to such low temperatures inhibiting the mosquito stage development of the malarial parasites. It was the debilitating effect of *malaria* caused by a series of years of deficient rainfall in the seventies of last century that appears to have caused *kala-azar* to spread up the Assam Valley, and my prophesy that some such debilitating effect might start a new outbreak was fulfilled about twenty years later by the recrudescence of the disease in Assam following the 1918 influenza epidemic. Later, in 1910, in connection with the Mian Mir Commission[5] I showed that high *malaria* in the troops stationed there occurred after unusually heavy and late monsoon rains, and ... Christophers [*see* Chapter 11] not long after showed that the precise areas of epidemic *malaria* in the Punjab could be foreseen some weeks ahead by the incidence of the rain. Colonel C A Gill [1878–?] put this to practical use by sending travelling dispensaries to treat the cases in the affected areas he had foreseen, and Sir Gilbert Walker [1868–1958], in a paper read before the Royal Society of Arts a few years ago, showed a chart illustrating high *malaria* after high rainfall in the Punjab, which was less evident in recent years, probably due, as I pointed out in the discussion to such dispensary treatment. I mention those early investigations because they led to the more extensive recent work on similar lines that I am about to describe, which I was only able to undertake after retiring from India while I still had some remaining energy and was unable in this country to obtain the necessary clinical material to enable me to continue the combined clinical and pathological investigations which occupied me fully during my twenty years' researches in Calcutta.

The first subject that now attracted my attention was the world incidence of *leprosy*, which I mapped out in relationship to rainfall with the aid of data collected during three years' study of several decades' literature and published in [the] *Transactions*.[6] I found that all the high *leprosy* rates occurred in areas with high rainfall and humidity, mostly in tropical and sub-tropical countries, and this was confirmed in a remarkable manner by the distribution in India revealed by the census returns.

I was next interested in the close similarity in many epidemiological points between the two acid-fast bacillus diseases, *leprosy* and *tuberculosis*, and worked out a map of the distribution of pulmonary *tuberculosis* in India[7] with a view to studying its relationship to climatic conditions especially rainfall, humidity and the direction of the winds, the latter of which had been shown by Dr [W] Gordon of Exeter to influence its distribution in Devonshire. I had worked out the rainfall data of my *leprosy* map from a large volume of Indian meteorological data, but fortunately, when starting on further laborious tabulation of data in relation to tubercle, I found from the letterpress of the volume that an *Indian Atlas of Meteorology* was being prepared and I found this at the India Office with maps for each month giving all the data, including rainfall, temperatures, winds and both the relative and absolute humidity or aqueous vapour pressure, the last being the actual amount of moisture in the air measured by its pressure in terms of mercury, and together with the direction of the winds, this proved to be the key to the differences in the distribution of *leprosy* and *tuberculosis* in India, and of crucial importance in my subsequent investigations as will appear presently.

In the same year I completed maps of the distribution of *pneumonia* in India in relation to the diurnal variations of temperature, low absolute humidity and the direction of the winds[8] all tending to produce chills predisposing the *pneumonia* in the winter months in the north-west of India where the pneumonia rate is ten times that of South India and Burma.

Sir Leonard focused his first in-depth observations in India on the role of climatological factors on the incidence of *smallpox*. It was clear, he claimed that '*smallpox* epidemics in India as a rule follow very material deficiencies in the monsoon rainfalls and absolute humidities …'. In fact, the better the monsoon and the higher the humidity the lower was the *smallpox* prevalence rate. However, he admitted that this technique for forecasting had failed in the Punjab and North-West Frontier Province and also in 1933 in the Central Provinces where the rates had not correlated with humidity in the way he was suggesting.

This was followed by a detailed discussion of the use of these meteorological indices for forecasting *plague* incidence; his experience, he claimed, led him to the conclusion that *plague* forecasting could be accurately made using his criteria.

And lastly, *cholera* was dealt with in a similar manner:

> *Cholera* is the most important epidemic disease in India as it annually carries off about 200,000 people and for a century it was believed that the epidemics of *cholera* spread from the endemic area of Bengal all over India (as it did in 1817 to 1818) until my studies[9] established smaller endemic areas on the Bombay coast and in South-East Madras from which the disease also spreads. … True *cholera* vibrios are more delicate than those generally considered to be non-pathogenic, so are likely to disappear first, and the longer the low temperature inimical to them persists the longer will be the decline or absence of *cholera* in any area, both being longest in the Punjab. This appears to be the most likely explanation of [a] relationship between climatic conditions and the seasonal incidence of *cholera* in different parts of India.

And after this detailed discussion of *cholera* forecasting – based on personal observations – Sir Leonard concluded his lecture:

> It should therefore prove possible to foresee the danger spots and to take … steps in good time to mitigate the disastrous epidemics of previous years with short winter rains following low monsoon ones.
>
> I have for some years been advocating the extensive use of *cholera* preventive inoculation of pilgrims going to and from infected or endemic areas, and something has already been done by voluntary inoculation measures to limit the importation of

cholera by pilgrims returning to the Central Provinces, but present conditions have not yet permitted of compulsion in the matter, even when the danger was clearly evident and had actually been foreseen as in 1930.

Taken as a whole ... I may fairly conclude that a case has been made out for further trials of my methods of forecasting epidemic diseases in India, and that my labours have not been altogether in vain.[10]

In retrospect, there seems little doubt that Rogers over-emphasised the use of his methods for forecasting epidemics. Climatological factors in the forecasting of epidemics had appealed to medical practitioners in the days *before* general acceptance of the 'germ theory' of disease. Rogers in fact spanned the pre-'germ theory', and 'germ theory' eras. His careful measurements and observations would in fact have been far more valuable in the nineteenth than twentieth centuries!

Bagshawe's address

On 17 October 1935, Sir Arthur Bagshawe CMG MB DPH (1871–1950)[11] (*see* Figure 9.2) (the fourteenth president) addressed the Society on **Problems of health and disease of some small tropical islands:**

I have long thought [he began] that interesting results would emerge from a study of disease in small tropical islands, especially those diseases which require for their spread an intermediate non-vertebrate host. Many such islands have, or had ... infrequent contact with other islands or the larger land masses and few of the inhabitants leave them in the course of their lives; there is in fact little migration to and fro, so that *clinical* observations can be relied upon to give a picture of the diseases or parasites peculiar to the island in question. ...

The major part of this address was devoted to *malaria:*

I begin with the Lesser Antilles and with the small island [of] Barbados, which has lately come into the limelight owing to its invasion by *malaria*. ...

Within the memory of living man Barbados has been free from *malaria* but the reason was not apparent till Ross's great discovery

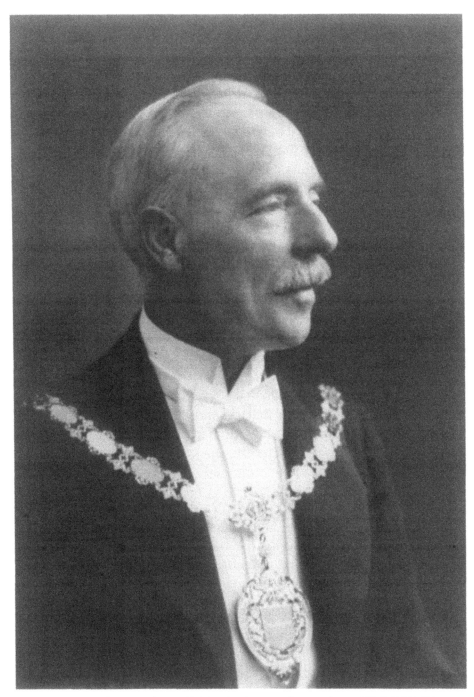

Figure 9.2: Sir Arthur Bagshawe CMG – the fourteenth president 1935–7 (RSTMH archive).

in 1897. In 1901 [George] Low[12] reported that *Anopheles* could not be found on the island, a conclusion in which the entomologist Lefroy concurred; Low noted the presence of a swamp 3 miles from Bridgetown, the capital, in which *Culex* was breeding. In a paper read at a meeting of the *British Medical Association* in 1913 Low attributed the absence of *anopheles* to the island's isolation ..., the distance of the above-mentioned swamp from town and harbour, and to the fact that vessels lay in an open roadstead a mile from the shore.[13] In the same year [Malcolm] Watson, fresh from his experience in Malaya, visited the island and attributed the absence of *anopheles* to the want of suitable breeding grounds;[14] it has since appeared that he was not far from the truth.

In 1927 a fever became epidemic in Barbados and was soon recognized to be *malaria*. ... From their distribution [Seagar] concluded that the *anopheles* had been there many months; they had probably been introduced by schooners carrying fruit, and ... it may be noted that Hanshell[15] on one occasion at Bridgetown found mosquitoes of undetermined genus in the forepeak of a schooner. ...

Some five years after the subsidence of the epidemic [in 1929–30], Haslam stated that malaria and *anopheles* were [both] absent. The mosquitoes had failed to make good their footing. Haslam[16] writes – 'Both indigenous malaria and its conveying mosquito continue to absent themselves from Barbados. The continued absence of *anopheles*, like its disappearance in 1930, must be attributed, along with many other advantages of this fortunate island, to the kindliness of Providence rather than to the sanitary efficiency of man ...'.

... there was [however] malaria in Barbados at the end of the 18th century, and in perusing the annual medical reports for the island I find the following [interesting] passage from the pen of Hutson[17], Public Health Inspector:-

> It is probable that malarial fevers occurred here as late as the middle of the eighteenth century at any rate. [William] Hillary [1697–1763], a pupil of Boerhaave, the celebrated Dutch physician, practised in the island from 1752 to 1758, and kept a careful monthly record of meteorological conditions and the various epidemics that occurred.[18] During these years he describes two or three outbreaks of malarial fever, and he says

'I must observe that intermitting fevers, especially quartans and tertians are very rarely or never seen in this island now, unless they are brought hither from some of the Leeward Islands, or some other places which are less cultivated, and not yet cleared of the woods; though it is said that they were more frequent here before this island was cleared of its wood and cultivated'.

Hillary's explanation of the gradual disappearance of malarial fever is probably correct, and a similar diminution of *malaria* resulting from cultivation has been seen in England and tropical countries, the haunts of the mosquito carriers of the disease being gradually abolished. The date of the last cases in Barbados is not known, and it is remarkable that the disease has never been re-introduced. It is interesting to observe that although the haunts of *anophelines* appear to have been destroyed by cultivation, there yet remain numerous collections of water, ponds, marshes, casual pools in the rainy season, which in other countries would be typical breeding places for *anophelines*, especially the permanent ponds more or less covered with water-lilies.

Hutson [*see* above]continues:-

Re-introduction would appear to be inevitable. For generations past numerous small craft of from 50 to 100 tons have traded between Barbados and adjacent malarious countries and colonies, going up the Orinoco to Bolivar, or lying in the rivers of British, French and Dutch Guiana, returning here with cargoes of firewood, charcoal, and such commodities, and discharging on the wharves of the inner harbour within the town. It is a matter of scientific interest to ascertain whether or not *anophelines* actually arrive in these vessels at Barbados. ...

Balfour's experience [*see* Chapter 7] at Khartoum has been that importation of *anophelines* by river boats and steamers, after mosquitos had been abolished in the town, was not infrequent.

I have consulted Hillary's book [*see* above] and feel that I am sufficiently familiar with the description of *malaria* by the old writers to be sure of the accuracy of the diagnosis; these old authors wrote a language which it is difficult for us ... to understand. He writes for instance:-

> The weather continuing to be wet and cool, several were seized with an irregular, ingeminated [redoubled or repeated], intermitting quotidian Fever; which at the first generally put on the appearance of a continual remitting Fever, but in two or three Days' time usually changed to an ingeminated Quotidian, with all the symptoms of that Fever, as usual in England. [After treatment, which is described] the Fever was generally carried quite off by a critical Sweat on the Seventh or Ninth Day; but in some few it came to intermit regularly after that time and then was soon cured by the *Cortex Peruv.*

If it be accepted that this was *malaria* it would appear probable that [it] is not new to Barbados, and that under exceptional conditions *A. albimanus* or another *anopheline* vector can temporarily establish itself, though this event is infrequent.

The subject of changes in the distribution of malaria, especially that of fresh invasions, is an interesting one ... Of the West Indies Hirsch[19] writes:-

> Among the West Indian islands those chiefly affected by malarial sickness are Cuba, Jamaica, San Domingo, Guadeloupe, Dominica, Martinique, St Lucia, Grenada, Tobago and Trinidad; while others such as Antigua, St Vincent and Barbados enjoy a relative immunity. ... In the Bahamas [it] is comparatively rare; in the Bermuda group it is almost unknown.

Instances are given of malaria in the two last groups in the sixties and seventies. Cameron[20] writes that [it] is now endemic in all the islands except Montserrat and St Kitts. Of the three islands described by Hirsch [*see above*] as relatively immune, in Antigua, according to McDonald[21] there is no question now of such immunity. In one year he saw 672 cases and states that it has a very serious effect on the quantity and quality of the labour supply; the predominant form is the subtertian [*P vivax*]. Here it would appear that conditions have altered since the period antecedent to Hirsch [*see above*] but whether an *anopheline* was introduced we have no means of knowing. In St Vincent the 1933 report records 14 deaths from *malaria*, and an earlier [one] mentions 532 notifications, so that this island also cannot now be described as relatively immune.

Bagshawe continued by relating a similar scenario in several other islands – although in some of them the available information was somewhat 'sketchy'. However, there seemed [he claimed] to be reliable data from Aldabra – one of the Seychelles islands where, although absent up to 1908, an outbreak of *malaria* coincided with the arrival of labourers from Madagascar, and lasted some ten months.[22] Although the island was free of *malaria* between 1908 and 1930, *Stegomyia* was present throughout. He then presented data from two other islands – Grand Comoro (north of Madagascar) and Rodrigues (365 miles from Mauritius). And then to the introduction of *A gambiae* into South America by a steamer or aircraft.[23] *Anopheles* was also absent from Polynesia despite the fact that 'for over one hundred years boats of all descriptions [had] passed freely ... 'from malarious islands.[24] ...'

Bagshawe then spoke of islands where 'an efficient malaria transmitter' was known to be present, but 'no indigenous disease [resulted]':

> Such in the West Indies are the isles of St Croix or Santa Cruz in the Virgin Isles ... and [also] St Barthelemy. ... Lowman[25] tells us that *A albimanus* was found in St Croix ... in a careful survey by Lieut Hayes, many infected Porto Ricans come in but the island is 'practically *malaria*-free'. St Barthelemy, Tara[26] states, has a population of 2,384, almost entirely white. The predominant insect is *A albimanus*, and infected persons come in from Guadeloupe. Nevertheless, of 400 children examined in two successive years only four had splenic enlargement, and when the author is called to a case of *malaria* it has nearly always been contracted in Guadeloupe. It seems improbable that there is any indigenous malaria. No doubt the absence could be explained if we knew all the facts. One of the chief industries of St Croix is ... cattle raising and it seems possible that the cattle provide blood for the *anopheles* but *A albimanus* is a notorious transmitter, its blood-thirstiness is generally remarked and it is described in the Canal Zone as semi-domesticated, occurring everywhere about houses and villages.

On *filariasis*, Bagshawe had this to say:

> I started with Barbados, and will now add a few words about *filariasis* in that island though the facts are fairly well known. Barbados was formerly notorious for elephantiasis, as the name

'Barbardos leg' indicates. [He then quoted Low's results for infection in 1901.[27]] But since then, the situation had improved markedly. … the tendency [Bagshawe concluded was] to attribute [this] improvement to measures of sanitation rather than to more natural if obscure causes. Siler attributed the decrease of elephantiasis to measures against *Stegomyia fasciata* initiated in 1908, the result of which again would be reduction of all domestic mosquitoes.[28] Whatever be the reason manifestations of filariasis are not infrequent in Barbados. Haslam writes:- 'Filariasis and filarial elephantiasis figure very inconspicuously in medical experience in Barbados now-a-days'.[29]

Of another West Indian island, Grenada, Low said that with apparently ideal conditions of climate and intermediaries filarial infection was practically non-existent.[30] And MacDonald stated that *Culex fatigans* was common, but filariasis 'in an acute form' was unknown; no microfilariae were found in 1,000 blood smears. [31] Later reports … confirm these observations.

And 'rectal *schistosomiasis*', which he considered was 'of particular interest in the West Indies':

Thanks to [both] Cameron and Jones we have a fairly complete account of [*Schistosoma mansoni infection*] in the island of St Kitts. [32] Cameron visited the island in 1928 and studied the schistosome infection reported by Jones. He found it to be restricted to the area of two permanent streams as had been shown in 1923 by Muench, who made the important discovery that the infection is shared by monkeys. … *Cercopithecus sabaeus*[33] the West African green monkey, [which] were introduced long ago as pets; and during the French wars escaped to the mountains and multiplied greatly, living in packs. Five out of seven [of them] were infected with *S mansoni* and one had severe dysentery. … the same monkey is found in Nevis, Grenada and Barbados, but fortunately *S mansoni* is not present in these islands. … Since Cameron's article I have seen no reference to his observations and I call attention to them because they seem of considerable interest and importance. … Other West Indian islands in which rectal schistosomiasis is found are St Martin, Antigua, Montserrat, Guadeloupe, Martinique and St Lucia. Manson's first patient (in 1902) is believed to have come from Antigua. The infection seems to be quite common in the two French islands, and ... is by no means always manifested by symptoms. ...

There can be little doubt [according to] Stitt[34] that schisto-somiasis was one of the diseases introduced from Africa with cargoes of slaves [see Chapter 11 – Scott]. Quoting Butler he writes:- 'It is reasonable to think that during 292 years of slave trade between 1512 and 1804 every type of disease that the continent of Africa might boast of was brought to the West Indies.' We must assume that the bladder infection [S haematobium] was also introduced but died out as did sleeping sickness for want of a suitable intermediary host.

Now reference to an ancient infection (a macro parasite) – Guinea-worm disease, or *dracontiasis*:

which [also] came into the West Indies with the African slaves. Hirsch writes:

'According to the ... the medical authorities for Guiana, Brazil and the West Indies ... *dracunculus* was imported into these countries ... by negroes from the West Coast of Africa; and it has almost disappeared again from them, excepting at one or two small centres since the importation of negroes has ceased. One of these ... is the island of Curaçao ... in which it is said there are still cases of *dracontiasis* occurring somewhat frequently among the native population'.[35]

... In America the guinea-worm is unknown, except in persons who have had communication with Africa or other parts where it is indigenous. ... Curaçoa is the only locality ... offering an apparent exception to this fact, which it would be highly desirable to ascertain the real state of in this instance.

... Pop, writing from Curaçao in 1859, however, makes no mention of the disease. At first sight it seems remarkable that guinea-worm should have been reported in Curaçao as late as the 40's for the slave trade came officially to an end early in the 19th century. However, Sir Harry Johnston [1858–1927] states that, between 1828 and 1878, 50,000 negroes were released from slave ships off the West Coast of Africa by the British Navy.[36] We may assume that at least as many slave ships got away undetected, so that Africans may well have been received in the Dutch West Indies as late as 1845. When the supply of slaves ceased guinea-worm disappeared, for its invertebrate host is absent. This is a sufficient explanation and one that should serve for the absence of guinea-worm from the Dutch East Indies also. However, it does not. Brug tells us that infected persons from India and Arabia have been coming in for centuries and *Cyclops leuckarti* is present, but guinea-worm infestation is very rare.[37]

... The freedom of the archipelago from guinea-worm is ... attributed to the preference of the inhabitants for running water for drinking, ... and Roubaud is quoted as stating that where in French West Africa the natives drink running water guinea-worm cases are absent – a good instance of the effect of native custom in determining the presence or absence of a disease.[38] In a book [written] by Richard Towne ... over 200 years ago, I find: 'The countries where this Distemper is discovered, are very hot and sultry, liable to great Droughts; and the Inhabitants make use of stagnatory corrupted Water, in which it is very probable that the ova of these Animalculae [guinea-worms] may be contained'.[39]

And finally, Bagshawe dwelt on a contemporary theme at the time of his lecture – *ie*, survival of the white race in the tropics:

... There is a small island not far from St Kitts in which white people have maintained not only purity of race but also their physical and mental vigour for 250 years and only now ... are being crowded out by their black neighbours. Price has written a valuable paper on the subject[40] ...

The history of ... colonization [of the Dutch island of Saba] is obscure, but it appears to have been settled from the neighbouring island [of] Statia before the middle of the 17th century by private persons under concessions from the Dutch West Indian Company. ... the whites [from 1665] hailed chiefly from the British Isles. The island is not easy of access, there are two regular landings where loads are carried up rugged paths ... by men and donkeys to the lowest and principal settlement [which is] at 800 feet. ... The total population is [now] 1,447 persons, but according to the *Encyclopaedia Britannica* it was, in 1911, 2,387. The people are mixed, white and black, but one cliff village, at 1,660 feet, of 231 persons is almost entirely white. Inbreeding among the whites is considerable but there is no intermarriage with the blacks. [However] inbreeding has not destroyed fertility, stamina or ability.

... The white Sabans are agriculturalists, and sturdy workers, carrying loads up gradients which no donkey could manage. ... during the Great War [1914–18] no less than 95 officers and one quartermaster of the United States Navy were Saban born. ... The purity of the race is an uncontested fact. The women are said to be the handsomest of the West Indians [and] distinguished by their slimness and fresh colour ... but Price tells us that the health of the women is much inferior to that of the men because from the traditions of the slave days they cannot work in the fields, nor become housekeepers, nurses or domestic servants; they spend their time indoors making Spanish lace. Price was favourably impressed with the white school children who were alert, well-dressed and clean.

... There is no *malaria* [in Saba] and [only a] 'few filarial or other tropical affections' and there is no trace of hookworm. Many white Sabans live to a great age. Price points to the great disproportion between the women and men – the census of 1932 showed 342 men, 655 women, 233 boys and 219 girls; ... 65 per cent [of the adults] were female, and 34 per cent male. ... [The young men] go abroad to increase the family resources and spend only brief periods in the island, which leads to what Price calls 'economic birth control'.

Between 1860 and 1920 two blows ruined the white settlers. The first was the emancipation of the 700 Saban slaves, after which production became difficult and the price of labour rose. The second ... was the change from sails to steam. Most of the energetic young men were drawn away to New York and other centres where they secured positions as commanders and officers of steamers. Thus the island lost her slaves, schooners and vigorous young people, so that the white population to-day consists largely of aged persons.

... Saba is clearly turning coloured as are almost all the islands and borderlands of the Caribbean. White settlers cannot compete with prolific negro families in which men, women and children are all workers [who are] prepared to accept a lower standard of life than the white. Scientific medicine is hastening the process by improving the vital statistics of coloured people. At present white and coloured are in equal numbers.

The conclusion reached by Price from his survey is that [:] whites can retain a fair standard for generations in the trade-wind tropics if the location is free from the worst forms of *tropical disease* and if the economic return is adequate and the community prepared to undertake hard physical work, but eventually such a community will fall before the economic competition of a coloured people. It seems a sad pity that such a race should disappear, or at least be scattered. The negro's 'disregard of sanitation, his miserable cabins, his dirt and carelessness and his neglect of the good 'white' houses he so frequently occupies ... contrast sadly with the standards of the people he is supplanting'.[41]

The Society in the mid-1930s

Honorary Fellows

Professor Richard P Strong (USA) was unanimously elected by *Council* in June 1936; he had contributed 'important work in *tropical medicine* since about 1903 in the Philippine Islands'. He was also, in fact, to give the first *Chadwick Lecture* on **21 January 1937** on '*Onchoceriasis in Central America and Africa*'. Professor Nocht of Hamburg was also made an Honorary Fellow on 21 October 1937, and a letter of congratulations was later sent to him on 4 November 1937 to mark his 80th birthday.

Ordinary meetings

Table 9.1 summarises the subjects and speakers at *Ordinary* meetings in the mid-1930s; the table includes the two presidential addresses (*see above*); that by S P James is recorded in Chapter 10.

Interest in intestinal absorption and the 'steatorrhoeas' was demonstrated at an *Ordinary* meeting in May 1936, when the speakers were:

> Dr N Hamilton Fairley FRCP of the HTD on '*Tropical sprue with special reference to Intestinal Absorption*', and C Wallace Ross of Birmingham on '*Intestinal Absorption in Coeliac Disease – with some remarks on the effect of Liver Extract upon carbohydrate metabolism*'.

Table 9.1: Communications at *Ordinary* meetings in the mid-1930s

Date	Subject	Speaker
1934		
18 January	Immunisation against yellow fever	G M Findlay
15 February	Erythrocyte regeneration	A E Boycott
	Treatment of non-tropical anaemias	J M (later Dame Janet) Vaughan
	Treatment of tropical anaemias	N H Fairley
17 May	Progress in leptospirosis	W Schüffner
21 June (27th AGM)	*Anopheles maculipennis*	L W Hackett
18 October	Medical services in Britain and abroad	W W Jameson
13 December	Electric charge and immunity	J C Broom
1935		
17 January	Chemotherapy and biological problems	Warrington Yorke, F Murgatroyd
21 February	Medical services in the Chaco War	J W Lindsay
16 May	Hot environments and *Homo sapiens*	D H K Lee
20 June (28th AGM)	Typhus fevers	J Megaw, W Fletcher, A Felix
17 October	Disease in tropical islands (*presidential address*)	A G Bagshawe
21 November	Rabies in bats in Trinidad	E de Verteuil
1936		
16 January	Malaria in Ceylon, 1934–5	C A Gill
20 February	Typhus-like fevers in Malaya	R Lewthwaite
21 May	Intestinal absorption in Tropical Sprue	N H Fairley
	Intestinal absorption in Coeliac Disease	C W Ross
18 June (29th AGM)	Yaws in Australian aborigines	C J Hackett
15 October	Human trypanosomes in Africa	H L Duke
10 December	Kala-azar in Sudan	Sir Robert Archibald, H Mansour
1937		
21 January	Onchoceriasis in Central America & Africa	R P Strong
18 February	Sigmoidoscopy in Tropical practice	P Manson-Bahr, A S Biggam
20 May	Bejel, the syphilis of the Euphrates Arab	E H Hudson
17 June (30th AGM)	Blackwater fever in Macedonia	H Foy, A Kondi
	Pseudo-methaemoglobin in blackwater fever	N H Fairley, R J Blomfield
21 October	Malaria – since 1914–18 War (*presidential address*) (see Chapter 10)	S P James
9 December	Leprosy epidemiology and control	E Muir
	Tuberculoid leprosy	W Hughes

Amongst the discussants at that meeting were: Dr H P (later Sir Harold) Himsworth FRS and Dr (Later Dame) Janet Vaughan.

Finances

The Society's finances were not assisted by a disappointing response to the *Manson House Fund* Appeal (*see* Chapter 8); therefore a substantial debt remained to be paid off. Bagshawe (knighted in June 1933) continued for a while as a successful Hon Treasurer. For example, he asked Fellows at the 26th AGM to help in letting out the Hall for meetings and social functions. However, on **19 October 1933**, he announced that recent donations to the *House Fund* amounted to a mere £40. Good news though was that the *British Society for the Study of Orthodontics* was happy with their deal (*ie* use of the Hall and *Council* room seven times annually), and wished to continue for the next 21 (later reduced to seven) years, at a rent of £50 per annum. He was also able to tell *Council* on **15 February 1934**, that Mr G P Joseph wished to continue renting the maisonette and garage at £820 per annum; the Society would continue paying rates and taxes, but Joseph was responsible for interior decorations and repairs. This income would more than cover both the mortgage interest (£552 10s) and the Charity Commissioners demand that £297 be set aside each year.

At a *Council* meeting on **14 December 1933**:

> The Treasurer explained that it would be necessary between the present date and 31st March [1934] to borrow certain sums from the Bank, which would be re-paid after receipt of the annual subscriptions at the beginning of the financial year on April 1st. [The previous] year a total of £1000 [had been] borrowed in this way but he hoped that this year £500 would suffice. He said that the Secretary had spoken to the Manager of the Westminster Bank and he had very kindly agreed to allow the Society to borrow up to £500 at 4½ per cent, in the form of an unsecured overdraft.
>
> [Bagshawe] then asked the *Council* to authorize this loan by passing the following resolution:
>
>> That the Society be at liberty to borrow from the Westminster Bank any sums that may be required from time to time, but the total amount outstanding shall not at any time exceed £500.
>
> The Treasurer's proposal was seconded by Dr Stanton and carried unanimously.

On **18 January 1934** he announced donations of only £76 to the *House Fund*; the total received in rents however, was more than sufficient [however] to cover the interest on the mortgage. In May, the president (Rogers) told of several donations to the *House Fund*, including a further £100 from Manson-Bahr. At that meeting, Bagshawe referred to the annual payment of £297 – towards redemption of the £13,000 mortgage; the first payment would be made in June 1934.

As was now customary, on **21 June** of that year, the excess of income over expenditure (£8 11s 2d) was transferred to the Manson House Fund. Also at that meeting, it was announced that Mrs Hill-Jones (a relation of Miss Wenyon) had left £500 to Manson House in her Will. It was also announced in October that total donations for the previous six-month period amounted to £649, and that £500 had been repaid to Manson-Bahr; furthermore, the first instalment of £297 for redemption of the mortgage had been paid. Sums received for letting the hall were 'steadily increasing', and further donations of £25 from the Lloyd Triestino Company of Bombay, and 10 guineas from Sir John Megaw were announced in November.

Excess of income over expenditure amounted to £476 5s 8d for the year ended 31 March 1935, and as usual this was transferred to the *House Fund*. During the year, no less than £967 had in fact been made available for reduction of the debt on Manson House. The retiring president (Rogers) later gave £10 to the *House Fund* – used for a new bookcase – in June 1935.

On **17 October 1935** Dr Oswald Marriott (who had taken over the Treasurership from Bagshawe, who was now president) reported that the final £500 had been repaid to Manson-Bahr, and that there was a 'balance in hand' of no less than £920.

In November 1932, *Council* had agreed that a British Broadcasting Corporation (BBC) appeal on behalf of the Society was a good idea, provided 'a suitable speaker could be obtained'. However, the minutes do not contain further mention of this matter!

Expenditure of 'a sum not exceeding £250' was authorised by *Council* to redecorate Manson House, on **19 March 1936**. Continued exemption from rates on Manson House had been granted by the St Marylebone Borough Council – *see CM*, 16 January 1936.

Tenants

Owing to its continuing unsatisfactory financial position, the Society was, until the disposal of Manson House in 2004, largely dependent on tenants. *Council* was informed on **19 January 1933** that Joseph had agreed to continue his tenancy of the maisonette for a further year – from September 1933 at an increased rent of £50. This event must have been good news. Another 'tenant' was the medico-legal Society which had agreed to pay £35 annually for the use of the library and hall (*see CM*, 17 October 1935).

The Library

By 1935, there seems to have been a major problem with lack of library shelf-space. The *Council* minute of **21 February 1935**, for example, reads:

> It was reported that the Library Committee had met to consider which of the various journals received regularly, it was desirable to keep permanently. The Committee [in fact] recommended that in addition to eleven already retained, it would be desirable to keep the following twelve journals, making 23 in all:
>
> 1. *Archives de l'Institut Pasteur d'algerie*
> 2.   "   "   "   *de Tunis*
> 3.   "   "   "   *de l'Indochine*
> 4. *Annales de la Société Belge de Méd Tropicale*
> 5. *Chinese Medical Journal*
> 6. *Indian Journal of Medical Research*
> 7.   "   "   "   "   *Memoirs*
> 8. *Indian Medical Gazette*
> 9. *International Journal of Leprosy*
> 10. *Kenya Med Jl*, [now *East African Med Jl*]
> 11. *Rivista di Malarialogia*
> 12 *Records of the Malaria Survey of India*
>
> After ... discussion the *Council* accepted [these] recommendations ... and decided to keep the additional twelve journals and to continue to keep, as had been done for some years, the following eleven journals also received as exchanges:
>
> 1. *Tropical Diseases Bulletin*
> 2. *Bulletin of Hygiene*
> 3. *Annals of Tropical Medicine & Parasitology*
> 4. *Philippine Journal of Science*
> 5. *Journal of Tropical Medicine & Hygiene*

6. *Veterinary Bulletin*
7. *Memorias do Instituto Oswaldo Cruz*
8. *Proc Royal Soc Med Section of Trop Med & Parasitology*
9. *American Journal Trop Med*
10. *Bulletin de la Société Path Exotique*
11. *Arch für Schiffs und Tropen Hygiene*

It was reported that in addition to these journals three copies of each volume of the *Transactions* and of each year book were bound annually. It was also agreed that upon the completion of each volume the previous [one] should no longer be kept, it being left to the officers of the Society to dispose of them by sale or otherwise.

At the same meeting Dr H H (later Sir Harold) Scott (to become the seventeenth president) was unanimously elected Honorary Librarian; in order to reduce the volume of 'dead-wood' he (and his Sub-Committee) removed a total of 151 'obsolete' volumes.

Secretarial salary

The question of the Secretary's salary was a subject for recurrent discussion in the 1930s; thus, at a *Council* meeting on **15 March 1934**:

The Hon Treasurer [now Marriott] said that now that a lease had been signed by the tenant of the maisonette and the Society's financial stability was [therefore] assured for [several] years the salary of the Secretary should be augmented. He pointed out that the income from Fellows' subscriptions had risen from £557 in 1921 (when Miss Wenyon was appointed), to £2388 in 1933. The sum spent on secretarial work had increased from £117 to £658: he did not think the latter sum at all excessive. Miss Wenyon had since 1930 received [a] salary at the rate of £350 per annum and a contribution of £35 to a pension scheme (to which she herself added £17.10 per annum) which at age 60 would provide a pension of £50=11=4. This arrangement he did not propose to disturb. Miss Wenyon was, in his opinion, an outstandingly efficient Secretary, excellent in all branches of her work. By her keenness and enterprise the Society's expenses were kept down while it was enabled to get the best value for its money. For these reasons, her value to the Society, her increased responsibilities in the management of Manson House and her experience, he proposed that as from April 1st 1934 her salary be increased to £400 per annum. Dr Stanton and Dr Fairley endorsed the Treasurer's remarks which were well received by the *Council*. The proposal was put from the Chair and … approved with unanimity.

Gifts to the Society in its permanent house

Now that the Society was well installed at Manson House, gifts were both welcome and plentiful. Not before or since has the RSTMH received so many presents as it did during this period. *Council* on **19 January 1933** thanked Mrs Fairley for her gift of a Persian Runner for the stairway. At a *Council* meeting in May, Manson-Bahr presented the diary kept by Sir Patrick Manson in China (now in Wellcome House – 183 Euston Road), together with 'some interesting photographs, papers and slides'. At the same meeting it was reported that Mrs Alcock (widow of Col A W Alcock FRS, a former vice-president, whose death was reported on 18 May 1933) had given three early volumes of *Transactions* (I, II and III) which were apparently very valuable. 'The History of Chinese Medicine' by K C Wong, and 'Recent Advances in Chemotherapy' by G W M Findlay, were also presented to the library on **18 October 1934**. Mrs Sidebotham donated three Persian rugs for the Library (*see CM*, 19 October).

On **16 November**, it was announced that the *Chadwick Trust* had donated £250 to the RSTMH for 'the encouragement of the study of *sanitary science*'; this should, they wrote, take the form of an annual prize or otherwise 'on terms to be arranged between the Trustees and the Society'. A great deal of discussion on the best use of the interest on this gift took place at a meeting of *Council* on 14 December; as there was no uniformity of opinion, the president (Rogers) decided to discuss the matter with the Officers and Chairman of the Chadwick Trust. After further discussion in January 1934, *Council* unanimously carried a resolution:

> That the sum of £250 presented to the Society by the Chadwick Trustees be devoted to the foundation of [a] Lectureship on subjects connected with *tropical medicine* and *hygiene*.

A later Council meeting (15 March 1934) decided that this should be entitled: *The RSTMH Chadwick Lecture*.

On 14 December 1933 Dr H H Scott (*see above*) presented a copy of *'The Child of Ocean'* by Sir Ronald Ross. Prof J W W Stephens presented: *'In exile'* and *'Fables and satires'* also by Ross, and Dr Fairley several volumes of the *Tropical Veterinary Bulletin* (*see CM*, **17 January 1934**). Dr R Row of Bombay presented a bound volume of personal reprints from 1898–1935. Dr Aranju of Bengal also presented a book for the library, and Col Crawford (Historian of the Indian Medical Service [IMS]) gave a collection of 'interesting and valuable books' written by officers of the IMS. Major (later General Sir) Neil Cantlie presented a photograph of Sir James Cantlie (his father) and Lady Leishman a photograph of her late husband (Sir William Leishman).

Council was informed on **16 January 1936** that Sir Robert Armstrong Jones (through the 'instrumentality of Sir Leonard Rogers') had presented, to the Society, five albums of photographs collected by his brother Col Lloyd Jones of the IMS. Further gifts to the library were announced by Scott at meetings on 16 January, 18 June, 1936 and 18 February 1937, and more were announced on 21 October and 18 November 1937; 19 May and 13 October 1938; and 19 January, 16 February, 15 June and 29 June 1939. A library bookcase was presented by Low (*see CM*, 21 October 1937). On 17 June 1937, Professor J W W Stephens presented a copy of his new book on *'blackwater fever'*, and at the same meeting, the retiring president (Bagshawe) presented a photograph of himself. An electric clock 'of Cromwellian design' for the Fellows Room was presented by Dr H M Shelley – the local Secretary for Nyasaland (*see CM*, 18 November). At a meeting of *Council* on **1 July**, the Will of Dr A S Burgess (*see above*), a Fellow since 1913 and formerly of the Colonial Medical Service (Gold Coast) had been presented; this was however, a complicated matter, but it was felt that the Society 'should eventually benefit to the tune of about £10,000'. A notable gift on **29 June 1939** was one, also from Scott – a copy of his two-volume work on *'A History of Tropical Medicine'*.

Dinners and receptions

Doubt about the level of interest in dinners had been aired on **16 January 1936**; when last held in 1930 only 58 Fellows and 70 guests had attended. It was agreed to circularise all Fellows in England in an attempt to decide whether a dinner would be welcomed or not. Intention to hold a dinner in 1936 was later scrapped owing to the recent death of the Society's Patron – King George V.

On **19 May 1938**, a *Council* minute indicates that the Colonial Office (Corona Club) Dinner was planned for the same day as the Society's AGM; this was regarded as an unfortunate clash of events.

Eighty-four Fellows and guests apparently attended an informal reception on 21 January 1937.

On 15 February 1934 *Council had* agreed to arrange a conversazione on 31 May of that year at Manson House – tickets were priced at 5s each; this was apparently a great success, about 120 Fellows and guests being received by the president and Lady Rogers.

Relationship with other societies

At the *Council* meeting on **16 February 1933**: Major E E Austen had been appointed to represent the Society at the *Entomological Society's* Centenary on 3–4 May; however, no action was taken regarding invitations to the *Royal Sanitary Institute* Congress, or that of the *Royal Institute of Public Health.*

Dr Balfour Kirk suggested to *Council* on **18 May** that the RSTMH should become affiliated to the *Fellowship of Medicine* (FM)[42] – which would only cost one guinea, and entitle Fellows to a reduction in fees for lectures. It was considered that 'such an affiliation was hardly appropriate for the Society'. However, on 19 October *Council* decided that affiliation with the FM would in fact be in the interest of both sides; both the president (Rogers) and Vice-president (Vice Admiral Sir Reginald Bond) testified to the useful work of the FM. Prof W W (later Sir Wilson) Jameson (at that time a member of *Council*) added that 'later on the opening of the new Postgraduate School might necessitate some adjustment'; affiliation was nevertheless 'a good idea', and Fellows could claim a reduction on fees for lectures arranged by the FM.

Council gave its approval for a lecture by a South-American scientist on a *tropical medicine* subject under the auspices of the *Ibero-American Institute of Great Britain* to take place at Manson House. Both the RSTMH and the RSM were approached regarding the visit of a Brazilian scientist; Prof Carlos Chagas would have been highly suitable, but he unfortunately had recently died. A dialogue continued, but there seems to have been a great deal of doubt as to whether or not the scientist considered was interested in *tropical* medicine! The RSM, it was decided, should however be left in command; and they later appointed Dr Torres to give a Lloyd Roberts lecture on 28 November 1934 on the 'pathology of Alastrim'.

On 17 May 1934, Dr G Basil Price was appointed to represent the Society at the Congress of the *National Association for the Prevention of Tuberculosis* on 14–15 June. The 21st annual conference of that association was held at Southport from 27–29 June 1935; it was left to the Hon Secretaries to identify a suitable delegate. Dr H G Earle represented the Society at the 9th Congress of the *Far Eastern Association of Tropical Medicine* at Nanking, China from 1–7 October 1934. Dr H S Stannus was invited on 15 March 1935 to represent the Society at the Congress of *Anthropological and Ethnological Sciences* the following July.

Dr A J R O'Brien of the Colonial Office represented the Society at the 1936 Congress of the *Royal Sanitary Institute;* he again undertook this task the following year, on 12–17 July. The 1937 Annual Conference of the *National Association for the prevention of Tuberculosis* was held in Bristol from 1–3 July; the Honorary Secretaries were left to decide the RSTMH's delegate.

Transactions

At a *Council* meeting on **8 December 1932**:

> A general discussion took place on the advisability of laboratory technicians' names appearing in the *Transactions* as the sole or joint authors of papers – this arose as a result of the following resolution proposed by Dr [H M] Hanschell and seconded by Mr [A T] Stanton:
>
>> That original papers, and laboratory reports by *laboratory technicians*, either as sole or as joint authors, may be accepted for publication in the Society's *Transactions:* provided that the Pathologist under whom the *technician* works consents to publication. While each contribution shall be considered on its merits, preference shall be given to those by *technicians* who are Registered members of the Pathological and Bacteriological Laboratory Assistants' Association.
>
> The result of the discussion was that it was felt that, in special cases, where exceptional merit had been displayed such authorship should be admitted; but that it would be highly inadvisable for it to become a general rule for the names of *laboratory technicians* to be placed at the head of papers as joint or sole authors. It was [also] noted that in the past such authorship had been admitted

in certain cases and it was thought that as in the future the same thing would probably occur again, the passing of any resolution was hardly necessary. It was finally agreed not to put the resolution to the meeting and the proposer of the resolution expressed himself as satisfied with the discussion.

On **18 May 1933**, Manson-Bahr suggested to *Council* that he 'had [formed] an impression that *clinical* papers were *not* welcomed by the Editors of *Transactions*'. However, the outcome of this comment is unclear!

Deaths and obituaries

Council decided on **19 January 1933** to 'continue the [current] practice of publishing obituaries only in special cases such as past presidents and Honorary Fellows'.

The death of Sir Havelock Charles, the fourth president, was announced at a *Council* meeting on 15 November 1934. Dr Theobald Smith's death was announced to *Council* the following month.

A plaque at the LSHTM to commemorate Sir William Simpson was announced in 1935 (*see CM*, 17 January 1935).

Council was informed in January 1936 that Dr Hockett had agreed to write an obituary of Professor Marchiafava – an Honorary Fellow. October 1936 was a particularly *bad* month for mortality; deaths of two more *Honorary Fellows* – Sir Arnold Theiler and Sir Henry Wellcome, and also Dr William Hartigan – the Society's first Treasurer, and for many years a Trustee, were announced. These deaths were all reported to both *Council* and an *Ordinary* meeting on 15 October 1936. Hartigan was replaced as a Trustee in November by Sir Thomas Stanton. The death of Sir Austen Chamberlain KG (an Honorary Fellow since 1932) was announced by the president (Bagshawe) on **18 March 1937**.

Royal Matters

The president (Bagshawe) referred on **20 February 1936** (when addressing both *Council* and the *Ordinary* meeting) to the death of the Patron (since 1923) King George V; a letter, signed by himself, had already been sent to King Edward VIII (and subsequently acknowledged by the Home Secretary) who had been proclaimed King on 22 January 1936, and it was hoped that he (a Vice-Patron since 1932, when he had officially opened Manson House as the Prince of Wales) would accept the patronage. It was announced (to both *Council* and an *Ordinary* meeting) on 21 May that he had indeed accepted. At a *Council* meeting on **21 January 1937**, the president read a memorandum received from the *Keeper of the Privy Purse* intimating that the new sovereign (King George VI) intended continuing patroncies granted by Edward VIII (who had abdicated on 10 December 1936).

A loyal address was later sent to King George VI on the occasion of his coronation on 12 May 1937; an acknowledgement (with thanks) was duly received from the Home Secretary, Sir John Simon.

The twenty-seventh to thirtieth annual reports

The number of Fellows 'on the register' increased from 1,622 to 1,682 during these four years.

The financial position of the Society continued to be satisfactory. The credit balance was £8 11s 2d for the year ended 31 March 1934, but that for the years ending 31 March 1935, 1936 and 1937 amounted to £476, £607 and £271 respectively. However, the remaining debt on Manson House continued to be a source of concern.

During this period, Bagshawe had stepped down as Treasurer after ten years' service (*see* above) and was succeeded by Oswald Marriott.

References and Notes

1   **Leonard Rogers** received his medical education at St Mary's Hospital, London, and after qualification joined the Indian Medical Service. He served as a pathologist at Calcutta (now Kolkata) from 1893 until 1920. He founded the School of Tropical Medicine there. Returning to London, he became extra physician to the Hospital for Tropical Diseases and also served on several committees. See: G McRobert, H J Power. Rogers, Sir Leonard (1868–1962). In: H C G Matthew, B Harrison (eds). *Oxford Dictionary of National Biography.* Oxford: Oxford University Press 2004; 47: 572–4; G C Cook. Leonard Rogers (1868–1962): the diseases of Bengal, and the founding of the Calcutta School of Tropical Medicine. *Tropical Medicine: an illustrated history of the* pioneers. London: Academic Press 2007: 183–95.
2   L Rogers. The etiology of malarial fever with special reference to the ground water level, and the parasite. *Indian med Gaz* 1896; 31: 49–55.
3   L Rogers. On the influence of variations of the ground-water level on the prevalence of malarial fevers. *Scientific memoirs of Medical Officers of the Army of India* 1897: 10: 53–8.

4   L Rogers. *Report of an investigation of the epidemic of malarial fevers in Assam, or kala-azar.* Shillong: Assam Secretarial Printing Office 1897: 223.

5   Anonymous. Malaria fever in the Punjab. *Indian med Gaz* 1911; 46: 354–5.

6   L Rogers. The world incidence of leprosy in relation to meteorological conditions and its bearing on the probable mode of transmission. *Trans R Soc trop Med Hyg* 1922–3; 16: 440–60.

7   L Rogers. Tuberculosis incidence and climate in India: rainfall and wet winds. *Br med J* 1925; i: 256–9. [*See also*: Anonymous. Gordon, William. *Munk's Roll* 4: 450–1; W Gordon. Wet winds and early phthisis. *Br med J* 1924; ii: 983–5].

8   L Rogers. Relationship between pneumonia incidence and climate in India. *Lancet* 1925; i: 1173–4.

9   L Rogers. The conditions influencing the incidence and spread of cholera in India. *Proc R Soc Med (Section of Epidemiology and State Medicine)*; 1926; 19: 59–93.

10 L Rogers. Presidential address. The methods and results of forecasting the incidence of cholera, smallpox and plague in India. *Trans R Soc trop Med Hyg* 1933–34; 27: 217–38.

11 **Arthur Bagshawe** was educated at Marlborough College and Caius College Cambridge. He initially served in the Uganda Protectorate. He later became Director of the Sleeping Sickness Bureau and also of The Bureau of Hygiene and Tropical Medicine at 25 Endsleigh Gardens, London from 1912–35. *See:* Anonymous. Bagshawe, Sir Arthur William Garrard. *Who Was Who, 1941–1950.* A & C Black 1952: 47.

12 G C Low. Malarial and filarial diseases in Barbados, West Indies. *Br med J* 1901; ii: 687. [*See also:* G C Cook. *Caribbean Diseases: Dr George Low's expedition in 1901–02.* Oxford: Radcliffe Publishing 2009: 229].

13 G C Low. Discussion on filariasis. *Br med J* 1913; ii: 1298–1302.

14 M Watson. Mosquito reduction and the consequent eradication of malaria. *Trans Soc trop Med Hyg* 1913; 7: 59–70.

15 H M Hanschell. The infection of Barbados with malaria. *Br med J* 1928; i: 157.

16 J F C Haslam. Barbados: Report of the Chief Medical Officer for the year 1933–34.

17 J Hutson. Barbados: Annual Report of the Public Health Inspector for the period April to December, 1913.

18 W Hillary. *Observations on the Changes of the Air, and the Concomitant Epidemical Diseases in the Island of Barbadoes.* 2nd ed. London: L Hawes, W Clarke & R Collins 1766: 276–97.

19 A Hirsch. *Handbook of Geographical and Historical Pathology: Acute Infective Disease* 1883: 1 London: New Sydenham Society.

20 T W H Cameron. Observations on a parasitological tour of the Lesser Antilles. *Proc R Soc Med* (Section of Tropical Diseases and Parasitology) 1929; 22: 933–41.

21 W M McDonald. The parasitology and clinical aspects of malaria in Antigua. *Br med J* 1922; i: 597–9.

22 L C D Hermitte. Occurrence of *Anopheles gambiae (costalis)* in Aldabra Islands (Seychelles). *Records of the Malaria Survey of India* 1931; ii: 643–54.

23 R C Shannon. O apparecimento de uma especie Africana de anopheles no Brasil. *Brasil-Medico* 1930; 44: 515.

24 S M Lambert. Medical conditions in the South Pacific. *Med J Australia* 1928; ii: 362–78.

25 K E Lowman. Health conditions in St Croix. *Military Surgeon* 1929; 64: 539.

26 S Tara. Sur l'emploi de la dihydroquinamine. *Rev Med et Hyg Trop* 1933; 25: 246.

27 *Op cit*. See note 12 above.

28 J F Siler. Medical notes on Barbados, British West Indies. *Am J trop Dis Preventive Med* 1915; 3: 46.

29 *Op cit*. See note 16 above.

30 *Op cit*. See note 13 above.

31 *Op cit*. See note 21 above.

32 T W M Cameron. A new definitive host for *Schistosoma mansoni. J Helminth* 1928; 6: 219–22; S B Jones. Report of a case of rectal bilharziasis. *Med Rep on the Sanitary Conditions of the Presidency (St Christopher-Nevis)* 1919: 8.

33 H Muench. Final Report of the Hookworm Infection Survey of St Christopher, BWI. [*See* Bagshawe's *presidential address*].

34 E R Stitt. Our disease inheritance from slavery. *U S Naval Med Bull* 1928; 26: 801.

35 *Op cit*. See note 19 above.

36 H H Johnston. *The negro in the New World*. London: Methuen.

37 S L Brug. *Dracunculus medinensis* in the Dutch East Indies. *Meded Dienst d Volksgezonheid in* Nederl-Indié 1930; 19: 153.

38 Reference *not* given by Bagshawe.

39 R Towne. *A treatise of the Diseases most frequent in the West Indies and herein more particularly of those which occur in Barbadoes*. London: J Clarke 1726: 192.

40 A G Price. White settlement in Saba Island, Dutch West Indies. *Geog Review* 1934; 24: 42.

41 A G Bagshawe. Presidential address. Problems of health and disease of some small tropical islands. *Trans R Soc trop Med Hyg* 1935–36; 29: 211–26.

42 G C Cook. *John McAlister's other vision: a history of the Fellowship of Postgraduate Medicine* Oxford: Radcliffe Publishing 2005: 178.

Chapter 10

The pre-World War II years

In the first half of 1937, Sir Arthur Bagshawe remained president. At the outbreak of war in late 1939, Sir Rickard Christophers occupied that position which he was to retain for much of the war (*see* Chapter 11). Between them however, was Sydney Price James – whose presidential address, devoted to *malaria*, is summarised in edited form below:

On 21 October 1937, Lt-Colonel S P James CMG MD FRS IMS (retd) (1870–1946)[1] (*see* Figure 10.1) gave his presidential address on **Advances in knowledge of malaria since the war.** This referred of course to the Great War, of 1914–18. He began with a general account of the present state of malariology:

> … everyone interested in *malaria* will agree that the 20 years … since the War were noteworthy first for the initiation and establishment of new and better arrangements for systematic research, second for some remarkable discoveries and additions to knowledge, [and] third for a lively renewal of practical anti-malarial efforts in many parts of the world.

'… the outlook for future success in the fight against *malaria* [he continued] is more hopeful' than it was 20 years ago when … 'faith in the efficacy of every prophylactic and therapeutic measure had fallen almost to zero'.

> … Everyone who had … taken part in efforts to deal with *malaria* in different parts of the world during the War came home with the uncomfortable feeling that we knew much less about the disease than we thought we did, and that it might be quite a good plan to sink our pride and [to] begin again, in all humility and with greater respect and reverence, to try to fathom some of its mysteries. Opportunities for this new beginning soon became available by the spread of the disease in eastern and western

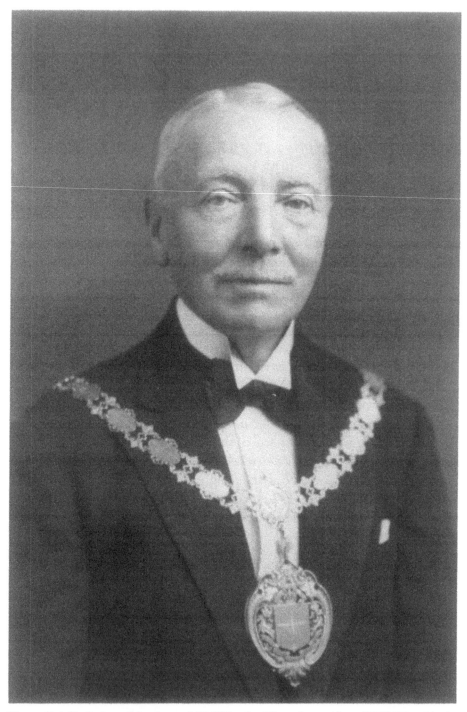

Figure 10.1: Dr Sydney Price James MD FRS – the fifteenth president (RSTMH archive).

Europe and by arrangements for … the internationalization of *malaria* research and control.

The idea of making *malaria* work a matter of *international* as well as of *national* concern had its origin in England in 1923 when various countries in Europe were beginning to recover from the effects of post-War epidemics and were trying to arrange for a continuous *public health* policy and a permanent medical and sanitary service for carrying it out. An initial difficulty in creating and developing the service was that the countries concerned were poverty-stricken and very backward in matters of medical assistance and *public health* arrangements. Doctors who had received a training in *public health* were few … and there was a great lack of subordinate personnel. *Malaria* was everywhere prevalent and severe and it was a question whether the *public health* policy should be based primarily on efforts to deal with this disease, or whether primary attention should be given to general medical and *public health* requirements which were equally of pressing importance. … useful advice [too] might perhaps be given by a group of workers who had had experience of similar conditions in the tropics.

In May 1923, a proposal to this effect was presented to [and accepted by] the Health Committee of the *League of Nations* [LN] [and] a small Malaria Sub-Committee [was appointed] and later the *Malaria Commission,* which in 1924 undertook [a] collective enquiry. …Seventeen members from eleven countries took part … and in each country and district visited, representatives of the local administration and medical staffs accompanied the Commission and took part in its discussions. Major Norman Lothian, … was Secretary to the Commission [both then and] in Palestine and part of Asia Minor in 1925. On this latter tour, the Commission had the advantage of the participation of an expert from the United States [in] Dr Samuel Darling, whose early work with General [W C] Gorgas [1854–1920] during the construction of the Panama Canal is so well known. [And] in Palestine he was at the zenith of his powers as an expert adviser on anti-malarial work. … Another collective study tour undertaken by members of the Commission in 1925 was to Spain and another to Sicily; in later years there were tours to the United States, British India and other countries.

[Other tours followed and they] afforded an opportunity of ascertaining and comparing conditions in a number of countries. … mutual discussions were the first occasion on which the collective thought of malariologists of different countries and different schools of teaching and practice were brought to bear on local *malaria* problems …

… the International Health Division of the *Rockefeller Foundation* … had [during the previous 15 years] financed the Commission's work. In addition to the international arrangements of the [LN], the Foundation [had] initiated and maintained from 1916 onwards an international arrangement of its own for systematic anti-malarial work in various countries [aimed at] reducing the incidence of malarial infection, such an anti-larval work, screening and the treatment of carriers … on a small scale in the field. The arrangements [were] made in collaboration with [numerous] Governments [in tropical countries on the American continent]. … In 1924 and 1925 they were extended to Italy, Poland, Palestine, and the Philippine Islands. … Each [one was] under the direction of a member of the staff of the Foundation's *International Health Division*. Some [were] called 'stations for the demonstration of methods of control' but perhaps 'research stations' would be a better name.

… during the 20 years [up to] 1935, the Foundation spent on anti-*malaria* work, exclusive of the cost of field services, about two and a half million dollars, of which one and a half million was spent in foreign countries. … There is hardly any item of *malaria* research, except perhaps chemotherapy, which has not received assistance directly or indirectly from its funds. The grant of [eighty] fellowships to enable medical graduates to become trained malariologists or to enable workers to see what is being done outside their own country is another beneficent activity of the Foundation. …

Changing tack, he then spoke about the establishment (both nationally and internationally) of mental hospitals – where 'malariatherapy' was practised, and of:

… research laboratories charged with the duty of cultivating malaria parasites in mosquitoes and of inducing [clinical] malarial attacks by [their] bites ... instead of by direct blood inoculation from patient to patient. ... The British Government, through its *Ministry of Health* ... were the first to make an official arrangement for this work by [establishing] a *malaria* research laboratory at the Horton Mental Hospital, Epsom, in May 1925. In March 1926 ... a report on the first results of the work was communicated to the [LN]'s *Malaria Commission* for presentation to the Health Committee ... Soon afterwards [similar] laboratories [to these] were established in ... Italy, Holland, the United States and Roumania [sic]. In the United States there are two [such] research centres [:] one maintained by the *Rockefeller Foundation* in Florida, the other by the *US Public Health Service* in Washington. Roumania also has two centres, one at Jassy, the other at Bucharest.

There has always been active co-operation between the several centres named. It is maintained by personal visits and [by] exchange of species and strains of [both] *malaria* parasites and mosquitoes with which the work is done. An interesting point ... was the finding that *anopheles* confined in cages invented by Captain Baraud in India travel well by sea and air. Between 1931 and 1933, batches of *anopheles* were received alive at Horton from ... British India, West Africa, Uganda and Trinidad, and on more frequent occasions from a number of countries in Europe.

And then to arrangements for research 'on other aspects of *malaria*':

... One [strategy] was the renewal of anti-malarial chemothera-peutic research by the chemical industries in Germany and France and [also] creation by the British Government of an organization for systematic work in England. For various reasons, arrangements made in this country were on a small scale but [nevertheless] some progress has [now] been made, particularly with arrangements for testing new synthetic preparations and for studying the biological and physico-chemical principles underlying the action of quinine and synthetic drugs. ... special units [are situated] in Liverpool, London and Cambridge. Recently, the *Medical Research Council* [MRC], in consultation with the Department of Scientific and Industrial Research, have made plans for promoting chemotherapeutic investigation on a larger scale, for which the Government have provided an annual grant of £30,000. ... the scheme includes the provision of a new Institute ...

Another [MRC] scheme is an arrangement by which [suitable] young graduates ... are given grants and facilities for [relevant] research [work] in the tropics [and] as qualified investigators become available under this scheme they will be eligible for permanent pensionable appointments for research work on *malaria* and other subjects of *tropical medicine* abroad and at home.

Lastly, I must not fail to mention arrangements made by particular societies and individuals. ... the Royal Society ... more than 35 years ago, followed up the discovery of the mosquito-cycle of the *malaria* parasite by sending research workers to Africa and India to study the new epidemiology of the disease and the life history and habits of the mosquitoes which transmit it. Last year the Society took a second step [by devoting] the major part of its Medical Research Fund to a scheme of *malaria* research consisting firstly of a study by modern experimental methods of the parasites and their relationship with human, animal and insect hosts, [and] secondly [involving] an intensive study of the ecology of one or more of the species of *anopheles* which spread malaria in the tropics. As a recent example I [will] cite the establishment of the *Dorothea Simmons Malaria Research Station* in Greece where the remarkable work on blackwater fever described by [Drs] Foy and Fairley [*see* Chapter 9] in June [1937] was done.

In the second part of his address, James spoke on 'the discoveries and additions to knowledge made during the period under review':

... the outstanding feature of the advance of knowledge ... was the discovery or invention of better ways of investigating the disease. After the war [an] uneasy feeling of ignorance ... caused workers to look about for new avenues of approach... Clinicians, epidemiologists and entomologists gave much thought to this matter. An early opportunity for new work was provided by the occurrence of cases of *malaria* in the families of soldiers who had returned to their homes. These ... were studied in detail with the object of ascertaining ... the sequence of events which led to their onset and the manner in which they multiplied to constitute local epidemics.

Attention was directed to the habits and behaviour of the insect vector in the adult stage, and to the circumstances in which it became infected and transmitted the infection in particular houses. In this way malaria began to be studied in individuals of selected families in their own homes as well as in the mass by random sampling in the village street, and *anopheles* began to be studied from the point of view of [the] behaviour of the adult female insect in these houses ... These studies were the starting-point of work which led to the discovery of biological races of *anopheles* indistinguishable morphologically in the adult stage, but with different habits and therefore, sometimes, with a different rôle in the epidemiology of the disease ... At first it was thought that the results of these household studies were of interest chiefly from the point of view of the epidemiology of *malaria* in Europe; later it was found that their application in the tropics gave equally fruitful results, so it is now generally recognised that a '*malaria survey*' ... must include [both] a clinical and parasitological study, over a considerable period, of selected individuals of particular age-groups in as many families as possible, and [also] a close study of the habits and behaviour of the insect vector in the adult as well as in the larval stage. A good example of studies of the first type was the investigation in Nigeria ... by ... J G Thomson ... Another is the investigation made by ... Bagster Wilson in Tanganyika [now Tanzania]. Results of the second type of study have led to ... a novel method of controlling malaria among uncivilized native races in South Africa.

Another avenue of approach ... was investigation into the circumstances and factors to which the apparent disappearance of *malaria* from England, Denmark and Holland may have been due. These enquiries showed that the apparent disappearance had come about without any reduction of the insect vector concerned. Malaria is essentially a house or family disease and its spread is greatly facilitated by circumstances which bring gametocyte carriers, insect vectors and non-immune persons into close and continuous association. [However,] in the countries named, this close association had been gradually broken in the course of years by progressive social, economic, educational, medical and *public health* improvements. Thus a way was opened which justified the application of other methods of dealing with *malaria* than those arising directly from the belief that *because mosquitoes transmit the disease their elimination must be the object of chief concern and expenditure* [author's italics].

Other methods of investigations devised during the early post-War years were [James considered] different ... In 1924, ... Roehl [developed] on a large scale at Elberfeld, in Germany, a method for seeking anti-malarial remedies by testing numerous quinine and quinoline derivatives to ascertain whether any of them were effective against the parasites of bird *malaria*. ... On the chemical side an epoch-making advance was the discovery of plasmoquine [pamaquine] and other synthetic compounds which promised to be effective anti-malarial agents. On the biological side additions to knowledge were no less important. ... It is now accepted [however] that the group comprises a number of species of which the morphological characters are quite distinct, and ... there are [also] a number of varieties of each species with lesser morphological differences, such, for example, as those described for the indigenous type of *Plasmodium vivax* endemic in Holland as compared with those of the tropical type from Madagascar. In addition, it is accepted that within each morphological species and variety there are many strains having different biological properties; they cannot be distinguished morphologically but can be separated by their clinical effects, immunological characters and [by their] reaction to anti-malarial drugs. Acquired tolerance or immunity as a result of repeated attacks was found to be specific not only as regards the various species of parasite ... but also as regards particular strains.

There were also notable advances [for example] on the therapeutics [for] although quinine is one of the most remarkable drugs ... it has several defects. In particular, it does not prevent infection of the human host or the insect vector, and [it] does not prevent relapses. Its merits and defects ... were for the first time clearly ascertained and described; and when this was done it became possible to justify anti-malarial chemotherapy on scientific grounds. Its aim is not to supplant the one and only remedy that has been available for 300 years, but to supplement it with additional weapons ...

[With the exception of] the practice of malariatherapy [*see* above] the study of avian *malaria* parasites and ... extensive use of canaries and other birds harbouring these parasites for laboratory work [has greatly increased knowledge]. ... MacCallum's discovery of the fertilization of the female gametocyte, Ross's working out of the mosquito cycle of the parasite, the early work of the curative action of quinine by Kopanaris, the ... Sergent[s], Giemsa and others, Roehl's drug-testing device which resulted in the discovery of plasmoquine, and the fundamental work of the Taliaferros on the mechanism of immunity [are examples].

About 1931 the knowledge which had been gained on human plasmodia by their study in the practice of malariatherapy was applied in new studies of the known avian species. Roehl's method of chemotherapeutic test was supplemented by using canaries infected by mosquito bites instead of by direct-blood inoculation and tests were made on birds harbouring the parasite *Haemoproteus* of which the schizogonic cycle is passed in endothelial cells instead of [erythrocytes]. Finally, new avian plasmodia were discovered and brought into use for experimental studies. One [example] is the ... parasite of the domestic fowl, which ... [Emil] Brumpt found and described in 1935 ... and to which he gave the name *Plasmodium gallinaceum*, another is a ... parasite of the Java sparrow which was apparently seen by Ziemann in 1896 and by Anschutz in 1909 and by several workers since, but was nameless until 1935 when Brumpt called it *Plasmodium paddae*. ... bird *malaria* [might solve problems which cannot] be investigated in the human subject. One [object] is the completion of knowledge of the schizogonic cycle of plasmodia in their respective vertebrate hosts. [Although] the sporogonic cycle of these parasites in the mosquito has been known [now] for nearly 40 years, ... we know only a part of the story of their life in the vertebrate host. ... we do not know [for example] what happens to the parasite during the interval between [the] inoculation of sporozoites by the mosquito and the appearance of trophozoites in the [erythocytes]. ... it was not until ... 1925 and 1927 that the question ... attracted [renewed] attention. [This] was due to the observation [of] Yorke and MacFie in Liverpool, and by ourselves at Horton, that the onset of a malarial attack ... cannot be prevented by giving quinine during the incubation period. I showed an example of this observation at a meeting of [the RSTMH] in 1931.[2] It is clear, in this example, that if the sporozoites which the thirty mosquitoes injected had immediately entered [erythrocytes] and had become trophozoites and schizonts the quinine would have killed them and no attack would have resulted. On the basis of these and similar experiments with plasmoquine the hypothesis was published in December, 1931, that what happens to sporozoites injected by the mosquito is that they are carried [first] to the internal organs where they enter reticulo-endothelial cells and go through a cycle of development resulting in the production of merozoites which are able to enter [erythrocytes]. Since then the problem of the destiny of sporozoites has been studied ... by many workers in different countries, [and] it seems ... that its solution may be close at hand. If so, it will provide an example of the manner in which advances of knowledge come about gradually as the result of observations made independently or collectively by many workers ...

Three results of experimental work are of outstanding importance. The first is the observation that very shortly after ... inoculation of sporozoites intravenously or intramuscularly, or by the bites of mosquitoes, the blood of the person or bird inoculated is not infective to other persons or birds, even when injected in large amounts, and that it remains non-infective for at least 2 or 3 days. This [observation] has been made repeatedly as regards the sporozoites of *P vivax* and *P falciparum*, and ... several species of avian plasmodia. The second is the observation [in] bird *malaria*, that during the latter part of the period of non-infectivity of the blood other birds can be infected by inoculating a small portion of the spleen, the liver or ... brain. Evidently these internal organs become infective earlier than the circulating blood. The conclusion drawn from these two observations is that sporozoites injected intravenously or by the mosquito are quickly cleared from the circulating blood and become lodged in the reticulo-endothelial [RE] system of the internal organs where they remain until they have developed to the stage which can become parasitic in the [erythocytes]. The third outstanding result of experimental work is the discovery that some avian plasmodia have two schizogonic cycles of development in their vertebrate hosts: one occurs in [RE] cells in the brain, spleen, liver, kidneys, lungs and bone marrow, the other in the [erythrocytes].

It is known that after infection by the bites of mosquitoes the cycle in the [RE] cells precedes [that] in [erythrocytes] because ... birds can be infected by inoculating them with a small portion of blood-free tissue from the spleen or liver or brain at a time when they cannot be infected even by inoculating a large quantity of blood. At the [March 1937] Laboratory meeting of the [RSTMH] [I showed] with ... Tate preparations of various stages of this endothelial cycle ... in ... *P gallinaceum* of the domestic fowl. ... Raffaele, of Rome, had previously discovered stages of the same cycle in canaries infected with *P elongatum* and *P relictum*, and [also] Huff and Bloom, of Chicago, had discovered what seemed to be the same stages in cells of the bone marrow of birds infected with *P elongatum*. ... Tate at Cambridge and ... Kikuth at Elberfeld, have confirmed Raffaele's findings with regard to *P relictum*, and ... Kikuth has obtained the same results with *P cathemerium*. ... Brumpt [et al] have confirmed the findings with regard to *P gallinaceum*. It has not yet been proved that the stages seen in endothelial cells are [those] of the growth and development of sporozoites taken up by these cells from the blood [soon] after their infection by the mosquito, but it is difficult to suggest any good reason against this view. It must be remembered ... that it is not yet justifiable to assume that sporozoites of the human plasmodia have to undergo the same kind of preliminary growth and development in endothelial cells of the internal organs before they can become parasitic in [erythrocytes], but if, ultimately, this should be found to be the case, we should be able to explain more satisfactorily ... the failure of ... quinine, plasmoquine and atebrin [mepacrine] to act as true prophylactics, and to [prevent] the occurrence of relapses. In the meantime ... the next step in anti-malarial chemotherapeutic research should be to search for a compound which will destroy avian plasmodia during their cycle in endothelial cells. ...

... systematic use of [monkeys] for experimental work dates only from 1932, when Napier and Campbell, and Knowles and Das Gupta in India described *malaria* parasites from the blood of naturally infected monkeys imported from Singapore. Since then several of these parasites have been the subject of intensive study particularly in relation to immunology, and one of them, *P knowlesi* is ... commonly used [in] the practice of human malariatherapy.

Most of the additions to knowledge have come from work done in British India by … Knowles and his collaborators, and by Sinton and Mulligan. The results of a remarkable collaborative study by … Taliaferro and … Mulligan, of the histopathology of malaria, based chiefly on work done on *P knowlesi* in India, have recently been published. During the last few years … Christophers [*see* Chapter 11] has used *P knowlesi* for an entirely new type of fundamental or basic research which is concerned with the physico-chemical principles underlying the mode of action of quinine and [also] synthetic anti-malarial compounds.

It was not until 1948 that the exo-erythocytic cycle in the liver of mammalian, and later human *P vivax* infection was demonstrated [*see* below and Chapter 12]; some studies leading to the elucidation were also carried out at the Horton Hospital.[3] In the last part of the lecture, James dealt with 'advances on work *in the field*':

> … An outstanding event … was the bringing to light of malarious conditions in Europe comparable with those in very malarious parts of the tropics. They had always existed, but their rediscovery attracted much attention. Medical men, *public health* specialists and entomologists from various parts of the world came to study them and many specific anti-malarial campaigns were started. The *Malaria Commission* of the [LN] played a large part in bringing the conditions to light, and the International Health Board of the *Rockefeller Foundation* are doing [much to assist] the Governments of affected countries to fight the disease. … The *Malaria Commission* … placed the creation and development of a permanent service first among their recommendations. They advised the establishment at the headquarters of the Governments concerned of a central official organization similar to that which is usual for *tuberculosis* and other social diseases. They suggested [that it should advise] the Governments on anti-malarial policy and measures, to arrange for *malaria* research, to arrange for training medical officers and subordinate personnel in malariology, to conduct *malaria* surveys and to give advice and assistance in the conduct of local measures. … But, … a chief post-War difficulty in European countries most affected by *malaria* was the absence of a health service of any kind and in many rural

areas the absence of effective arrangements even for treatment of the sick. ... the goal [must be] the development of a general rural medical and health service which provides for adequate medical attention in sickness of all kinds, for improvements in housing, water supply, conservancy and general welfare, and ... organization of educational campaigns designed to get the people to understand and to co-operate in the measures taken for their benefit. When this general service has been organized, arrangements for dealing with *malaria* will take their rightful place ... in accordance with the relative importance of this particular disease in comparison with [that] of other diseases and conditions affecting the *public health*.

In some other countries, where medical and *public health* arrangements are more advanced, it has been possible to begin ... organization of a special anti-malarial service at the centre rather than at the periphery. British India is a notable example ... and it is a country, too, in which definite advances in practical anti-malarial arrangements were made during the period under review. A few years after the War [of 1914–18] an official central organization called the *Malaria Survey of India* was inaugurated and financed by the Central Government to the extent of 2 lakhs of rupees a year. Its primary function was to conduct research into all branches of malariology, to act as an information and advisory bureau, to prepare and issue bulletins for the use of executive malariologists and *public health* officers, to train medical graduates in laboratory and field *malaria* work, to maintain a reference library, to identify specimens sent for opinion and to undertake special investigations in various parts of India for the purpose of carrying out measures of control. ... Many major field enquiries were conducted by research workers ... as well as an investigation lasting from 1923 to 1931 into the therapeutics of *malaria* with reference to the efficacy of the cinchona alkaloids in comparison with quinine. Apart from this official organization ... the different Provincial Governments have their own organizations, acting partly through institutes such as the *Institute of Hygiene* and the *School of Tropical Medicine at Calcutta*, the *King Institute at Madras* and the *Assam Institute at Shillong*, [and] partly through the *Public Health* Departments ... In addition there are many local organizations for research and anti-malarial measures, such as the branches of the Ross Institute ... chiefly occupied with industrial *malaria* in the tea gardens, the special organizations for railways in Bengal and for reclamation and construction works in various parts of the country, the organizations in Indian native states, Mysore, Travancore, Patiala, etc, and the special anti-*malaria* staffs maintained by large cities, such as Bombay, Calcutta and Delhi. The campaign in the Delhi urban district is being conducted over an area of 55 square miles and is under the direct control of the *Malaria Survey of India.* The cost of the permanent works included in the first year's programme of measures was 14.75 lakhs of rupees and [that] of the temporary measures Rs. 75,000.

... the most striking advances of knowledge on malaria since the War were on the therapeutics of the disease. ... The first [aim] is to provide a remedy that ... can be obtained so cheaply that it can be made readily available to the whole population of malarious countries. The second is to find preparations which, regardless of their cost, will be effective for purposes for which quinine is known to fail. On the first aim the chief advance was the finding that for the treatment of the great majority of cases of *malaria* occurring among the indigenous inhabitants of malarious regions quinine has little or no practical advantages over the mixture of alkaloids known in India as *cinchona febrifuge* and in Europe as *totaquina*. Both are cheaper ... than quinine. On the second ... was the discovery of plasmoquine, atebrin [mepacrine] and various other synthetic anti-malarial remedies. The *Malaria Commission*'s second general report describes the results of clinical trials [which were] made in various countries between 1933 and 1936 with the object of comparing the efficacy of these synthetic preparations with that of quinine. ... One [unanswered question] was whether a short course of plasmoquine ... after cure of the attack by quinine reduces relapses or not. This is now answered definitely in the affirmative. ... this practice was introduced some years ago in a standard plan of treatment adopted for the British Army in India, and [the remarkable decline of admissions to hospital] was attributed largely to it. ...

... Many inventions for killing larvae, for preventing *anopheles* from breeding ... and for killing adult insects were made [during this period], but most is expected from the new knowledge on what are called biological or natural methods of control ... The successful employment of these measures in several campaigns are described [in] L W Hackett's ... book, *Malaria in Europe*. ... Increased attention is also being given to ... 'species-sanitation' although like most methods its practical application [is] difficult, particularly in the United States where the idea (as first put forward by Carter and Darling for dealing with *Anopheles quadrimaculatus*) did not get a favourable reception. ... To be rid of mosquitoes of all kinds is what the people want. No *public health* department in the United States can afford to neglect this desire ... This makes it difficult to do selective control work on the different species. ... in some parts of the world, killing adult mosquitoes by the use of insecticidal sprays in houses appeals more to the inhabitants than anti-larval work. The practice has been applied systematically on a large scale in native huts in Natal and Zululand, and has been reported ... as being willingly and enthusiastically received, as costing only about a third of the cost of anti-larval work and as being more effective in controlling *malaria*. The same method is being tried in campaigns in India.

On the whole [the] existing anti-mosquito measures are still very crude and [it is likely that] no striking advance can be expected until we know more of the life history, habits and behaviour or these 'pestiferous insects'. ... [Alternative] advances in other anti-malarial methods [include, according to James] reclamation of land, bonification, housing, screening and propaganda ...[4]

The Society in the pre-World War II years

Ordinary Meetings

The *Ordinary* meetings immediately before and during the war, became more diversified than hitherto. *Malaria, trypanosomiasis*, and *beri-beri* of course all continued to be featured, but that on **19 January 1939**, for example, was largely devoted to plant viruses. Table 10.1 summarises the subjects and speakers at these meetings.

Financial matters (including the Manson House Fund)

Council meetings in the pre-war years were dominated by financial matters; paying off the sizeable debt accrued when the Society purchased

Table 10.1: Communications to *Ordinary* Meetings – 1938 and 1939

Date	Subject	Speaker
1938		
20 January	Treatment of cardiac beri-beri	R B Hawes
	B_1 deficiency	R A Peters
	Biochemical changes in Beri-beri	B S Platt
17 February	Lymphogranuloma inguinale	H M Hanschell
	Lymphogranuloma in African natives	C C Chesterman
	Investigation of lymphogranuloma inguinale	G M Findlay
19 May	The placenta in malaria	P C C Garnham
30 June (31st AGM)	Nutritional macrocyctic anaemia in Macedonia	N H Fairley, *et al*
13 October	Yellow fever in South America	F L Soper
8 December	Endemic malaria in East Africa	D B Wilson
1939		
19 January	Plant and animal viruses	K M Smith
16 February	Tuberculosis in tropical natives	C Wilcocks
18 May	African trypanosomiasis	H M O Lester
15 June (32nd AGM)	Sulphanilamide in tropical diseases	G A H Buttle
19 October*	Malaria in War (presidential address) (see Chapter 11)	Sir Rickard Christophers
16 November	The louse – present and future	P A Buxton

* The first *Ordinary* meeting after the beginning of the Second World War (*see* Chapter 11).

26 Portland Place in 1931 remained of serious concern, and financial statements were therefore numerous.

Professor R P Strong (an Honorary Fellow) donated £20 to the Fund in 1937 (*see CM*, **18 February 1937**). Several relatively trivial donations, as well as £250 from Mr W J Courthauld a month later were also received about this time.

After discussion, *Council* unanimously agreed on **9 December** to a motion put by the Treasurer – Dr Oswald Marriott – and seconded by Col Sinton FRS VC:

> That the Council authorizes the Treasurer to repay to the Mortgagees of Manson House the sum of £3,000 (three thousand pounds) reducing the Mortgage from £13,000 (thirteen thousand pounds) to £10,000 (ten thousand pounds) on Midsummer

quarter day, June 24th 1938 utilizing for this purpose the *Mortgage Redemption Fund* and the *Manson House Fund* and if necessary a sum borrowed from the Society's *Accumulated Fund.*

This was agreed by the Charity Commissioners (*see CM*, **20 January 1938**), but they also felt that 'in view of the lower rates of interest now prevailing, the annual payment to the sinking fund for mortgage redemption should be increased from £297 to £300'.

In order to minimise legal costs (whenever there was a change of Trustees) associated with Manson House, Low (Senior Trustee) proposed, and Marriott (Treasurer) seconded, a motion (*see CM*, **13 October 1938**):

> That steps be taken to have the legal estate in the Society's leasehold premises Number 26 Portland Place and Number 4 Cavendish Mews South, London and any other real or leasehold property if and when required by the Society vested in the Official Trustee of Charity Lands upon trust for the Society and that the Secretary be and is hereby authorized to sign the formal application to the Charity Commissioners for a vesting order to that effect.

At the same meeting, Marriott indicated that the Westminster Bank was now willing 'to take over the mortgage on Manson House at a rate of interest of 4%, which was [a fraction] lower than the 4¼% the Society had been paying for the past six years'. The following motion, proposed by Marriott was then carried unanimously:

> The Executive Committee having reported that the Society's Bankers (Westminster Bank Ltd) are willing to lend to the Society the sum of £10,000 at interest at the rate of ½% above bank rate with a minimum of £4% per annum upon security of the Society's leasehold premises Number 26 Portland Place and Number 4 Cavendish Mews South annual reduction of principal to be made in accordance with the order of the Charity Commissioners authorizing the transaction the Society also giving an Undertaking that the fund eventually available under the Will of the late Dr A S Burgess will be utilised for the repayment of the loan: 'That as soon as arrangements can be made to repay the existing Mortgage of £10,000 in favour of The Roffey Trust Co and the Innes Trust Co Ltd without duplicating interest payments

such sum shall be borrowed for that purpose from the Society's Bankers (Westminster Bank Ltd) on the terms above mentioned and that the Official Trustee of the Charity Lands be requested and he is hereby authorized to execute in favour of the Bank the Instrument of Charge requisite to give effect to the arrangement. Such Charge to include a provision that no personal liability shall be imposed upon the Members of the Society the Trustees or the Official Trustee of the Charity Lands as the case may be for the payment of the principal moneys and interest thereby secured.

On **17 November**, Low proposed vestment of the Society's funds in the *Official Trustee of Charitable Funds*, so that 'investments would be inscribed in the Books of the Bank of England in the name of the Official Trustee who act under the direction of the Society's three Trustees'. The following proposal was carried unanimously:

> That the Officers of the [RSTMH] be authorized to take the necessary steps to vest the Society's funds in the *Official Trustee of Charitable Funds* upon trust for the Society and that the Secretary be and is hereby authorized to sign the formal application to the Charity Commissioners for an Order to that effect.

This move thus avoided correspondence with the income tax authorities and consequent renewed investigation of claims for exemption, when the Trustees changed.

The Treasurer (Marriott) announced on **19 January 1939** that the 'amount now required to pay off the debt on Manson house [had fallen to] £10,482'.

On **18 May**, the Treasurer explained to *Council* that in order to complete the repayment of £3,000 of the £13,000 mortgage it had been necessary to borrow £534 3s 9d from the Society's General Accumulated Fund. He also proposed that a similar sum be transferred to the House Fund; this too was again approved unanimously.

Two pieces of good news were recorded on **19 October**: A donation of 50 guineas from the Committee of the *West African Medical Journal* (which had ceased publication in October 1938) to the House Fund was announced to *Council*, and a letter from Professor R P Strong (an Honorary Fellow and now entitled to receive *Transactions* gratis) was read, in which he instructed that his annual subscription to *Transactions* be directed to the House Fund.

By this meeting (*ie* about six weeks after the outbreak of World War II), the debt, after paying all fees for redecoration, and legal fees in connection with transfer of the Society's property, and funds to the official Trustees had been paid, was £9,582, *ie* less than £10,000!

The two resident tenants continued paying rents during these years; income from letting the hall had, for example, risen by £35 over the year ended 21 October 1937.

Preservation of another Portland Place property

The Society agreed to *oppose* the building of a block of offices at 34 Portland Place; an appeal was currently being heard against refusal of the LCC's Town Planning Authority to allow this building to be erected (*see CM*, **16 March 1939**).

The Fellowship

On **16 March** also, *Council* was informed of a letter from Professor R T Leiper (a long-standing Fellow) resigning from the Society; *Council* decided to postpone consideration but, on 15 June 1939 his resignation was duly accepted.

Death of distinguished Fellows

Council, on **21 October 1937**, confirmed their previous decision (*see* Chapter 9) that it was customary to publish *only* obituaries of Honorary Fellows and past presidents in *Transactions*.

Deaths of two original Fellows were announced to *Council* on **20 January 1938**: Professor G H F Nuttall FRS (Cambridge) and Major E E Austen (a former vice-president, and Trustee). Sir Thomas Stanton's death – he had been a founder member and a Trustee of the Society – was referred to at length by the president (James) at a *Council* meeting on **17 February**, and it was resolved to insert a note referring to his services to 'advancement of *public health* in the tropics' in *Transactions*. The death of another Honorary Fellow (since 1921) – Professor Mesnil – was announced to *Council* on **17 March**. Dr Fletcher's death (he had been a member of Council and of the editorial panel, and former vice-president, 1933–5) was announced on **13 October**, and that of Professor Danilewsky (an Honorary Fellow since 1907) of the USSR on **18 May 1939**.

Transactions

Transactions had always been a major topic at *Council* meetings. This publication continued to be an important 'money spinner', and 'exchanges' with other *tropical* journals were also important. Approval that *monographs* be sent *gratis* to all Fellows was given on **18 June 1936**; the first of the Society's monographs was titled 'Boomerang legs and Yaws in Australian Aborigines'. This was the first recognition that some papers submitted to *Transactions* were too long for inclusion in that journal.

Relationship with other Societies

The *3rd International Congress of Tropical Medicine and malaria* in 1938 took place at Amsterdam and Rotterdam; members of *Council* of the RSTMH formed the 'National Committee' for the UK.

Other invitations to send delegates to Congresses were recorded at a *Council* meeting on **9 December 1937**:

- *International Congress of Leprosy* – Cairo (March 1938) – Dr Ernest Muir.
- The *Royal Sanitary Institute* – Portsmouth (July 1938) – O'Brien was nominated, although Professor D B Blacklock did in fact represent the Society from 3–8 July.
- *International Congress of Anthropological and Ethnological Science* – Copenhagen (August 1938).

Other matters

ALTERATION TO THE SOCIETY'S LAWS

Several alterations to the laws were made during this pre-war period. Also, amendments to 'the Instructions for local Secretaries' had been adopted on **19 March 1936**.

DONATIONS

Council narrowly voted on **17 June 1937** to make a donation (£5) to the *Freshwater Biological Association* because it was felt that it might increase 'understanding and bionomics of arthropod vectors and parasites which had aquatic stages of development'.

PRIZES

On **17 November 1938**, Council was made aware of two prizes for 'original research in leprosy' awarded by the Instituto Oswaldo Cruz.

HERPETOLOGY

Council was *not* solely interested in 'domestic' matters. For example, in response to a letter received from the Natural History Museum, the following resolution was carried unanimously (*see CM*, **20 January 1938**).

> The *Council* of the [RSTMH] views with alarm the proposal to substitute the generic name *Cobra* Laurenti 1768 for *Bitis* Gray 1842. Having regard to the established meaning of the word Cobra in the English and other languages for proteroglyphous colubrine snakes, the use of a similar generic name for a viperine snake must result in great confusion which may have serious practical consequences in medicine. They are of the opinion that this is an occasion when the strict application of the Rules of Zoological Nomenclature will 'result in greater confusion than uniformity' and that a suspension of the rules under the power conferred on the Commission by the 9th International Congress of Zoology is desirable.

The thirty-first and thirty-second annual reports

Although the number of Fellows was to decline during World War II, the number 'on the books' in the immediate pre-war years showed a significant increase: 1,709 in the 31st, and 1,713 in the 32nd annual report.

The financial position remained satisfactory. An excess of income over expenditure was recorded as £589 10s 0d for the year ended 31 March 1938, and £404 13s 11d for that ended 31 March 1939.

References and Notes

1   **Sydney James** had a distinguished career in *tropical* medicine. In his earlier days, from 1896–1918, he had served in the Indian Medical Service in which he rose to the rank of Lieutenant-Colonel. He became a member of the *Malarial Commission* of the *League of Nations* (LN), of the *Chemotherapy Committee* of the MRC, and of the *Tropical Diseases Committee* of the Royal Society. He also represented the British Government on the LN. James also served on the Local Government Board. In later years, he researched on induced malaria at the Horton Hospital – near Epsom; his work there had an important bearing on elucidation of the exo-erythrocytic cycle of *Plasmodium vivax*

infection. Apart from malaria, James was an expert on Kala azar and Yellow Fever. *See*: S R Christophers. Sydney Price James 1870–1946. *Obituary Notices of Fellows of the Royal Society* 1947; 5: 507–23; Anonymous. James, Lt-Col Sydney Price. *Who Was Who, 1941–1950*. London: A & C Black 1952: 596–7.

2   S P James. Some general results of a study of induced malaria in England. *Trans R Soc trop Med Hyg* 1930–31; 24: 477–525.

3   H E Shortt, P C C Garnham, B Malamos. The pre-erythrocytic stage of mammalian malaria. *Br med J* 1948; i: 192–4; H E Shortt, P C C Garnham, G Covell, P G Shute. The pre-erythrocytic stage of human malaria, Plasmodium vivax. *Br med J* 1948; i: 547.

4   S P James. Presidential address. Advances in knowledge of malaria since the War. *Trans R Soc trop Med Hyg* 1937–8; 31: 263–78.

Chapter 11

The Society during World War II (1939–45) and the future of *clinical* tropical medicine

The Society's 33rd Annual Report, for the period 1 April 1939 to 31 March 1940 began:

> The clouds of war were gathering over Europe when the year under review began. Well-attended meetings were held at Manson House in May and June; and in August a number of ... Fellows journeyed hopefully across the Atlantic to New York to represent their respective countries at the *Third International Congress of Microbiology* (September 2nd to 9th); but the declaration of war on September 3rd 1939 found many of them already on the high seas *en route* for home.

Presidential addresses

There were only two presidential addresses during these long war years – those of Christophers and Scott.

The beginning of the Second World War had been announced by the British Prime Minister Mr Neville Chamberlain (1869–1940). Some six weeks later (on 19 October) the presidential address, delivered by Sir (Samuel) Rickard Christophers CIE OBE FRS, Colonel IMS (retd) (1873–1978)[1] (*see* Figure 11.1), was appropriately titled: **Malaria in War:**

> Recent events [he began] have modified the choice of a subject for my address ... I had originally intended to deal with certain aspects of the chemotherapy of malaria. It seemed to me, however, that whilst we are not bound to think of nothing but the war, most of us are naturally more concerned at the moment with this than with anything else and are therefore not in the most suitable frame of mind to give attention to such a relatively

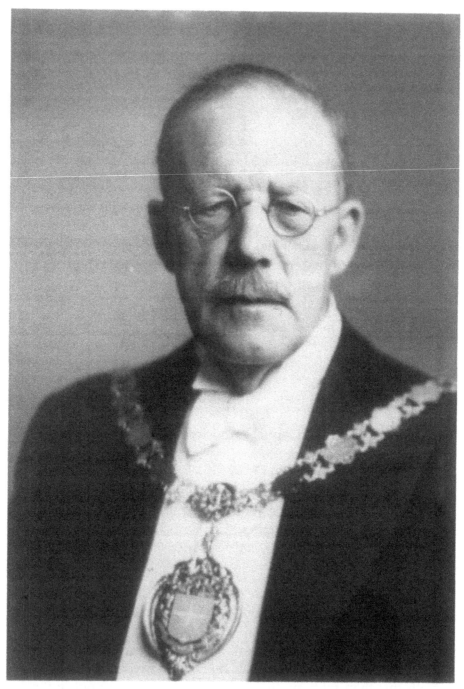

Figure 11.1: Sir Rickard Christophers KCMG FRCP FRS – the sixteenth president (RSTMH archive).

abstruse subject … Also [he considered] the subject … might serve a useful purpose in drawing attention to certain matters in which we as a Society have some responsibility. …

Christophers continued:

That there is a connection between *malaria* and war is [widely] recognized and though we need not suppose that the aetiological fundamentals are essentially different from those with which we are accustomed to deal in civil life, yet there are features of *malaria* [in] war which are interesting and important enough to merit special consideration. …

[*Malaria* in war] may modify or even determine the results of a campaign as history has several times shown. [Although] the essential aetiology may not be different, the epidemiology … in an army in the field is likely to have features which are by no means necessarily those with which we are most familiar in our usual dealings with this disease. [Importantly] questions of prevention [and] treatment are quite special in such a setting. There is a certain justification therefore for the term *'war malaria'* [which] includes aspects of [both] incidence and control [affecting] other than those in the fighting forces. And even the *control* of *malaria* in the fighting forces involves many considerations other than those at first sight most obvious.

… as [C A] Gill[2] …points out, troops are not always engaged in active operations. They are employed even in peace-time to garrison stations and are maintained in large numbers in cantonments. Even if we do not consider the prevention and treatment of sickness in such circumstances a direct war measure, it has an indirect importance to war. It is not merely that such troops, if seriously affected with *malaria*, are likely to be useless when sent on a campaign. There is the even more important question … of them being a danger and distributing infection among other troops in the theatre of war. In fact failure to *control malaria* in stations and cantonments in peace-time and in troops in reserve may be a most serious matter in war. … experience in *control* of *malaria* in stations and cantonments and the maintaining of troops in peace-time is actually therefore very definitely related to control in war.

[An] important aspect of *malaria* in war is the provision of the immense quantities of quinine and other anti-malarial drugs that may be required ... If drugs other than quinine have also to be employed it has to be considered how they are to be obtained or produced in war-time. It may be that drugs now familiar have to be replaced by other compounds with which we shall have to become familiar ... Policy in respect to cinchona growing and quinine storage, as well as knowledge of and ability to produce in large amounts anti-malarial synthetic drugs are matters therefore which, developed in peace-time, would have an important bearing on *control* of *malaria* in war.

Other issues which bear upon *malaria control* in war [involve] the supply of suitable stains (this was a serious difficulty in the early stages of the [Great] war), the supply of suitable forms of Paris green and of apparatus suitable for spreading this possibly on an unprecedented scale, the sources from which personnel trained in *malaria* work in the laboratory and in the field are to be provided ...

An aspect of war *malaria* which ought to be mentioned is the liability for *malaria* to be transmitted in theatres remote from the war due to the introduction in large numbers of infected returning soldiery. Numerous instances are to be found in the literature of cases of *malaria* contracted in this country from infection introduced from abroad; and even the possibility of local epidemics due to this cause has to be considered. Over and above such local effects may be a flare up of the disease from the direct and indirect effects of the war upon civil populations. A very marked example of this state of affairs occurred during the last war [1914–18] in the Emden district in north Germany. Since 1890 *malaria* cases ... had been seen only in sporadic form, but during the war enforced neglect of canals and even of important drainage systems and other changes (brought about by the war) led to this area becoming seriously malarious with many thousands of cases of the disease. Even more wide-spread and serious effects followed the war in Russia and some other European countries: a state of affairs which led to the formation of the *Malaria Commission* of the *League of Nations* [LN] [*see* Chapters 10 and 13]. ...

Christophers proceeded to give an historical account of *malaria* in wars apart from that of 1914–18:

> ... Some writers have [incorrectly] suggested that *malaria* is a relatively recent introduction in many countries. This, however, is very improbable. The most probable explanation is that the idea of *malaria* [particularly] as a definite disease entity, is comparatively modern ... Torti[3] must have known more than anyone else in his time, or before his time, of *malaria* as a single disease, but his figure of [the] 'fever tree' well indicates the absolute confusion [existing] up even to the eighteenth century and later in the diagnosis of fevers. ... [Early workers] must have seen and been struck by tertian and quartan periodicity. But that they attributed these to '*malaria*' as we do is doubtful. Certainly the name '*malaria*' does not go back very far and we should be careful in interpreting old writers ... The following extract [which comes] from [Harold] Scott[4] has ... a very familiar ring to those of us who have had occasion to study war *malaria* ...:

>> Celli has endeavoured to trace the history of *malaria* in Rome and the Campagna from ancient times, obtaining his information, not from medical writers only, but from historians, poets, [and] archaeologists ... Though the disease became prevalent in Rome after the second Punic War, about 200 BC, Celli does not believe it was imported from Carthage. It declined again during the days of the Empire until the end of the 4th Century AD and early in the 5th, when Rome was sacked by the Goths. The sacking of Rome in 1527 was followed by another recrudescence.

> Even accounts of more recent wars are not very helpful and it is perhaps not without interest to recall that it was only in 1881 [sic] that Laveran discovered the parasite [and] many of the wars we know well by name were before this time. It is only since about 1900 that the mosquito cycle has been generally accepted or recent ideas of the nature of malaria transmission developed. Hence up to and including the time of the South African War [1899–1902] we need not expect to learn much from writings on the subject. [Table 11.1 gives a list of wars since the Napoleonic]. ...

Table 11.1: The *malaria* situation in historical military campaigns

War*	Date	Remarks
Napoleonic	1793–1815	Included the Walcheren Expedition, 1806.
Russo-Polish	1831	Cholera most noticeable feature.
Crimean	1854–6	Exposure, improper food and cholera chiefly noted. 'Fever' also referred to in connection with shortage of quinine.
China	1860	
American	1861	So-called 'typho-malarial' fevers prominent.
Abyssinian Expedition	1867	Twenty-five weeks in country, British force of 2,674. Malaria only about 10% of strength.
Franco-Prussian	1870–71	
Soudan [sic] Expedition	1884	February to April.
Nile Expedition	1884	March to July.
Ashanti Expedition	1896	Average strength, 5,213; 1,401 admissions for malaria in six months; 40% officers went to hospital.
Chinese-Japanese	1897	Malaria chief cause of sickness; 41,734 cases.
Nile Expeditionary Force	1898	10 months.
South African	1899–1904	Enteric [typhoid] main problem. Little malaria.
Spanish-American	1898–99	May to February. American losses from disease, 5,277.
Soudan War	1904	Expeditions up Blue and White Nile suffered severely from malaria.
Russo-Japanese	1904–5	Twenty-one months, 20 battles, 220,812 casualties; 2 per 1,000 malaria.
Italian-Abyssinian	1935–6	Apparently little malaria.

* Major wars in bold.

On the whole, *malaria* does not figure very largely except in the famous Walcheren episode and the Chinese-Japanese war of 1897. In the case of some of these wars one would not have expected much *malaria*, but it is [nevertheless] surprising that there appears to have been so little ... in the South African War [and] the recent war in Abyssinia [1935–6].

It is only when one comes to operations in certain countries during the [1914–18] War that one begins to be given information of much utility. The experiences in [the Great War] are [certainly] worthy of the closest study since they constitute the basis upon which we must form most of our ideas regarding war *malaria* and its prevention.

During the 1914–18 war, Christophers outlined several examples:

- *Taranto**came into prominence because it was early realized that troops proceeding … to Egypt and other theatres of war were becoming infected even by a short stay [there].[5] … Attempts to provide protection by mosquito-proofed huts … met with difficulty [because those] provided were unsuitable for mosquito-proofing and if so protected were almost untenable in the climate of Taranto. Eventually the operations carried out had to be largely of an anti-larval type.

- The *Macedonian*** experience was one of the greatest medical surprises of the war. Both British and French troops were affected, the total casualties from *malaria* being enormous and quite unanticipated. A very complete account [has been] given[6] … but [many] other writers have also dealt with different aspects of *malaria* as seen in this theatre of war. Altogether the operations covered [about] three years occupation by the troops of a tract of country lying to the north of Salonica … Prior to June 1916 [they] were in position mostly on the line: Monastir Road, Salonica, Langaza and Bezik, and [during] the first five months of the year there [were] fifty cases only. In June the line began to move forward into the low lying valley of the Struma, extending up this river past Lake Tachinos to Lakes Bulkova and Doiran and thence to the River Vardar … a distance of about 60 miles. The French continued this line further to the west. After some ninety cases in June the incidence rose rapidly and in 1916 there were [about] 30,000 cases of *malaria*. [According to] Wenyon at least a quarter of the whole force [was probably infected in the winter of 1916–17].

  … measures taken included every known means of combating the disease; yet in spite of an amount of work … Wenyon gives it as his opinion that 'it is doubtful if any appreciable reduction in infections took place during our stay in the country'. After the formation of

---

*Sea-port and naval base in South-eastern Italy, which was founded by Greeks in the eighth century BC.
**Republic north of Greece, in South-eastern Europe, and bounded by Albania, Yugoslavia and Bulgaria.

a special *Malaria Enquiry Laboratory* … there was undertaken the drainage of swamps, clearing of streams, oiling and other methods of treating breeding places, fumigation and spraying, the mosquito-proofing of huts and dug-outs and the carrying out of quinine prophylaxis. The antilarval type of operations began with operations early in 1917 and were carried out [on] at least ten times as great [a scale], in 1918. … [According to] Wenyon [the] consensus of opinion was that quinine administration had little or no effect in controlling the disease. The only doubt this observer had was whether if quinine had not been given an even heavier incidence might have occurred. A very interesting feature [is in] the use of mosquito-nets. Two forms were used: a bivouac net modified and altered until in 1918 a serviceable pattern was evolved, and a bell net pattern. [Charles] Wenyon states that in his opinion *'the mosquito net did more to prevent infection than all the other methods of prevention* [author's italics].

- … operations in *Mesopotamia** are described by Christophers and Shortt.[7] The army [there] numbered approximately 400,000, of whom about one quarter were British. The [occupied] area … included the plains of the Tigris and Euphrates and parts of Persia [now Iran] and Kurdistan, a tract possibly about the size of England … The troops which at first were located in the lower parts of the Tigris and Euphrates plain moved up after the taking of Kut to Baghdad and Mosul and eventually extended into Persia. At the Base at Busra [sic], however, where a new port was created extending 7 miles along the river, railways constructed and other works undertaken – there were encamped throughout the period some 100,000 men. Nothing was previously known regarding *malaria* in this tract. The only authority mentioning it appears to be Hirsch[8] … As was ascertained during the early stages of the war we now know that there is a moderately endemic tract in the palm grove belt about Mohammerah and Busra [sic] where *Anopheles stephensi* is the vector, then a great belt of swamp and river extending up to Baghdad and beyond which is practically non-endemic, and then severely endemic tracts when the Persian and Armenian hills are reached.

  … The outstanding problem was *control* in the large Base area at Busra [sic]. The greater part of the area was palm grove land with its

---

* The tract of land situated between the Tigris and Euphrates rivers (now Iraq).

characteristic network of deep irrigation ditches. It was not, however, only the conditions natural to the country which had to be considered, for in the course of the necessary [excavations, etc] leakage from the river became [an] extensive sources of *anopheles*. No other decision was possible in the Base area therefore but to undertake large scale anti-larval operations chiefly of a protective nature. Troops, up country in Baghdad and elsewhere [were] relatively safe from any heavy incidence and it was only on entering the hilly country ... that *malaria* once again became a problem. [Morbidity] from *malaria* was considerable, though not to be compared with the incidence in Macedonia. That the anti-larval operations at the Base had at least some effect is suggested by ... figures for September to December 1918, *ie* for the chief fever season in that year (*see* Table 11.2).

In 1916–17 all units were supposed to be receiving prophylactic quinine [regularly]. Every effort to secure actual administration was made. As information was gradually acquired and systematized it became evident that whilst some units were suffering from *malaria* and exposed to infection others were not to [anything like] the same extent. In 1918 [owing to] early notification of cases and visiting of different units those which seemed in little danger of infection were

Table 11.2

Type of Area	No. Troops and Followers	No. Cases of Malaria	Admissions per mille per week
Well protected:			
Magil	22,810	407	1.1
Makina West	9,637	221	1.4
Total	**32,447**	**628**	**1.2**
Imperfectly protected:			
Makina East	4,810	336	4.4
River Front North	8,379	494	3.7
Total	**13,189**	**830**	**4.0**
Unprotected or [only] partially protected			
Base Transport	2,880	143	3.2
Hospital area	8,040	280	2.2
Ashar	6,345	296	2.9
Tanooma	2,440	103	2.6
River Front South	3,701	537	9.0
Total	**23,406**	**1,359**	**3.6**

taken off the compulsory quinine roster and attention [was] directed to such units as showed a heavy incidence or appeared to be in danger of infection.

One fact brought out was that admissions to hospital [played only] a small part [for in] 45,846 examinations [carried out] in the different hospitals about 19 per cent were … positive [for *malaria* parasites]. [And] in men on duty … the following percentage infection rates were[:] British troops, 13.7; Indian troops, 27.4. If this rate [was] general there should have been on any one day, 1,000 British and 8,000 Indians (excluding cases in hospital) with [a parasitaemia]. On an average, however, those actually admitted to hospital for *malaria* in a day were 27 and 31 respectively. Admissions therefore did not represent the same thing as infections.

Most of the 'specially affected units' were found to have previous 'histories'. They had been serving in East Africa or stations on the Persian Gulf. In an effort to trace infections to local conditions, 60 per cent of admissions after investigation had to be returned … as 'casual', *ie* the case was difficult to trace to any definite source. At one time many units coming from India were more heavily infected than those who had been some time in the country.

In regard to the value of quinine prophylaxis … as in Wenyon's experience in Macedonia, the incidence might have been even heavier if it had not been carried out. Mosquito-nets were issued but their erection and use was beset with difficulties. …

- Regarding operations in *East Africa* little need be said [other than] they involved an average strength of about 50,000 allied troops and [total] admissions for *malaria* in the two years 1916, 1917 [were] estimated at 120,000.

- [An account has been given of] the *Palestine* operations.[9] The capture of Gaza took place on 7th November 1917. In December *malaria* began to assert itself in the Summeil and Sarona area about the mouth of the river Auja. A mosquito survey in January 1918 showed that the vector was chiefly *A bifurcatus* breeding in wells, not *anopheles* from pools etc and the troops in the orange groves were [overall] most affected. In April 1918 the intended advance was postponed and the troops became stationary. The position occupied from this time to September was a line about 25 miles long stretching north of the Auja … The country occupied was notoriously malarious with marshes, streams, wadis and many sources of *anopheles*. The main efforts at *control* were of the anti-larval type ... Mosquito-proofed huts were used in dangerous places and wherever possible the sites of the camps selected. Evacuation of cases and quinine prophylaxis were also adopted. The anti-mosquito operations appeared to ... have reduced breeding to a minimum at a time when it might have been optimum. On 19th September, 1918, the ... Corps moved forwards into country that had previously been in occupation by the enemy. [From then on] the troops suffered severely from *malaria*. To what extent this was due to infection contracted after the move or the result of moving troops already infected [is impossible to deduce].

Following this fascinating historical narrative, Christophers continued with a survey of 'Preventive measures applicable to troops in the field'; he concentrated on anti-larval measures and quinine prophylaxis: Then, to other *preventive* measures:

> ... *Mosquito-proofed huts.* – Robertson[10] states that at Taranto [*see above*] he regarded mosquito-proofed huts [if ones of a suitable pattern could be obtained] as the most effective measure against *malaria* ... As this might again be an important method of control ... the possibility of devising suitable types of hut would be worth careful consideration. [This] should be given before the occasion for their use actually arises.
>
> *Mosquito-nets* – Wenyon's[11] remarks about mosquito-nets in Macedonia are not to be lightly dismissed. The mosquito-net is the method of prevention effective vastly beyond all others ... The difficulty of utilizing the method in the case of troops is, however, admittedly very great. ... Merely to issue nets, leaving it to someone in the field to devise methods of using them and to get them used is no way to proceed. ... The proper type of net is a matter that requires the most serious consideration, as also do the means by which it is to be supported and the method in which it is to be used. ... It is not supposed that such protection could always be provided in the front line, but experience shows that in an army there are usually troops at the base and lines of communication where protection of this kind is extremely desirable.
>
> Ideas regarding the care of troops have changed [markedly]. With electricity and modern facilities there is nothing preposterous in the idea that men might be accommodated in mosquito-proofed

huts with electric fans or provided with mosquito-nets ... all this requires a good deal of [thought], preparation and experiment *before* the event. Again the Higher Command must ... appreciate the importance of the measure. Officers and men must be taught the importance of using the nets properly, just [as] they must be taught the use of a gas mask ...

And the value of a well-equipped laboratory:

... It is impossible that any one laboratory organization can make all the examinations necessary for *clinical* purposes [as well as] notification of cases. [All] hospitals must themselves have the necessary equipment. Not only must microscopes be available, but the necessary slides and stains as well as at least one technician fully familiar with the technique and detection of parasites. ...

These are the main methods of *prevention* [which are] employed under war conditions. As regards any choice or selection it seems certain ... that in the event of an army operating in a malarious country all [these] methods [should] be prepared for. We dare not neglect quinine prophylaxis and must attempt to get it properly carried out. ... in some of the theatres of war the desirability of anti-larval operations should never be ignored. We must be prepared to use [all of] these methods and [also] others ...

And finally, Christophers stressed the problem(s) of 'planning ahead':

I now come to the most important of the points I have raised ... How is [planning ahead] to be achieved. ... I do not know what probability there may be that operations may again be undertaken in which large bodies of troops are employed in malarious areas, but if there is such a probability, then time should be taken by the forelock and an effective advisory organization ... established well ahead.

We know that personnel and equipment for one or more *Malaria Inquiry Laboratories* will be necessary, that hospitals will be required to make large numbers of blood examinations and ... be in a position to do so adequately. We know that mosquito-proofed huts will be asked for and mosquito-nets tried out. All these things could as well be thought out beforehand as at the time they are required. Paris greening will be required on an enormous scale.

What are the requirements for such large scale application? What is the programme as to quinine and atebrin [mepacrine] or substitutes for atebrin? What teaching in practical matters for subordinate staff will be necessary? What subordinate staff is actually available? Who are the people who might be thinking, planning and experimenting about these things and how are they to come together and collaborate?

It is most desirable [Christophers concluded] that all these matters should be dealt with well in advance and whilst the going is good.[12]

On 21 October 1943, Sir Harold Scott KCMG MD FRCP FRSE (1874–1956)[13] (*see* Figure 11.2), a notable pathologist and historian of *tropical medicine*, delivered the second war-time Address on: **The influence of the slave-trade on the spread of tropical disease.** After indicating that he had not been involved in research into *tropical medicine* for many years, he asked his audience to 'go back ... to a romantic period of *tropical medicine* [and to recall] with what delight we read, as boys, tales of the sea and the chase of slave-ships'. He began:

Slavery and slave-trading go back to the dawn of history. [This lecture is] confined to the trade which brought slaves from West Africa to the New World.[14] [It does not contain] anything of those who voluntarily became slaves in times of insolvency, famine or scarcity, just as some peculiar people in this country commit a small crime about the middle of December to ensure warm housing, good fare and entertainment at Christmas time at Government expense, amid conditions better than they would find in their own homes. I [dwell on] the slave by capture; his lot was very different. ... The prospective dealer would go into the country of peaceable negroes – militant tribes would give too much trouble – taking a few muskets, some spirits and a little merchandise, say calico. He visits the most powerful chief of the district, gives him presents, keeps him in a happy state of semi-drunkenness, tells him he wants more slaves and doles out the muskets. The chief without much difficulty recalls an old-standing quarrel with a neighbour and war is declared. The

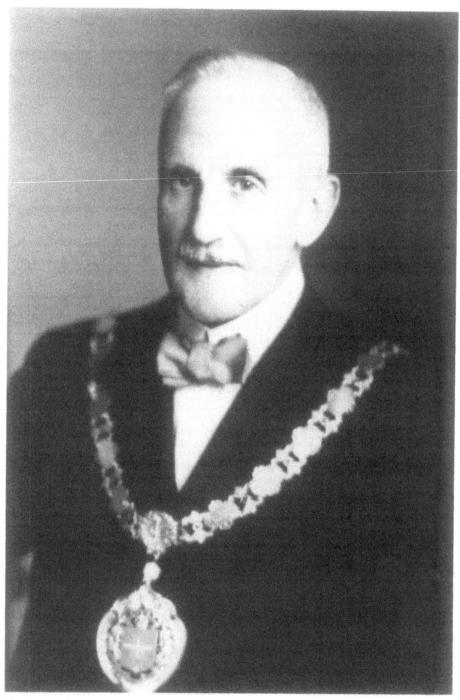

Figure 11.2: Sir (H) Harold Scott KCMG FRCP – the seventeenth president (RSTMH archive).

enemy's subjects are captured, the ground, their own as well as that of the enemy, is left untilled, scarcity and famine ensue and both chiefs will sell large numbers of their subjects and the captives at a cheap rate. Another method, much favoured by the Portuguese, was to exchange slaves for ivory in the interior, to use human porterage – in fact [this] was a necessity, there was no other way – to get the ivory to the coast and then sell the porters with the ivory to the greater gain of the ivory trader. At other times there would be raids for slaves without any declaration of intertribal war and without warning.

In the course of capture there was often much cruelty. Many villages might have to be raided to obtain the number wanted, many of the natives would die from injury, starvation and disease in the jungle. Those captured would be chained to prevent their escape, with slave-forks round their necks, hands fastened behind their backs and attached by a cord to the master's waist, and sometimes gagged by a wooden snaffle. The heavy mortality among them on their journey to the coast was evidenced by the skeletons, slave-clogs and forks strewn along the way. Underfeeding, overworking, exhaustion, disease and cruelty might lose one-third of the total. Much of the hardship was due to natural attempts at escape. Lovett Cameron observed at one time a gang of fifty-two women tied together in three lots; some had children in their arms, others were far advanced in pregnancy, all were laden and covered with weals, and scars – sheer wanton cruelty.

Yet a further loss, perhaps as much as another third, might occur at the barracoons where the slaves were collected on the beach before transportation. Here, too, the fatality would be high owing to insufficient food, overcrowding, dysentery and fevers, for they were kept in irons and roped in fours, legs fettered, chains round their necks.

The 'middle passage' [*ie*] the journey from Africa to the New World … might be fairly easy, but in many cases entailed much suffering. The food was usually good and if the weather was fair they might come on deck for air and exercise, perhaps a hose-bath, the exercise consisting of dancing to a drum. All this was arranged, not primarily for the benefit of the negro, but because sickness and mortality among them would reduce the owner's profit. On a 'bad ship', and later, when the trade was being made illegal, all slave-ships were bad ships, conditions must have been truly frightful. If one cargo in three got through the adventure paid, so overcrowding was disregarded. In the hold were stored provisions, powder, rum and so forth; in the 'tween decks the slaves were stowed in hundreds, the men forward, shackled at the start of the voyage, the women and children aft, unchained. They would be thrust in till they were packed actually in contact and might stay there, if the weather was bad, for many days together. Some would die and the living and the dead would lie chained together in the dark, and hunger, thirst, misery and disease, in particular dysentery, might, on a bad voyage, kill off 70 per cent; the average mortality on a favourable voyage was 11 to 12 per cent. Stories have been told of where the packing was so close that some would have to sit between the legs of others, and the boarding above them so low – they might be in two tiers – that even sitting upright was not possible, and on arrival every conceivable distortion might be observed, as a result of the long cramped posture. If lying down, each adult was allotted a space of 5 feet 6 inches long, 16 inches wide, and 24, occasionally 26, inches between the tiers.

Woe betide any who fell sick! According to the terms of insurance, if a death occurred on board the loss had to be borne by the owner, whereas jettisoning alive came under the head of 'sacrifice of cargo' and insurance was paid; so those seriously ill might be thrown overboard. After the trade became illegal [in 1833], a slaver when chased would jettison her living cargo to delay the pursuer, or cast the slaves manacled into the sea to prevent their being rescued to give evidence against their captors. ... The filth and stench of the vessels on reaching port were sometimes such that no one could be got to clean them and they had to be abandoned. Most of the slaves on arrival were very emaciated, often deformed from restricted posture, half-blind from the dark and ophthalmia and, possibly, onchocerciasis and months might elapse before they were fit for sale. ...

Obviously the slave-trade and conditions under which it flourished afforded potentialities for the spread of disease ... The study is a fascinating one, for we are often too ready to assume that because a disease is, or was, common in West Africa and was recorded for the first time in the New World in the seventeenth and eighteenth centuries, therefore the latter was infected by importation from the former – a very fallacious line of argument. …

Scott began an account of disease with *yellow fever* [YF]:

> … the place of origin [of YF] has been the subject of much discussion. … Historically, the value of the evidence of American origin must depend [very] largely on the meaning of terms used and the accuracy of translation of ancient records. We may dismiss … the view of Augustin that its origin was *Asiatic*, for he based his view on the Martinique outbreak of 1688–90, when the *Oriflamme* brought the infection, *la maladie de Siam*, or … *typhus miasmatique putride jaune*, on its voyage from Bangkok, disregarding the fact that the ship, blown [off] course, called at a port in Brazil where [YF] was raging before [sailing] to Martinique. Augustin affirms also that Smyrna was an original focus because remittent fevers of antiquity devastated the Grecian Archipelago and the shores of Asia Minor.
>
> The chief supporters of the American origin are [Carlos] Finlay, Caizergues, Kermorgant, Jorge, and Rubert Boyce [of Liverpool]. … The reasons [for the pro-American view] are:
>
> - After the battle of Vega Real, in March 1494, a serious outbreak [of disease] took place among Columbus's men, with loss of one-third [of them] Finlay, by a process of exclusion, maintains that this was [YF] because other diseases with [a] high mortality – *typhus*, *plague*, *smallpox* and *cholera* – were known to Europeans and would have been recognized by Columbus.
> - New colonies established by survivors of the San Domingo epidemic of 1493 … namely, Porto Rico and Jamaica in 1509, and Cuba in 1511, did not suffer any loss [because they were 'immunised'].
> - The term *xekik*, a name given to a Mexican disease in pre-Columban days, means 'vomiting of blood' and is translated, after 1648, as 'black vomit', and an old Mayan manuscript, says a translation of the seventeenth century, contains a medicine for 'Xekik, with black blood like an infusion of soot'. *Cocolitzli* is another Mexican disease, or

an alternative name for the same disease, and is referred to before the coming of Europeans.

- The *coup de barre* epidemic in Guadeloupe in 1635 is regarded by Finlay and Bérenger-Féraud as [YF].
- Expeditions to tropical America often suffered a high mortality.
- Navigators make no mention of any disease like [YF] on the West coast of Africa prior to the discovery of America. Accounts begin to be suspicious in the middle of the sixteenth century and [are] more certain in the seventeenth.
- Communication between Europe and West Africa was … frequent in the sixteenth and seventeenth centuries, and the disease, if it had existed in Africa, would have often been imported into Europe.
- The slave-trade was not well established till the seventeenth century, whereas [according to] Finlay and Bérenger-Féraud, [YF] has [existed] in America … since the fifteenth and sixteenth centuries.

[Many descriptions] were [however] by laymen, … and we have, therefore, to rely largely on epidemiological factors and data – mortality, climatic conditions, acclimatization, etc.

Scott then assembled a vast amount of historical evidence with a clinical, biological and entomological basis, supporting both the theory that *YF* originated in South America and *not* Africa, and *vice versa*. The major problem in assessing old descriptions is of course confusion with other febrile diseases, eg *malaria* and even *smallpox*. Records of the disease in the New World undoubtedly preceded accounts in West Africa, but this certainly does not establish its site of origin. Summing up the historical evidence, Scott was of the opinion that:

[We must] conclude … that positive evidence is not sufficient for us to affirm beyond all doubt where human [YF] originated. Owing to paucity of records, confusion of diseases, to the writers being non-medical, we really cannot say what actually were the pestilences before the arrival of Europeans. The statement that *America* was probably the primary site because jungle yellow fever occurs there and not in *Africa* is [totally] unwarranted.

... Whether [YF] had its origin in West Africa or in the New World is important [however] in so far as the incrimination of the slave-trade as *introducing* the disease into America is concerned, but it is immaterial as regards the wider question whether the trade was the cause of the spread of infection, for whether it was carried from Africa to America or brought back in ships returning from America to Africa, to the West Indies, to Europe, the slave-trade was the means of effecting the extension.

The next disease discussed was *leprosy*. Scott again began by questioning where the disease originated; by examining the available evidence he considered that Africa seemed the most likely continent, probably in:

... The belt of land extending across the Continent from Nigeria to Abyssinia, the country where its endemicity is greatest today. Brugsch, in his *Histoire d'Egypte*, mentions that it was prevalent in Egypt in the reign of Husapti, 2400 BC, and ... it has [certainly] been common in Africa, Egypt and India for the past 3000 years and [was] re-introduced into Egypt by negro slaves brought from the Sudan in the time of Rameses II, 1350 BC ...

... America became infected from four sources: Europe, Asia, Africa and the West Indies. Chico, the only writer ... who affirms that the Spaniards at the Conquest of Mexico in 1519 found cases among the natives, was probably misinformed; Juliano Moreira, who has gone deeply into the question, has concluded that these were more likely cases of *mal del pinto*. It is now generally admitted that America was free from the disease until the Spaniards and Portuguese introduced it; and when the slave-trade became a thriving industry the negroes who were brought over included hundreds, perhaps thousands, of lepers, and after emancipation of the slaves indentured Indians and Chinese introduced yet more. ...

... In the case of the West Indies the story [Scott considered] is very similar to that of South America – primary introduction by Europeans, Spaniards and Portuguese, when the islands were colonized and traffic arose between the islands and the mainland. The actual introduction is supposed to have taken place from Martinique or Cuba about 1776. Later [however] much wider extension was brought about by the slaves imported directly from Africa.

Yaws was the next disease to be included in the Address:

It was the widely, if not generally, held opinion at the beginning of the nineteenth century that *yaws* originated in West Africa and that the slave-trade was the means of importing [it] into other places where it [was then] endemic. Even at the end of the [nineteenth] century Wallbridge and Daniels[15] ... stated categorically: 'The disease, as far as the West Indies are concerned, is of African origin', but Daniels goes on to say that the West Indian *yaws* is identical with the *coko* of Fiji, and he saw many cases of both. Deeper investigation throws much doubt upon this; in fact, from all the evidence I have been able to obtain [Scott continued], it would appear that, when tropical medical history began, pian, framboesia, *yaws* existed in many regions of the world as far apart as the east is from the west. ...

... The fact – it appears to be factual – that the disease was present in the West *before* Columban days concerns, of course, the question of its primary introduction only; there can be no doubt that importation of infected slaves would contribute much towards spreading the disease, for it is known that epidemics ... occurred on slave-ships. During [the] slavery days fresh cases were ... constantly imported and [cases] became so numerous that they were segregated in '*yaws* houses' in many West Indian islands. (There was some confusion at times between *yaws* and *leprosy* and the same houses were used for both). After emancipation these houses were abandoned, the inmates scattered [to become] foci for other cases all over the country. [In conclusion] *yaws* was [therefore] probably autochthonous in Hispaniola, Brazil, Fiji, Samoa and West Africa, and imported into the West Indies by slaves.

Scott then gave brief accounts of the history of two protozoan infections – *trypanosomiasis* and *leishmaniasis*:

African trypanosomiasis, negro lethargy, was certainly carried to the West Indies by slaves, but the ... creoles were never attacked, only the negroes, and of these only ... as had themselves been brought over as slaves, that is, others born in the islands, even if their parents were victims, were not attacked, though the disease might not show itself until the subjects had been in the islands for a considerable time. The natives … in Africa were aware of the significance of … enlarged glands in the neck … Winterbottom's sign – for the Mandingoes in the Gambia used to 'cut the neck-stones of the boys to prevent the occurrence of sleeping-sickness later in life'. … The slave-trade, therefore, was responsible for transporting cases, but not for spreading [it] in the West because, fortunately, there were no suitable vectors … in the New World. …

… *American trypanosomiasis* was *not* brought from South America to Africa, bearing in mind … that until Sierra Leone was founded as a slave settlement and Liberia established for repatriated slaves in 1820 the traffic in slaves was … one-way traffic only.

… we must guard against the inference that because a morbid condition, or a causative organism, is found in Africa and also the New world the latter became infected by importation from the former. A good example is *cutaneous leishmaniasis*. It is present as *bouton d'Orient* in the East, in Asia Minor, along the Mediterranean littoral, in Southern Russia, India, China (Hunan), in Africa, Tunisia, Egypt, the Sudan, the French Congo, Nigeria and the West Coast down to Angola; in the New World it occurs in Brazil, Peru, Guiana, Paraguay, Bolivia, São Paulo, the Argentine and Mexico. … Though the dates [of these records] in the New World are of the [twentieth] century, the condition must be of old standing in South America, for ancient Inca pottery depicts figures with the facial mutilations of *espundia*.

Mal del pinto has a [very] wide distribution in the New World – Mexico, Colombia, Venezuela, Ecuador, Chile, Peru, Guatemala, Brazil, Cuba – and some have thought that, as a spirochaetal disease, it might be grouped with *yaws*, prevalent among slaves brought to America. There [is] little to support this, for [there were no reports] in the negroes of Africa. It may well be that the slave-trade did assist in its spread by transporting from one part of the New World to another slaves who had already acquired the disease, from Cuba to Brazil for example …

And a brief reference to two viral diseases apart from *YF*:

> We are usually given to understand that the earliest account [of *dengue*] is that by Gaberti of the outbreak in Cairo in 1779, but [there is no convincing evidence] that this was dengue. He calls it *mal de genoux*, but mentions neither secondary fever nor rash. Though these may not always be present, it is unlikely that they would be absent from all, or even the majority of cases in one outbreak. Rush, of Philadelphia, was the first to describe it clearly under the name 'break-bone fever' in 1780. From the early ... nineteenth century outbreaks were reported from many tropical and subtropical regions – India, Spain, Tripoli, North and South America, the West Indies. ... one suggestion in support of the possible transference of the disease by a slave-ship and this is the Guadeloupe outbreak in 1635, which, if it was *dengue*, antedated Gaberti and Rush by nearly a century and a half. ...
>
> Mention may be made ... that according to [Colin] Chisholm [1747–1825] *smallpox*, whether mild or confluent and malignant, has 'in every instance been introduced [into the West Indies] from the coast of Africa by slave ships'.

Finally, a brief survey of helminthic diseases:

> ... *Wuchereria bancrofti* is very widespread. Rhazes and Avicenna, Arabian physicians, wrote of it in the ninth and tenth centuries, and it [was probably] known to Hindu writers 1,500 to 1,600 years earlier. It is found in North and South America, in Australia, India, South China, Japan, the Dutch East Indies, Samoa, and in West and Central Africa. [J N] Demarquay [1814–75], in Paris, was the first to demonstrate the embryo in the hydrocele fluid of a patient from Havana in 1863; [Otto] Wucherer [1820–73] three years later found it in the chylous urine of a man from Brazil; [Timothy] Lewis [1841–86], in 1872, in the blood of a Hindu in India; the adult worm was seen by [Joseph] Bancroft [1836–94] in Australia in 1876–77, and [Patrick] Manson [1844–1922] in Amoy worked out its life-history ...
>
> Daniels [*see* above] discovered the adult of another filaria, *Acanthocheilonema* [now *Mansonella*] *perstans*, in British Guiana, and Manson the embryo in the blood of Congo natives in 1891. (For a time he was inclined to regard it as the cause of negro lethargy.)

It is very common in the Congo, Nigeria, Sierra Leone, the Gold Coast, the Ivory Coast and the Cameroons; also in Rhodesia and Uganda [and] it has been reported in South America, Venezuela and Trinidad, in the Amazon Valley and northern Argentina. [Therefore] there is a high degree of probability that the [slave] trade initiated ... spread of infection.

Loa loa we may certainly regard as slave-imported. *Loa loa*, the eye-worm of Africa, was known to Pigafetta in the Congo at the end of the sixteenth century, and Mongin in 1770 removed one from the eye of a negress in Haiti. Other cases, all in imported African slaves, were seen in Brazil, French Guiana and Haiti. [It was] imported but whether it spread after importation is less certain because all cases reported in the New World are thought to have contracted the infection in the endemic areas of Africa.

Dracontiasis has been known for a long time. It is believed that the 'fiery serpents' which attacked the Israelites when Moses took them from slavery in Egypt were *Dracunculus medinensis* and, according to Stitt, it was suggested that Moses taught the sufferers how to extract them by winding round a piece of stick. His pupils, if so, do not seem to have been very apt because the fiery part comes when the worm is broken by over-zealous or unskilful attempts at extraction... Pigafetta ... saw it in the Congo and illustrates it in the account of his travels. The endemic foci of *Dracunculus* are widespread; the Nile Valley, Uganda, Equatorial Central Africa, West Africa, Persia, India. After [introduction] into the New World cases [were] reported in the Guianas, the Caribbean, West Indian Islands, San Domingo (by Peré and Pouppé-Desportes), Jamaica (by Sloane), Barbados (by Hillary) and Martinique (by Saravésy) and in Southern Brazil. These records all come from the time when negroes were imported from West Africa. Since ... importation ceased there have been practically no more reported cases, except from a very few centres of which Curaçao appears to be one and Feira de Santa Anna in the Province of Bahia another. This last is particularly interesting because in 1849 two caravans encamped by a stream there and, though warned against it by the natives, the travellers used the water for drinking [and] a few months later all the party fell ill except a negro who had refrained from drinking the water. All writers on this [infection] in Brazil, Guiana, the West and East

Indies and Egypt agree that dracontiasis was unknown there before negro importation and after that time most [of the] cases recorded are in Africans. When the trade ceased ... cases became fewer and from many of its former haunts none was reported. [Infection in] Bombay is attributed to imported negro troops; similarly, Madras in 1834, but these have no connection with the slave-trade ...

Schistosomiasis – For a time after [Theodor] Bilharz [1825–62]'s discovery of *Schistosoma haematobium* in 1851, the lateral-spined ova were thought to be due to accidental distortion of the terminal-spined when passing through the tissues. Then, in 1903, Manson thought it must be a distinct species when he found these eggs in the faeces of a patient from the West Indies who had never suffered from haematuria. ... the distinction was eventually proved in 1916–18 by [the work of] R T Leiper [who showed] that the intermediary snail of the lateral-spined variety was a *Planorbis*, a different genus from that of the terminal-spined ... *Bulinus*, and that the two species of schistosomes differed morphologically. *S mansoni* ... was originally a West African species [where it is widely distributed]. Slaves brought from Africa have introduced it into Brazil, Venezuela, Dutch Guiana, St Kitts and other West Indian islands – St Lucia, Nevis, Montserrat, Antigua, Guadeloupe and Martinique. ... in St Kitts [it] is far from uncommon in *Ceropithecus sabaeus*, the ... 'green monkey', itself an importation from ... West Africa.

Scott concluded:

... there are other [diseases], such as ackee poisoning due to ingestion of a fruit native to West Africa, brought thence to Jamaica in a slave-ship in 1778 [and] evidence in favour of the African origin of alastrim and amoebic dysentery would provoke [an] interesting discussion ....[16]

Future of *clinical* tropical medicine

Brigadier Fairley was present at a *Council* meeting on **14 December 1944**. He had recently arrived from Australia and *en route* had attended a meeting of the *American Society of Tropical Medicine* (ASTM) at St Louis. He spoke of the ASTM as a 'thriving Society' (membership had risen from 500 to 1,500 during the previous four years), and he brought greetings from the president, Dr [W A] Sawyer. He also alluded to the establishment of several centres of *tropical medicine* (*see* below) and felt that if something was not done *urgently* in London, the British Empire would lose its position at the forefront of *Tropical Medicine*.[17] *Council* asked Fairley to prepare a memorandum on the subject 'in a form suitable for transmission to the Secretary of State for the Colonies'. At the next *Council* meeting (in January 1945) Fairley's memorandum, which contained an erudite account of the status of *clinical* tropical medicine throughout the world, was presented. It seems worthwhile to report most of this in full, as it contains much of importance both then, and even today:

> ### The present and future status of Tropical Medicine in England, The Dominions and the USA
>
> Throughout my association with the American and Australian Armed Forces in the South West Pacific Army, and during a recent tour in the [USA] and Canada [Fairley wrote], I have been impressed by the steadily increasing interest in *Tropical Medicine* and Tropical problems created during the War.
>
> #### I. *USA*
> #### AMERICAN SOCIETY OF TROPICAL MEDICINE
> From November 13th–16th 1944, I attended the meetings of the [ASTM] at St Louis. When I had last attended this gathering in 1934 the membership was about 500; today, it exceeds 1,500, the increase largely [having occurred] since the entry of USA into the War. The membership of the [ASTM] has thus practically trebled itself and now approximately equals that of the [RSTMH], London, the membership of which has decreased by about 200 since 1939. At their Annual Luncheon on November 15th 1944, Dr Wilbur A Sawyer, the President, asked me to convey the good wishes of the [ASTM] to the [RSTMH].
>
> On the same day I attended the 12th Annual Dinner of the *Academy of Tropical Medicine*, when the President, Colonel E B Vedder, read a paper on *'The Present Status of Tropical medicine and some Future Problems'*. This body is comprised of scientists and medical specialists whose aim is to assist scientific research and *clinical* study of tropical diseases, and to supply financial aid for

this purpose. Working in close conjunction with the [ASTM] its activities and sphere of influence are steadily extending.

Many of the papers read at the Annual Meeting of the [ASTM] were of ... interest and merit, and the advancing standard attained in *tropical medicine* since the War is reflected in recent publications in the official Journal of the Society.

Research in Tropical Diseases

Much research is being done in USA on insect repellents and the chemotherapy of tropical diseases. Special efforts are being directed to *malaria, dysentery, filariasis, scrub typhus* and *dengue* which are causing heavy casualties in the Pacific. By far the largest experimental investigation in chemotherapy ever attempted is at present being undertaken in the USA in bird *malaria*. Some 11,000 new compounds have been screened in *malaria*-infected birds, and a few of the more promising of those have been selected for testing therapeutically in man. Hundreds of chemists are giving their whole time to the synthesis of new compounds and almost equal numbers of pharmacologists to biological testing. New methods of estimating the concentration of anti-malarial drugs in plasma are being constantly devised. Investigations concerning the value of various antimony compounds in *filariasis* and of amoebicidal drugs are also being undertaken. At the end of the War there will be in the USA a considerable body of scientists and scientifically trained personnel peculiarly fitted for investigation and research in tropical diseases. In addition there will be large numbers of medical specialists and pathologists returning to America after several years of intensive study of tropical diseases occurring in members of the Armed Forces in the South Pacific, South-West Pacific and South-East Asia Commands.

Present or projected centres for post-graduate teaching of tropical medicine in USA

(1) *Tulane University*

At the present time there is a Tropical School for postgraduate teaching of *Tropical Medicine* at the Tulane University, New Orleans, which is under the Directorship of Dr Faust. Dr L Everard Napier, formerly of Calcutta, is visiting Professor of *Tropical Medicine*. This centre is based on the Port of New

Orleans, drains the Caribbean area and the East coast of South America, and during the War has been actively engaged in post-graduate teaching of army and civilian doctors. There is a Field Station at Vera Cruz working in association with Tulane.

(2) *Tropical Medical School, University of California, San Francisco*

The President of the University of California has agreed that there will be a School of *Tropical Medicine* associated with the University. Its primary function will be post-graduate teaching in *Tropical Medicine*. No Tropical Diseases Hospital is contemplated, but there will be a special tropical diseases ward in the new extension wing which is being added to the present hospital. This, in addition to clinical cases available in the new Naval Hospital of 1,500 beds and other local hospitals, should afford abundant material for *clinical* teaching. This School will cater for the Pacific Basin, the West coast of South America, China, Australia, etc. It would work in conjunction with the new State School of Hygiene, for which 15,000,000 dollars is available, and be closely associated with Dr Carl Meyer (Bacteriology) and Dr Hamilton Anderson (Pharmacology) at the University of California.

(3) *Tropical Medical Centre, University of Columbia, New York*

For many years the Presbyterian Hospital, University of Columbia, has handled a limited number of tropical cases from the Port of New York and Puerto Rico. It has now been decided to build a 300 bed Hospital for Tropical Diseases to cater for the Port of New York, and to create a School of *Tropical Medicine* associated with the University of Columbia for post-graduate teaching on a world-wide basis. The Mayor of New York, Mr La Guardia, at the dinner of the 52nd Annual Meeting of the *Association of Military Surgeons of the United States* held in New York on November 3rd 1944, stated that the object of this and other projects was 'to make New York City the medical centre of the world'.

II. *Canada*

Though the facilities for teaching *clinical tropical medicine* must be strictly limited, a course of instruction was opened at McGill University, Montreal, for the first time during the session 1944–1945. Its object was to train medical graduates to deal with medical problems peculiar to tropical areas. A diploma is granted to graduates of any recognised medical school after completion of three out of four of the following [3 month] courses –

(a) parasitology, medical entomology and bacteriology.
(b) public health and tropical hygiene.
(c) study at an approved hospital in the tropics. (Exemption can be given to candidates who have been engaged for at least 12 months in the treatment of tropical diseases in any tropical or sub-tropical country.)
(d) care of ambulatory patients in syphilology, dermatology, tuberculosis, child welfare clinics or paediatrics and haematology.

Professor T W H Cameron – formerly of the London School of Hygiene and Tropical Medicine [LSHTM] – is specially interested in this project. He informed me the course was designed largely [for] West Indian graduates ... unless the University of McGill is prepared to supply specially trained tropical physicians to staff a hospital in the tropics, it will have little or no control of the standard of *clinical* teaching adopted there.

III. *Australia*
A well staffed School of Hygiene and *Tropical Medicine* is located at the University of Sydney under the Directorship of Professor Harvey Sutton, and a Diploma in *Tropical Medicine and Hygiene* is granted after a 6 months' course. Additional short courses in *tropical medicine* and hygiene for medical officers from the Navy, Army and Air Force were held in 1942–44, the diseases dealt with being those met with in the South-West Pacific Areas. No tropical disease hospital is associated with the School, and before the War the course was undoubtedly weak on the *clinical* side.
   Research: In June 1943, a large medical research unit for the study of anti-*malaria* drugs in volunteers experimentally infected with *malaria* was established in Northern Australia; information of ... military importance has been already gained regarding the control of *malaria* in the Field, and new anti-malarials are continually being tested on a scale not hitherto applied to man. Over 500 volunteers have been used in these experiments to date.
   A new vector of *dengue fever*, *Aedes variegates*, has been found in New Guinea.

Other successful researches have included (1) the effects of anti-mite fluids like dimethyl-phthalate and dibutyl-phthalate on mites carrying *scrub typhus*, and (2) the chemotherapeutic control and cure of *bacillary dysentery* in the Field by sulphaguanidine.

Considerable stimulus has been afforded by the War to the study of tropical diseases by the medical profession of Australia and … physicians, pathologists, entomologists and sanitarians have had extensive training and experience in the Middle East, New Guinea, etc. This should strengthen the hygiene and medical services in Australia, Papua and the Mandated Territories after the War.

IV. *India*

The School of Tropical Medicine, Calcutta, gives a Diploma of *Tropical Medicine*. The post-graduates include private practitioners, medical officers of hospitals and dispensaries, tea estate doctors, medical officers to the railways and civil and military assistant surgeons. *Clinical* teaching is carried out at the Carmichael Hospital for Tropical Diseases. Research work is undertaken by special research staff under the Endowment Fund (Leonard Rogers' Laboratories), the Indian Research Fund Association, the British Empire Leprosy Relief Association, etc.

V. *South Africa*

A Diploma of *Tropical Medicine* is given by the Witwatersrand University, Johannesburg.

VI. *Europe*

It is possible that the various tropical teaching centres on the Continent, including the Tropical Institute at Hamburg and those at Brussels, Antwerp and Rotterdam, may no longer be functioning at the end of the War. … *a new Tropical Institute has suddenly sprung up at Basle in Switzerland which has neither ports nor tropical possessions* [author's italics].

Notorious Nazi medical authorities are amongst the advertised collaborators in their new official journal, *Acta Tropica*, which is a review of tropical science and *tropical medicine*. Is anything more probable than that German tropical scientists, backed by big chemical industries in Germany, are already planning ahead so as to lose no time in re-establishing their dominant position in the control of chemotherapy of tropical diseases? …

VIII. *Great Britain*

Today no Hospital for Topical Diseases [HTD] exists in London, and the wing of the bomb-damaged [LSHTM], which was specially concerned with the teaching of parasitology, is no longer serviceable.

- *Temporary measures to meet the coming emergency.*
  Apart from the usual floating population on leave from the tropics which passes through Harley Street or its adnexa, there will be large numbers of people with tropical disease such as refugees, ex-prisoners of war, discharged members of the Armed Forces, who will be returning to Great Britain during the next two or three years. If they are to be properly investigated and receive appropriate treatment, a large sized, well-staffed and equipped [HTD] should be made temporarily available in London to meet this expediency, and centralize patients from the tropics so that they can be under the care of tropical medical specialists and available for teaching purposes. ... in Liverpool ... Dr [A R D] Adams, a full-time teacher at the *Liverpool School of Tropical Medicine*, has been appointed to take charge of 300 beds.
- *Permanent measures to re-establish tropical medicine on a stronger basis*
  In the past many medical graduates from this country, India, Egypt, the Dominions, the Colonies and USA have come to the [LSHTM] and the [HTD] London, to obtain the D T M & H (London), or to the *Liverpool School of Tropical Medicine* or to Edinburgh for their diploma. If this country is to retain its former lead in the post-graduate teaching of *tropical medicine* in competition with new tropical centres in USA, especially that contemplated in New York, a co-ordinated effort on the part of all interested bodies will be necessary to centralize teaching by building a modern Imperial [HTD] not far removed from the renovated [LSHTM] and the Wellcome Research Institution with its unique museum facilities for the study of tropical diseases. Thus all teaching of *tropical medicine* would be centralized and the closest possible association established between clinicians and heads of departments. The collection in one centre of all patients suffering from tropical diseases

would increase the scope and value of *clinical* teaching, which is such an important aspect of *tropical medicine* to the average post-graduate seeking a diploma in this subject.

The formation of a tropical centre so efficient that it will attract post-graduates from all countries is feasible with Government assistance, provided the various interested bodies will co-operate and reach agreement. Co-ordination of the teaching of tropical medicine with the *Liverpool School of Tropical Medicine* and throughout the Empire should be aimed at, and, as a corollary to this, it would not be difficult to arrange interchange of professorial staff within the various Schools and Institutes of Tropical Medicine within the Empire.

The creation (at the earliest possible moment compatible with the non-interference with the War effort) of a select and influential central committee representative of all tropical interests would appear to be essential for dealing with this matter on a high plane. The various bodies interested might include the Government, the Colonial Office, the Seamen's Hospital Society [SHS], the *London* and *Liverpool Schools of Tropical Medicine*, the Royal Society, the Medical Research Council, the Wellcome Research Institution, the India Office, the Navy, Army and Air Force, Dominion representatives Missionary Societies and Banks and Business Firms in the City with vested interests in the tropics, etc.

... advancement of *tropical medicine* in this country [should be assisted] by grants such as that given by the *Rockefeller Foundation* for the building of the [LSHTM]. In the future, assistance on this scale can hardly be anticipated. With the establishment of large modern tropical schools in New York and San Francisco the USA will become a formidable competitor for post-graduate teaching in *tropical medicine* on a world-wide basis.

From an Empire viewpoint it is pertinent to consider whether medical graduates from the Dominions, Colonies, India, Egypt and elsewhere, interested in tropical problems will complete their general education in an American environment, or will be afforded facilities for high-standard post-graduate tropical training in this country where, in addition to technical knowledge, they will make personal contact with the peoples of Great Britain and learn something first-hand of their history and culture.

- *Future Tropical Research*

Time will not permit a review of the important research activities into tropical medical problems undertaken in the UK during the present War. What can be stressed, however, regarding the future is the pressing need for tropical research workers stationed in Great Britain to go out to the tropics from time to time to investigate tropical problems in their local setting. The limitations imposed by animal experiment have been strikingly demonstrated in the present War in relationship to the chemotherapy of *malaria* and *filariasis*, and in the future it would appear that the country which possesses the best organised clinical facilities for co-ordinated team work in the tropics will be most favourably situated for chemotherapeutic and allied investigations.

There is urgent need for adequately staffed and well equipped laboratories built *in association with hospitals in the tropics* for the long-term study of the prevalent local diseases with accommodation adequate to provide for individual workers or teams of research workers sent out from Great Britain to solve specific problems arising in the course of such studies, especially with reference to chemotherapy, vitamin deficiency and the like.

In peasant and native populations all *clinical* investigations are best conducted in association with the institutions which have an established reputation regarding the diagnosis and treatment of such diseases. This is well exemplified in the Wellcome Trust Research Laboratories attached to the Refugee Hospital, Salonika, in regard to blackwater fever, where facilities have been built up which are superior to those existing in any country, The establishment of similar laboratories, sited in the first place for research on a specific disease, would save valuable time and materially assist any research unit investigating that particular problem. Finally, in the investigation of rarer diseases in native villages and communities where such centres could not be built up, the more extensive use of field laboratories, mobile radiological units etc would on occasions permit collection of scientific data on a scale rarely attainable by other means.

VIII. *Recommendations*

With the object of strengthening the position of this country in regard to (1) the care of its tropical sick, (2) post-graduate teaching in tropical medicine, (3) the furtherance of research in tropical diseases, the following recommendations are made –

(1) The Government, the Colonial Office, the *London* and *Liverpool Schools of Tropical Medicine*, the [SHS], the Navy, the Army, the Air Force, the India Office, the Royal Society, and certain other bodies, be formed as soon as possible with the object of founding an Imperial [HTD] in London, serving all tropical interests and all strata of society – re-establishing and expanding those facilities for the treatment of patients from the tropics which have been lost as a result of the War.

(2) That preference be given to building such a hospital in a central position, as near as possible to the [LSHTM] and the Wellcome Research Institution, so as to centralize tropical post-graduate teaching in London, and create a tropical medical centre which would be worthy of the British Empire with its vast tropical responsibilities.

(3) That, as occasion demands, a chain of adequately staffed and well-equipped tropical research laboratories be built in different parts of the tropics in association with selected hospitals with the object of affording facilities for research on specified diseases. In addition to serving the requirements of the permanent staff, such laboratories should be built and equipped so as to afford accommodation for individual research workers or a selected team sent out by the British Schools of *Tropical Medicine*, Hospitals for Tropical Diseases, the Royal Society, the Medical Research Council or other bodies to study specific problems requiring for their solution highly trained experts. Any such research laboratories built in the Colonies would need to be linked [to] Colonial Medical Development schemes and Colonial Office plans for medical schools in the Colonies.

N Hamilton Fairley
Brigadier
Director of Medicine AMF
16.1.45

A copy of this memorandum was then sent from *Council* to the Secretary of State for the Colonies, other Government departments, the Royal Society, the Medical Research Council, the SHS and others likely to be interested – for information.

Fairley reported to the next meeting of *Council* that in response to his memorandum, the president of the Royal Society had convened a meeting of people interested in the re-establishment of an HTD in London. However, little seems to have been done, and Col Drew (an Hon Secretary) stressed at the following *Council* meeting (**13 December**) that 'the subject should not be allowed to drop'. The then president (Wenyon) added that the Colonial Office had appointed a Sub-Committee, but 'there the matter rests'. Manson-Bahr later referred to the 'small nucleus of an HTD recently established [at Devonshire Street]'.

The Society during the War (1939–45)

During this War, the Society lost numerous Fellows; many were killed by enemy action. Also, many overseas Fellows fell into 'enemy hands'. This obviously resulted in a great loss of income in subscriptions. Also, Manson House sustained damage on several occasions during the 'Blitz' of late 1940. (*see* below).

Meetings during the War

The first meeting of *Council* after the outbreak of hostilities was on **19 October 1939** when the president, Sir Rickard Christophers (who had recently recovered from a serous accident) took the chair. First indication that the war was in progress came in the Treasurer's (Marriott) report:

> ... All bookings for the use of the Hall had been cancelled and the garage tenant had notified his inability to make any further payments for the present. [However,] the *Buddhist Association* had applied for use of the Hall every Sunday for 1½ hours and [they] were willing to pay £150 per annum; Council agreed ... but only for one year.

The first *Ordinary* meeting of the War took place later that day, when Christophers delivered his presidential address on 'Malaria in War' (*see above*). No less than 34 new Fellows were elected at that meeting.

At the next *Council* meeting on **16 November**, several [Councillors] offered to resign due to 'difficulties created by the war', but this was considered unnecessary. The Hospital for Tropical Diseases (HTD) (still under the aegis of the Seamen's Hospital Society), it was announced, was *not* available 'owing to the War' and could *not* therefore host the customary annual *clinical* and *laboratory* meetings.

According to the minute books, the next meeting of *Council* took place on **15 February 1940** at 3.00pm (*ie* some five months later); AGMs took place regularly every June/July.

During the War years, most of the Society's business was in fact enacted by an *Executive Committee* – consisting of the president, the Treasurer (Marriott), the Hon Secretaries (Col N Hamilton Fairley and Dr C M Wenyon) and Dr G Carmichael Low, who was co-opted. They in fact met no less than 23 times between 20 June 1940 and 17 July 1941*.

It was decided by *Council* on **17 July 1941** (and ratified at the 34th AGM later that day) that 'those now in office should continue'; Sir Rickard Christophers therefore remained president until the following election. *Council* also recommended at the next (35th) AGM that the same officers should [continue] for the present; this was unanimously accepted.

The next meetings – of both *Council* and also an *Ordinary* meeting – were on **23 July 1942**. As the previous year, the *Executive Committee* was keeping the Society afloat – there having been fifteen meetings of this body between 17 July 1941 and 23 July 1942. It was now estimated that the total cost of air raid damage to Manson House (*see above*) amounted to £3,266 16s 8d.

At a *Council* meeting on **24 February 1943** it was recorded that between 23 July 1942 and then, the Executive Committee had met nine times, although Fairley's attendance had been limited to two meetings on account of Service commitments. They had little to report on that occasion, other than that minor repairs had been effected at Manson House and the Assistant Secretary – Miss Mann, who had been with the Society for twelve years – had married; as Mrs Enfield, she left in late 1945 after 'nearly fourteen years' in order to 'devote herself to her family'; the Society gave her £50.

At a further meeting of *Council* on **1 July**, the *Executive Committee* reported on its seven meetings since 24 February 1943; the only items of

---

* These meetings were not well documented. However, brief notes were recorded in two small 'exercise' books – for the periods 1940–42 and 1942–44.

interest related to local Secretaries and relatively trivial financial affairs. However, they recommended to the 36th AGM that Scott become the next president; he duly gave his presidential address on 21 October (*see* above).

Council decided on **14 July** to continue with *the Executive Committee* despite the fact that the Laws did not provide for its existence. At this meeting, they also suggested more frequent *Ordinary* meetings (*see* Table 11.3) than of late, and further that they be held in the afternoon rather than the evening. They were to return to evenings (at 8.00pm) in 1945; this alteration was announced at the 38th AGM. On **21 October 1943** a report from the *Executive Committee* (27 July–7 October 1943) was tabled; the new tenants (*see* below) were approved, permits to let Manson House having been obtained from both the Howard de Walden Estate and the LCC.

On **21 October**, also, *Council* was made aware of a letter from Dr A G H Smart, Chief Medical Adviser to the Secretary of State for the Colonies asking whether the Colonial Office could join the RSTMH. It transpired, however, that there was no provision in the Laws for corporate fellowship, and an alternative solution was that the Secretary of State for the Colonies be made an *ex officio* Honorary Fellow; however, this was *not* accepted. It was decided that while association with the Colonial Office seemed highly desirable, any solution to the dilemma would be postponed.

For most of the War years, *Ordinary* meetings were thus few and far between. Following a paper by Professor Warrington Yorke on **15 February 1940**, amongst the discussants was Sir Henry Dale FRS. The next few years were devoid of most *Ordinary* meetings, proceedings being confined to *Executive Committee* meetings (*see above*) with the occasional *Council* meeting and of course, the AGMs. However, an exception occurred on **4 November 1942** when Col Hamilton Fairley and Col J S K Boyd presented a joint paper on the modern treatment (sulphaguanidine chemotherapy) of bacillary dysentery (shigellosis). Although attendance at those meetings which did take place declined a little during the War, the average 'stood up' fairly well; on **24 February 1943**, for example, 77 Fellows and their guests were present.

During the War, addresses of Fellows and Society Laws were omitted from the *year-book* for obvious reasons.

Gifts to the Society

Gifts to the library, although fewer than heretofore, were announced on 28 March 1940, 17 July 1941, 1 July 1943 and 16 March 1944. On **16 May**

Table 11.3: Communications at *Ordinary* meetings during World War II

Date	Subject	Speaker
1940		
15 February	Chemotherapy of protozoan infections	Warrington Yorke
28 March	Diagnosis of shigellosis	J S K Boyd
	Treatment and prophylaxis of shigellosis	R A O'Brien
16 May	Immunization against Rickettsial infections	F Murgatroyd
20 June (33rd AGM)	Sulphanilamide drugs in southern Sudan	J Bryant
1941		
17 July (34th AGM)	Yellow fever in Africa	G M Findlay
1942		
23 July (35th AGM)	Drugs against Malaria	S R Christophers
	Treatment of Malaria in a hyperendemic zone	W Hughes
4 November	Treatment of bacillary dysentery	N H Fairley, J S K Boyd
1943		
24 February	Medical problems in the colonies in War-time	A G H Smart
1 July (36th AGM)	–	
14 July	Modern drugs in tropical diseases	S P James
21 October	Slave trade and tropical disease (presidential address)	Sir Harold Scott
18 November	Tropical disease in soldiers in the Middle-East	E Bulmer
1944		
20 January	Disease in West African native troops	R M Murray-Lyon
16 March	Heat effects in British Service personnel in Iraq	T C Morton
18 May	Blackwater fever anuria	B Maegraith
15 June (37th AGM)	–	
20 July	Cholera in India	Sir Leonard Rogers
19 October	Malaria control in the Gold Coast	L G Eddey
16 November	Treatment of amoebiasis	A R D Adams
14 December	'The Manson Saga'	Sir Philip Manson-Bahr & others
1945		
18 January	Chemotherapy and prophylaxis of malaria	N H Fairley
15 February	DDT in tropical medicine	P A Buxton
17 May	Kala-azar in India	H E Shortt
21 June (38th AGM)	–	
16 October	Tropical Medicine in War and Peace (*presidential address*) (see Chapter 12)	C M Wenyon
13 December	Teaching *tropical medicine*	L E Napier

1940, Manson-Bahr was thanked by *Council* for a gift of the new (11th) edition of *Manson's Tropical Diseases*, which he had edited.

Manson House

At a meeting of *Council* on **20 June 1940**, in reply to a question from Dr C C Chesterman concerning *provisional* accommodation in the event of the Society being compelled to evacuate the Manson House offices, it was decided that the Secretaries were authorised to make suitable arrangements.

Owing to a possibility of letting the Society's vacant premises, *Council* decided on **24 February 1943** to carry out further repairs to make the upper floors of Manson House habitable; the £556 already spent on temporary repairs had by then been refunded by the War Damage Commission.

THE BLITZ

Manson House was first damaged by blast from a bomb which fell in Portland Place (opposite the Langham Hotel); *urgent* repairs to the roof and windows were immediately carried out – the cost (£200) being included in the first War Damage claim for £1,412. On **16 April 1941**, more extensive damage was sustained from bombs in Hallam Street (behind the BBC building); the claim for this damage was £1,534. Lesser destruction was sustained on 10 May 1941. However, the Lecture Hall was not harmed in any way.

Despite these events, Manson House remained open, and the Hall was let many times for meetings during 1941 and 42. Meanwhile, the Society's furniture was insured for £2,000, and the books and records removed to the strong rooms in the basement.

TENANTS ETC

Mr G P Joseph, the long-standing tenant of the maisonette gave notice that he would be leaving at Christmas 1940 (*see CM*, **28 March 1940**); search for a successor at £825=00 per annum was begun immediately. (The maisonette incidentally consisted of eleven rooms, four bathrooms and the garage; it also contained a four-room flat).

The following document (copies of which had been pre-circulated to *Council* members) entitled *Question of tenants at Manson House* was debated on **1 July 1943**:

The Society occupies the ground floor and basement of Manson House, the three upper floors and the garage premises at the back having been let until soon after the outbreak of war. Leases which then terminated were not renewed with the result that the annual loss to the Society [was] in the neighbourhood of £800 per annum. In spite of this loss, by reason of strict economies and [a] publication grant of £200 per annum from the *Rockefeller fund* at the disposal of the Royal Society, the Society has not only paid its way but has been able to some extent to reduce its debt.

Efforts have been made to secure tenants and … there is now a distinct possibility of letting the upper part of Manson House and the garage premises again if it is decided to do so. One enquiry from a Medical Insurance Society is for a lease of not less than 21 years.

This raises the question of the future development of the Society. If soon after the war more space than that at present occupied by the Society should be required then it would be inadvisable to tie up the premises by a lease of a number of years. For instance it might be desirable for the Society to use for its receptions before or after meetings in the large room on the first floor. There is [a] kitchen on this floor so the serving of refreshments could be easily carried out. This would avoid any clashing with meetings of the *Council* and would give Fellows and visitors more space for talking and [taking] refreshments etc. Another suggestion was that at some time it might be possible to provide bedroom and breakfast accommodation for Fellows visiting London for a few days – whether such a scheme is feasible or not it is difficult to decide.

It would seem therefore that a decision has to be made as to whether the premises should be let either wholly or in part; and if let, for how long. In this connection it has to be remembered that before the war the premises were let without interference with the progress of the Society.

This document in fact provoked a great deal of discussion, after which Sir Leonard Rogers moved the following resolution which, with the exception of one dissident – Col S P James (the next president), who felt that even five years was too long, and that 'Manson House should be made as soon as possible a really nice house for the Society's Fellows' – was carried:

> That the *Executive Committee* be authorized to let the upper floors of Manson House and the garage premises to a suitable tenant or tenants for a period *not exceeding five years*, on condition that safeguards are ensured for regaining possession of the premises on the expiry of the lease if the premises are then required by the Society.

Dr C M Wenyon (an Hon Secretary) reported to *Council* on **14 July 1943**, that negotiations were in progress for a five-year lease with the *British Chemical Plant Manufacturers Association* for the three upper floors of Manson House at £750 per annum (they were to take up occupancy on 11 October 1943), and also with Messrs William Page and Co Ltd for the 'garage premises' at £275 per annum for a similar period also inclusive of rates. On 16 November 1944, meetings in the Hall – organised by the *Progressive Businessmen's Forum* and the *Oil and Colour Chemists Association* were announced by the Treasurer; rent from these would bring in about £150 in 1945.

The Fellowship

During the war years, many Fellows died on active service (*see above*). However there were numerous other deaths, and many of these were reported at *Council* and/or *Ordinary* meetings. For example, Professor Ziemann's death (an Honorary Fellow since 1911) was reported to *Council* on **15 February 1940**. Dr A J R O'Brien's death (a vice-president) was announced to *Council* on **28 March**; he was replaced by Air-Vice-Marshal Sir Harold Whittingham. The death on active service of the Society's architect – Major J N R Vining FRIBA – who had re-joined the Royal Engineers, was also reported in 1941 (*see CM, 23 July 1942*). Professor Warrington Yorke's death was announced by the retiring president (Christophers) at the 36th AGM, as well as that of an Honorary Fellow, Professor C A Stiles. The death of Col Mackie, an original Fellow of the Society, was noted on **20 July 1944**.

The Society's finances

Owing to the War, many overseas Fellows had difficulty in paying their subscriptions (*see above*); however, the Society was understanding and tolerant.

After several minor donations, the deficit on the Manson House Fund had fallen to £8,889 2s 3d by 1 July 1941. A 'windfall' occurred in early 1943 when it was reported to *Council* that Mrs M K Coldwell (totally unknown to any *Council* member) had left £5,000, free of duty, to the Society in her Will;

this sum was subsequently placed in the House Fund, further reducing the debt to £3,093. On **18 May 1944** the debt on Manson House was further reduced to £2,564 and a transfer of £1,000 from the General Accumulated Fund lowered this (now in the form of a loan from the Westminster Bank) to £1,559 (*see CM,* **15 June**). The Treasurer (Marriott) reported on **17 May 1945** that the debt on Manson House had been reduced to £1,012 4s 4d but that by utilising £600 of the previous year's balance – in the accumulated funds – and £420 4s 4d from the income from subscriptions and rents, the debt would soon be paid off in entirety. Marriott gave special recognition of the contributions of Low and Wenyon, who had done so much in connection with the House Fund which had been inaugurated in **1923**; total expenditure had by then been nearly £30,000.

Relations with the RCP and GMC

At the **23 July 1942** *Council* meeting, a letter from the Royal College of Physicians (RCP) was read, asking the Society to 'appoint an advisory committee of tropical consultants'. This was however considered unnecessary, and it was decided that the RCP should channel any enquiries to the Honorary Secretaries who would 'set the necessary machinery in motion'.

Later in the war, on **20 January 1944**, the Society formed a Sub-Committee of *Council* consisting of the Officers together with Manson-Bahr, Biggam, Hawes and Chesterman to look into the GMC's request for credentials of a *Consultant in Tropical Medicine*. As a basis for future discussions, this Sub-Committee reporting on **16 March**, laid down the following criteria:

> *Consultants in Tropical Medicine:*
> - ... shall have a minimum of 7 years approved training and experience after qualification of which at least 5 shall have been spent overseas in localities affording special opportunities for the study of tropical diseases
> - ... must have passed the membership examination of a [Royal] College of Physicians and hold a diploma or degree in *Tropical Medicine*
> - ... must hold, or have held, a recognised appointment in a hospital where special facilities are available for the study of tropical diseases
> - ... must not engage in general practice.

Also in March 1944 *Council*, at the request of Lord Moran PRCP, appointed Sir Harold Scott to serve as the Society's delegate on the Royal College of Physicians *'The Nomenclature of Diseases'* Committee. A later letter from Moran, referring to the new edition, requested the names of two Fellows who would be willing to work with Scott and revise the section on *Animal Pathology and Tropical Medicine*; Dr C Wilcocks and Col W R M Drew were nominated.

Other matters

In June 1944, a circular letter suggesting formation of a *Society for General Microbiology* was circulated, and comments from the RSTMH were requested. However, I have *not* been able to find views on this matter in the minutes.

On **19 October 1944**, *Council* resolved that the centenary of Manson's birth should be commemorated with a lecture; Manson-Bahr was identified and he agreed to give the lecture on 14 December 1944 (*see* Table 11.3). A later meeting (16 November 1944) was told that Low would also give a talk on this occasion. In the event, 91 Fellows and guests were present.

Hostilities cease

World War II came at last to an end in 1945; although the German surrender was signed on 8 May (Hitler had committed suicide on 30 April), Japan's formal surrender was not announced until 2 September of that year.

The thirty-third to thirty-seventh annual reports

During the War (1939–45) the number of Fellows fell from 1,663 (50 less than the previous year) to 1613, 1617, 1635, 1645 in the four succeeding years.

The Treasurer's (O Marriott) report for the year ended 31 March 1940 showed a balance carried forward of £506 10s 9d and that at the end of the War (during which both subscriptions and rents from tenants plummeted spectacularly) was £79 8s 6d for the year ended 31 March 1944.

References and Notes

1   **Rickard Christophers** received his medical education in Liverpool, where he came under the influence of Sir Charles Sherrington FRS. He then served in South America, Central and West Africa, and India, where his researches with J W W Stephens centred on malaria. Joining the IMS, with which he remained for some thirty years, his research on malaria continued. On return to Britain, he was appointed to a chair at the LSHTM. He later pursued entomology at Cambridge. His centenary was celebrated by the RSTMH. C Garnham. Christophers. Sir (Samuel) Rickard (1873–1978). In: H C G Matthew, B Harrison (eds). *Oxford Dictionary of National Biography.* Oxford: Oxford University Press 2004; 11: 559–60.

2   C A Gill. The prevention of malaria in war, with special reference to the Indian Army. *J R Army Med Corps* 1917; 29: 439–56.

3   F Torti. *Therapeutice specialis ad Febres quatdam perniciosas, in opinard, ac repente lethales, und verd china china, peculiari Methodo ministrata, sanabiles.* Bartholomaei Soliani Impress 1712: 736.

4   **Harold Scott** received his medical education at University College, St Bartholomew's and St Thomas's, qualifying in 1897. Three years later, he joined the RAMC and served in the South Africa War. He was later government pathologist in Jamaica, and there carried out research on the 'vomiting-sickness'; in Hong Kong, and the Zoological Society of London, his research was mainly on tuberculosis in man and animals. He was then assistant-director and subsequently director of the *Bureau of Tropical Medicine and Hygiene.* Scott was a notable writer and medical historian. G C Cook. Scott, Sir (Henry) Harold (1874–1956). In: H C G Matthew, B Harrison (eds). *Oxford Dictionary of National Biography.* Oxford: Oxford University Press 2004; 49: 386–7.

5   J C Robertson. On the anti-malaria campaign at Taranto during 1918. *J R Army Med Corps* 1920; 34: 444–67.

6   C M Wenyon, A G Anderson, K McLay, T S Hele, J Waterston. Malaria in Macedonia, 1915–1919. *J R Army Med Corps* 1921; 37: 81–108, 172–92, 264–77, 352–65.

7   S R Christophers, H E Shortt. Malaria in Mesopotamia; Incidence of malaria among troops in Mesopotamia, 1916–1919; Antimalaria operations at Busra, 1916–1919. *Indian J Med Res* 1920–21; 8: 508–52, 553–70, 571–92.

8   A Hirsch. *Handbook of Geographical and Historical Pathology.* London: New Sydenham Society 1883; 1: 202.

9   E P Sewell, A S M MacGregor. An anti-malaria campaign in Palestine: an account of the preventive measures undertaken in the 21st Corps Area in 1918. *J R Army Med Corps* 1920; 34: 85–100, 204–18.

10   *Op cit.* See note 5 above.

11   *Op cit.* See note 6 above.

12   S R Christophers. Presidential address: Malaria in War. *Trans R Soc top Med Hyg* 1939–40; 33: 277–92.

13 *Op cit.* See note 4 above.

14 H Thomas. *The Slave Trade: the history of the Atlantic slave trade 1440–1870.* London: Picador 1997: 925.

15 G C Cook. Charles Wilberforce Daniels FRCP (1862–1927): underrated pioneer of tropical medicine. *Acta Tropica* 2002; 81: 237–50.

16 H H Scott. Presidential address: The influence of the slave-trade in the spread of tropical disease. *Trans R Soc trop Med Hyg* 1943–44; 37: 169–88.

17 G C Cook. *From the Greenwich hulks to Old St Pancras: a history of tropical disease in London.* London: Athlone Press 1991; 338; G C Cook. *Tropical Medicine: an illustrated history of the pioneers.* London: Academic Press 2007: 215–7.

Chapter 12

The early post-war years – 1946–50

The 39th annual report (for the year ended 31 March 1946) began:

> In looking back over the past year the outstanding event has been the end of the war. Manson House stands secure. It was never closed down in spite of many nearby hazards. Permanent repair of blast damage is now taking the place of temporary work carried out during the emergencies of the last five years. Well-attended meetings are again being held in the evenings (instead of afternoons) and the last four have been preceded by an informal dinner for Fellows. This has proved a popular innovation, affording those on leave an opportunity of meeting Fellows at home.

Future of the *clinical* discipline

There was by now a great deal of concern regarding the future of *clinical tropical medicine* in London (*see* Chapter 11). Fairley's memorandum, Dr [L E] Napier[1]'s recent paper on the teaching of *tropical medicine* (*see* Chapter 11), and the latter part of Wenyon's presidential address (*see* below) had all made the point that London *must* have a Hospital for Tropical Diseases (HTD). As a result the RSTMH appointed a *Tropical Medicine Policy Committee* with Dr George Macdonald as its Secretary.

At a meeting of *Council* on **17 January 1946**, Macdonald claimed that 'the *Colonial Office* and some others were taking steps to provide beds at University College Hospital (UCH), but he knew nothing of the details of the scheme'. It was also agreed that Macdonald, who had produced a memorandum on the future of *clinical* tropical medicine (*see* below), should form a *Policy Committee*. His recommendations were:

> *General.* At the beginning of 1945 the President and Council expressed their opinion, by sponsoring Brigadier Hamilton

Fairley's memorandum, that facilities for the study, teaching and practice of *tropical medicine* are inadequate in the United Kingdom, particularly in London, and overseas, and also that it was in the *urgent* national interest that the defects should be remedied. Twice since then public discussion of the subject has been stimulated, by Dr Wenyon's presidential address [*see* below] and by the discussion opened by Dr Napier on 13 December [1945].

The initial expression of opinion achieved its immediate object. At a meeting convened by the President of the Royal Society it was agreed to, and the then Secretary of State for the Colonies expressed his personal conviction of the need for the *tropical medical* centre in London, stating that he hoped to find the necessary finance for its erection and no public appeal for funds was therefore needed. From that time, however, the project passed into the control of a Sub-Committee with which the *Council* has no communication and which has not since reported. It appears, from the failure even to formulate a concrete scheme at a time when Government support was promised, that the matter has been shelved.

The two subsequent measures have received wide Press attention which must have stirred public interest and attention. There is, however, no reason to suppose that their material effect will be greater than that of the first effort unless the Society establishes machinery to ensure continuity of this interest, the formulation of detailed proposals, and their consideration by executive bodies capable of implementing them.

The Committee. An appropriate form for this machinery would be a permanent Policy Committee, with a continuing general instruction to concern itself in matters of policy, as well as periodical instructions to concern itself with matters specially referred to it. It should be elected by the *Council* (though it should not be necessary to elect *Council* members only), and should have the power to co-opt members or invite occasional attendance by individuals. The President of the Society should be *ex-officio* a member and Chairman. A Vice Chairman should be appointed to take the Chair in his absence. A total membership of eight would form a workable Committee. It should be laid down that the Committee should meet not less frequently than the *Council*, to facilitate the calling of *ad hoc* reports at *Council* meetings. It should be recognised as a means of speeding business that it should for sub-committees to consider any purely local matters, or other special matters, though any report to the *Council* should carry the support of the full Committee.

Terms of Reference. The following general terms of reference are suggested:-
(1) To consider and report to the *Council* on (a) matters relating to the study, teaching, and practice of *tropical medicine and hygiene*, and particularly the steps necessary [and] their appropriateness to the needs of the United Kingdom and the tropical countries dependent on it, and (b) any matter specially referred to it.
(2) On receiving approval of a recommended policy from the *Council* of the [RSTMH], to take any action necessary and feasible to further it, by the formulation of exact proposals, representations to Government Departments, Universities, Tropical Schools, and other bodies or individuals or by any other means.

It will be noted that these terms are general, and do not refer specifically to the proposals raised by … Fairley, which would, only be the first of several subjects it should consider and should therefore consider the subject of special reference, as outlined below.

Matter for Immediate Special Reference to the Committee. The first function of the Committee should be to prepare detailed proposals embodying the substance of … Fairley's and … Wenyon's recommendations, but in such form that they could achieve general support not only in the *Council* but also in the [LSHTM] which is directly affected, and the *Liverpool School of Tropical Medicine* which would be affected by any exclusive function of London. To this end the relationship of the proposed London centre to other centres at home and abroad, and to the London School, should be clearly stated. An outline of the desirable provision for the United Kingdom, the Colonies and Dependencies should be drawn up, and the Scheme for London drawn up in full detail, in such a form that it fits into the general and larger one. Two matters should therefore be immediately referred [*ie* Britain and the Empire generally, and London specifically]:-

1.   To prepare outline proposals for the organisation of the study and teaching of *tropical medicine* in the United Kingdom and overseas within the Colonial Empire, including a statement of:-

- the desirable number and approximate location of research centres devoted entirely, or mainly, to this subject.
- the most suitable form of clinical facilities for this purpose, and whether in the United Kingdom wards should preferably be in independent hospitals, or attached to general hospitals.
- the sufficiency of present clinical facilities in the United Kingdom to the needs of patients other than those cared for by Government Departments, and their appropriateness to existing research and teaching institutions.
- the form in which overseas laboratory accommodation should be made available to research workers from the Schools of *Tropical Medicine* in the United Kingdom.
- the form in which the Schools in the United kingdom could best make accommodation and other facilities available to visiting workers from the Colonial Empire.

2.

- To report on the scale on which arrangements for the study, teaching, and practice of *tropical medicine and hygiene* should be available in London in the best national interest, and the sufficiency of existing arrangements for this purpose.
- To prepare, in a form which could be incorporated in a general scheme such as that asked for in the first reference, detailed proposals for any supplementation of existing arrangements, or provision of new ones, necessary to bring facilities in London up to an adequate standard.

The Committee should be asked to submit at least a brief *interim* report on these subjects for consideration by the next *Council* meeting, so that they could be considered and action on them authorised with the minimum of delay.

G Macdonald [1903–67]

The Ross Institute of Tropical Hygiene
17th December 1945.

Macdonald subsequently wrote a letter to *Council* which was read on **21 February**, containing the following:

I suggest that Dr C M Wenyon – President of the Society – Brigadier N Hamilton Fairley – originator of the memorandum of 1945, and Sir Philip Manson-Bahr – the senior teacher of clinical *tropical medicine* in the Society, should be members.

After these three I think that members should be chosen, not as 'representatives' of institutions, but to secure a fair balance of knowledge of the requirements of Liverpool, London, Edinburgh and the Services, and also wide general knowledge of *Tropical Medicine and Hygiene*. My nominations with this object are:

> Dr C M Wenyon
> Brigadier Hamilton Fairley
> Sir Philip Manson-Bahr
> Professor B Maegraith (Chairman of the Professional Committee, Liverpool School)
> Professor T H Davey (Professor of Tropical Hygiene, Liverpool)
> Professor P A Buxton (Professor [of] Entomology, London School)
> Dr G Macdonald (Director of [the] Ross Institute of Tropical Hygiene)
> Lt Col W R M Drew (Asst. Professor of Tropical Medicine R A M College)

However, perhaps surprisingly and without adequate explanation, on **11 December 1947** *Council* decided that the *Medicine Policy Committee* probably served no useful purpose and should be 'allowed to lapse' and that any question that might arise, perhaps under the new [NHS] Health Act or otherwise, should be referred to the *Council*.

Presidential Addresses

The three addresses in this chapter are valuable in depicting the 'state-of-the-art' in these years, and they also summarise the contemporary position regarding understanding of the diseases of warm climates at this time.

C M Wenyon CMG CBE MB BSc FRS (1878–1948)[2] (*see* Figure 12.1) gave his Address entitled: **Tropical medicine in war and peace** on 18 October 1945. This lecture was an overview of the then current state of knowledge of the major *tropical* diseases between 1939 and 45. He began by recalling events during the 'last war' (*ie* 1914–18) which had, of course, already been eclipsed by that of World War II:

Many of us here have had the experience of two wars, and some of us, no doubt, of other wars as well. I served in the 1914–18 war and saw something of medical progress during its 4 or 5 years, and [I] was led to wonder what outstanding advances in *tropical medicine* had been made during that period.

Many of these [changes] were more of a negative than of a positive nature. Thus, it was finally realized that quinine was not such a good drug as we had supposed it to be. Even in maximal daily doses it failed to prevent attacks of malaria in a large proportion of those taking it, though [it is probable that] under *prophylactic* quinine these attacks were fewer and generally less severe than they otherwise would have been. When quinine was given in larger doses for *treatment* of malarial attacks there is no doubt that the fever was controlled and parasites banished from the blood.

Unfortunately relapses were very common and ... cases diagnosed as malignant tertian malaria [*Plasmodium falciparum* infection] and treated as such, frequently had relapses of benign tertian malaria [*P vivax*]. So striking was this that the suggestion was made [that they] were merely different phases of one species. Those who made this suggestion failed to realize that originally both infections had been present, though only one had been detected because of the tendency of the [*P falciparum*] parasite to keep in abeyance that of [*P vivax*]. Quinine had cured ... one infection but not the other ...

In the case of the dysenteries ... there gradually came about a realization that emetine [also] too often failed in the chronic *amoebic* infections. To overcome this difficulty emetine bismuth iodide [EBI] was introduced. Given [orally], it [brought] about a greater percentage of permanent cures than other methods of emetine administration. As regards *bacillary* dysentery, no great improvement in treatment occurred ... Even anti-dysentery serum [in fact] really appeared to have little if any influence on the disease.

... a diagnosis of *amoebic* dysentery [was erroneously] made in nearly all cases of dysentery contracted in Gallipoli, in Egypt and

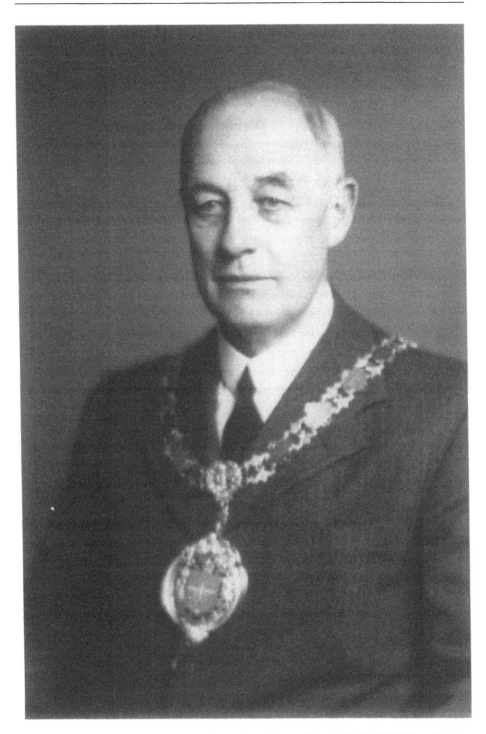

Figure 12.1: Dr C M Wenyon FRS – the eighteenth president 1945–7 (RSTMH archive).

elsewhere ... during the last war [WWI]. It was first discovered that *amoebic* infection was [widespread] amongst apparently healthy individuals [however, and] the policy was adopted of dealing only with those showing *clinical* signs of ... infection. ...

During [WW1] one of the most striking advances in *tropical medicine* was the solution of the bilharzia problem in Egypt. ... shortly before the war [the] Japanese helminthologists had given a complete account of the life history of *Schistosoma japonicum* ... Soon after this announcement the London School of Tropical Medicine [LSTM] arranged for [Robert] Leiper to go out East to [validate] these claims' ... The war had then started and ... Leiper realized the importance of schistosomiasis to our troops in Egypt. He was dispatched to Egypt by the War Office and there, applying the Japanese technique to both *S haematobium* and *S mansoni*, he and his co-workers [soon] showed that the method of infection was identical with that of *S japonicum* and that contrary to the claims of the German helminthologist Looss, who had studied the subject for many years in Egypt, snail intermediate hosts were involved in the life cycles and that infection resulted from bathing or wading in water in which cercariae emerging from these snails were swimming.

Another subject which received much attention [during WWI] was *Weil's disease*. ... Much information was accumulated amongst the troops in France. It is interesting to note that this disease [also] had been thoroughly studied by the Japanese before the war.

During the war active research had been carried out on *typhus fever* in several countries. The chief outcome of this was the ... Weil-Felix Reaction [which] has been extensively used in connection with the typhus fever of the tropics.

Then followed a brief account of *tropical medicine* between the two Wars (1919–38):

... at the outbreak of war in 1939 the means at our disposal for the handling of tropical disease [were similar to those at the close of WWI]. [Exceptions were] introduction by the Germans in 1933 of atebrin (mepacrine) for the treatment of *malaria*, and [of] the [American] discovery ... of a practical method of immunization against *yellow fever* [YF]. ...in 1940 [there was a serious epidemic] in the Nuba mountains in the Sudan, when [YF] broke out in a non-immune population.

And on to *tropical* disease *during* the 1939–45 war. He began:

I think it will be evident that [it] will ... have been more productive of new knowledge than the last.

Malaria

... With the stoppage of the world's supplies of quinine, owing to the seizure of the East Indies by the Japanese, a most serious situation presented itself [and] if no substitute for quinine were forthcoming the difficulties of carrying on [campaigns in the Pacific and West Africa] might [have been] insuperable.

... there was the German drug atebrin [*see above*], the manufacture of which, however, was shrouded in mystery. At the outbreak of war the value of atebrin as an anti-malarial drug was fairly well recognised ... For the treatment of malarial attacks it was agreed that one pill ... three times a day for a week, was sufficient in nearly all cases to reduce the fever and clear the blood of parasites. It was recognized that in the case of *P falciparum* infections this treatment [usually] brought about a complete cure, not followed by relapse; whereas in the case of [*P vivax* infection] relapses commonly occurred. Also as a prophylactic atebrin ... appeared to show that it was superior to quinine. ... though it produced ... yellow staining of the skin it could be taken daily over long periods, sometimes amounting to several years [and] without any harmful effects ... It was [however] thought that the evidence that atebrin could be taken regularly over long periods without undermining ... health through injury to the liver, or other cause, was inconclusive. However ... reliance had to be placed at first on what quinine supplies there were, while field trials of atebrin were being carried out in Africa [and] strenuous efforts were made by chemists to discover a method of preparing it on a large scale. [Trials] were highly successful [and] adequate supplies were [ultimately] forthcoming ...

Matters were in this somewhat unsatisfactory state when [Neil] Fairley [*see* Chapter 13], then with the Australian Army in the South West Pacific, realized that it was imperative to obtain more precise information about the properties of atebrin and other possible malaria remedies.[3] Accordingly, the Experimental Malaria Centre was set up at Cairns [Queensland] under his direction, and there volunteers … were infected with *malaria* [via] mosquitoes imported by air from New Guinea, while atebrin, quinine and other drugs were administered for varying periods and in varying doses before and after exposure to infection. … Frequently groups of men on prophylactic … treatment were submitted to violent exercises and exposure, with a view to simulating strenuous active service conditions in order to see if attacks of *malaria* could be induced. … The main outcome of [Fairley's] work was the clear demonstration that persons taking [one tablet] of atebrin [daily], did not suffer from *malaria*, though exposed under active service conditions to the most intensive infection by the bites of mosquitoes, and that the daily dose could be continued practically indefinitely with no more inconvenience … than the slight yellow coloration of the skin. … this demonstration [ultimately] altered the whole course of the war in the Pacific. [The] incidence [of *malaria*] fell rapidly [from 750 per 1,000 per annum] to 26 per 1,000 …

… In other localities where malaria is hyperendemic, such as West Africa and Burma, the enforcement of the one pill a day rule under strict military discipline [was] followed by similar reductions in the incidence of malaria. … Whether there exist strains more resistant to atebrin cannot be stated till a greater number have been tested … Though atebrin is better than quinine [as a prophylactic] it has its limitations, as relapses are not infrequent after its use. In dealing with troops returning from malarious areas in New Guinea the procedure was adopted of continuing the daily dose for about 3 weeks after the malarious area had been left. In spite of this, within a few weeks of ceasing to take the drug attacks of *malaria* occurred. These attacks, however, were invariably due to [*P vivax*] malaria: the daily dose of atebrin had entirely eliminated [a *P falciparum*] infection … This selective action of atebrin was amply confirmed by controlled experiments carried out at Cairns. It is in some respects similar to the experience of the [1914–18] war … the cases of [*P falciparum* infection] which had been treated with quinine in Macedonia and presumably cured, after return to England suffered relapses not of [*P falciparum*] but of [*P vivax*] *malaria*. Though atebrin fails to cure [*P vivax*] *malaria* entirely, the demonstration that it is an effective prophylactic – even in areas where the infection rate … is very high indeed [and] is one of the outstanding achievements of the war.

… It seems that the loss to the Japanese of the main cinchona plantations of the world was a blessing in disguise, for it was the chief stimulus which led to the production of atebrin on a large scale. As [Leonard] Rogers [*see* Chapter 9] [has] remarked … it is paradoxical that a German-invented drug was one of the chief means of our defeating their ally, the Japanese [and] without the use of atebrin in Burma it would have been impossible to have prevented the Japanese from overrunning India.

Exoerythrocytic development
… significant observations were made at Cairns on the infectivity of … blood taken from volunteers on whom infected mosquitoes had been allowed to feed. Blood taken from one arm 7 minutes after mosquitoes had fed on the other arm was infective to fresh volunteers, showing that sporozoites were circulating in the blood. After 30 minutes the blood was no longer infective and it remained so in the case of *P falciparum* till the 7th day, when it again became infective, and in the case of *P vivax* till the 9th day. When the experiment was repeated on volunteers taking one pill of atebrin a day the blood in the case of *P falciparum* infections was again negative till the 7th day, when it became infective, though parasites could not be … demonstrated in thick films. It remained infective on the 8th and 9th days and then became persistently negative if the daily dose of atebrin was continued for the prescribed period of about 3 weeks. In the case of *P vivax* infections, on the other hand, a period of non-infectivity of the blood was almost invariably followed by attacks of *malaria* some time after the daily dose of atebrin had been stopped.

The [sum] result of these observations is that after an infective mosquito bite sporozoites are present in the blood for a few minutes only: [it] is then negative for 6 to 9 days, when it again becomes positive. If atebrin is being taken daily this positive phase still occurs but it lasts only 2 or 3 days in the case of *P falciparum* infections. …

Another important advance ... has to do with the development of sporozoites of *Plasmodium gallinaceum* of chickens. ... [despite earlier work] it was left to Huff and Coulston to give the most complete account in ...1944 of what happens to the sporozoite when it is injected into the chicken. They have found that in the skin the sporozoites quickly penetrate the mononuclear phagocytic cells of the connective tissue. There they increase in size and in about 42 hours break up into 100 to 200 merozoites when the cryptozoic generation is completed. These cryptozoic merozoites enter other cells, either local or more remote, and commence the first metacryptozoic generation. This is very similar to the first or cryptozoic generation and, like it, ends in about 42 hours with ... production of the first metacryptozoic merozoites. These merozoites are scattered [widely] throughout the body and a few apparently ... start the erythrocytic phase of development. Others enter macrophages or endothelial cells of various organs to commence the second metacryptozoic generation. Shortly before this it has become possible to distinguish two types of mature schizont ... One produces from 100 to 200 large merozoites and the other from 500 to 1,000 small merozoites. They are termed macro- and micro-merozoites respectively. As development proceeds, more of the latter and fewer of the former are produced, while with each succeeding metacryptozoic cycle larger numbers of ... merozoites enter the [erythrocytes] ...

Now that the early stages of development of the malarial parasite of fowls has been so clearly demonstrated it is very tempting to suppose that a similar development exists in the case of the human malarial parasites. ...

[Fairley's work at Cairns] is highly suggestive of a development in some part of the body other than in the [erythrocytes]. In this connection I was reminded ... by ... Manson-Bahr of a paper ... on the subject of [*P falciparum*] malaria in Macedonia, by Gaskell and Millar [which was] published in 1920 [indicating] that even then the possibility of ... hiding places was being considered. They stated that they had seen malarial parasites in the trabeculae and supporting cells of the spleen pulp, in stellate cells in the liver, and in the heart in lymph spaces between the muscle fibres and, most remarkable of all, in the sarcoplasm which immediately surrounds the nuclei of the muscle fibres themselves. These forms contained no pigment but were small solid bodies with a single granule interpreted as chromatin. ...

Insecticides and Repellents
... The most important [aspect of mosquito destruction] relates to DDT, an up-to-date account of which [has been] given [recently] by Buxton ... No doubt in due time DDT will be tried out against sandflies and other vectors of their larvae, as a means of prevention of many tropical diseases.

As regards *malaria* prevention ... Simmons from the United States [reports] that the spraying of a room with DDT, using 20 mg per square foot, will cause the death of 60 to 90 per cent of all wild mosquitoes which enter the room 20 weeks later, while the spraying of water, using 1/10 lb of DDT per acre, will kill all mosquito larvae, and this at one-fifth the cost of the amount of oil necessary to give the same result. Already DDT has its competitor in the gamma isomer of benzenehexachloride (666) or 'Gammexane' recently introduced by the ICI.

The question of insect repellents is one which has occupied the attention of investigators in this war, particularly from the point of view of the louse and the mosquito. This work was commenced in the Entomological Department of the [LSHTM] under Buxton ... Christophers ... has been responsible for the major part of what we now know under this heading. A great deal has also been done in the United States and [also] Russia. ... the phthalates – dimethyl, diethyl, and dibutyl phthalate – are very much disliked by many insects, so much so that dimethyl phthalate has been employed very extensively for rubbing on the skin to ward off biting insects, particularly mosquitoes ... They repel insects when applied to the skin, drive them away or even kill them when introduced into clothes and bedding; and when sprayed on to mosquito netting, as observed by American and Russian investigators, will set up a barrier which insects are reluctant to pass, even though the mesh is wide enough to admit them easily.

Having spent a high proportion of his time on *malaria*, Wenyon then proceeded to deal with the present state of knowledge of several other tropical infections.

Typhus

[This disease] has threatened our troops in Burma and [also] the islands of the South-West Pacific. [*Scrub typhus*] is the Japanese river fever, or *tsutsugamushi* disease, which [was] thoroughly studied in Japan long before the war and later in the Malay States. The vector, ... a mite, is a most insidious creature which it is practically impossible to avoid in those localities ... It seems that the sudden termination of hostilities will have interrupted [a] large scale experiment [involving a vaccine] which was just commencing.

Louse-borne *typhus* has also been a menace in North Africa, Irak [sic], Persia [now Iran] and other places. ... Though the full results [of immunisation] have not yet been assessed, I believe the general impression is that some degree of protection has been conferred.

In the prevention of *typhus* there can be no doubt that DDT has given the most remarkable results. Apart from the fact that the dusting of individuals already lousy will quickly clear them, the observation that garments can be rendered louse-proof by impregnation with this insecticide has been of the utmost service in the prevention of *typhus* and other louse-borne infections. A soldier's shirt once impregnated will retain its insecticidal properties through a number of launderings – practically during the whole life of the shirt. If this were the only property of DDT its discovery might rightly be regarded as one of the most important hygienic advances of the war. ...

Dysentery – bacillary

... during the first year or two it seemed to be just as prevalent [as it was during the 1914–18 war] and there was ... every gradation of severity between the serious Shiga cases and the mild forms of 'gippy tummy'. Treatment was by salines and serum, but I do not think anyone had much confidence in the latter. ... Matters were in this somewhat unsatisfactory state when there appeared the papers by Marshall and his co-workers of Johns Hopkins University, announcing a new sulphonamide, namely, sulphanilylguanidine, or *sulphaguanidine*, which though soluble in water was not so readily absorbed from the intestine as some of the other derivatives, so that saturation of the intestinal contents could be obtained. ... [It] proved to be [non] toxic even in large doses and as the blood concentration was relatively low there was less danger of ... kidney damage which is associated with some of the other more readily absorbed sulphonamides. These preliminary results were confirmed in Egypt by Fairley[,] and Boyd and Buttle, who had received a small supply from the US, and soon demands ... came ... from many theatres of war.

A period had to elapse before supplies [of sulphaguanidine] became adequate, and efforts were made meanwhile to improve the anti-Shiga serum. ... The results of treatment of bacillary dysentery and of what might be termed ... pre-dysentery diarrhoea were so satisfactory that [it] ceased to be a war problem. Other sulphonamides are known to exert a favourable action ... and it seems probable that sulphaguanidine may not be the last word in the treatment of this disease ... Some claim that succinylsulphathiazole, or sulphasuxidine ... is better, as not more than 5 per cent of the dose is absorbed ... as against 30 to 60 per cent of that of sulphaguanidine.

Dysentery – amoebic
At the outbreak of [the 1939–45] war *amoebic* dysentery was ... in the same position as it was after [WWI]. ... emetine hydrochloride by injection would control the acute dysenteric condition and it [was] also effective for *amoebic hepatitis* and *liver abscess*. In the more chronic cases, however, it ... often failed ... Better results were obtained with [EBI], especially in healthy, or relatively healthy carriers, but even this [preparation] might be inactive in ... chronic cases where there had been a long-standing colitis.

[Other remedies] fall into two groups – the arsenicals, such as stovarsol and carbasone, and the iodo-compounds, like chinofon or yatren, diodoquin and vioform. ... There still remain far too many [cases however] which appear to be absolutely resistant, and it is in connection with these that one of the most important developments in regard to the treatment of *amoebic* infections has been made. ... Hargreaves [has] reported that certain cases which were resisting all anti-amoebic treatment ... improved dramatically when given a course of penicillin. The *amoebic* infection, however, persisted and it appeared that the improvement was due to the elimination of bacterial infections. The striking observation was then made that after this improvement the *amoebic* infection responded readily to the routine anti-amoebic treatment. [In a more recent study, he] finds that the initial improvement may be even greater if, in addition to penicillin, one of the sulphonamides is also given. [This] disproves the [widely held] view … that such cases are resistant [primarily] because the amoebae are emetine-fast [for which there is no] satisfactory evidence …

Leishmaniasis

During this war [it has been proved] that *kala azar* in India is transmitted by the bite of the sandfly, *Phlebotomus argentipes*. At first [it] was incriminated on epidemiological grounds, then it was shown that development of the parasite took place in the stomach and proboscis of the fly. This was followed by the discovery of a method of feeding and keeping alive the infected flies which led to the successful transmission of the infection by their bites to hamsters. Finally, there was the human experiment in which infected sandflies were allowed to feed on five volunteers from an area where *kala-azar* did not occur; [and] all five volunteers contracted the disease. …

Another interesting development in our knowledge of *leishmaniasis* is due to investigations carried out by Russian workers, Latyshev and Kriukova, in Middle Asia. In certain rural settlements bordering on the desert the incidence of oriental sore is very high. … It was proved that the gerbils were acting as reservoirs of the human virus … transmitted to man chiefly by *Phlebotomus papatasii*, the other sandfly, *Phlebotomus caucasisus*, being responsible for maintaining the infection in the rodent population in the burrows. It was found that within the burrows atmospheric conditions remained constant throughout the year, so that amongst the rodents there was not the seasonal incidence which characterized the infection in human beings on ground level. Another aspect of this work is that a distinction is drawn between the oriental sore of the desert areas and that which is common in towns. The former is said to be a moist variety and it is of this that the gerbils and sousliks are the reservoirs. In towns oriental sore is of a dry type but so far evidence of a reservoir host has only been outlined. … Hoare [has reviewed] this and other

Russian work on *leishmaniasis* in the *Tropical Diseases Bulletin* for May [1944].

Helminthic infections

... There have been outbreaks of *schistosomiasis* amongst the troops and attempts have been made to find a better treatment for this [than] tartar emetic or fouadin, but without any definite result ...

Similarly, there have been a number of cases of *filariasis* from the South-West Pacific area and a great deal of work to find a cure for this condition has been carried out in the United States.

... one or other of the sulphonamides, or penicillin, [might] have a curative action [in] *plague, cholera, relapsing fever, yaws* and other tropical diseases [and] workers in Madagascar have isolated from a plant ... a glucoside named asiaticoside, which they claim to be of value in the treatment of *leprosy* ...

In the last part of his Address, Wenyon dwelt on three controversial themes: *'The future of tropical medicine'*, *'Tropical medicine in Great Britain'*, and *'The urgent need for a tropical medical centre in London'*. Regarding the first, he spoke of the stimulus which the war had exerted on the development of *tropical medicine* in the USA (a theme that Fairley had outlined to *Council* – *see* Chapter 11); it had acted as an incentive to establish Schools of Tropical Medicine, and also research into tropical diseases. He briefly surveyed other centres where 'tropical medicine' was developing – emphasising those of India in particular. He then referred to Manson's pioneering work in establishing *teaching* of tropical medicine in Great Britain; 'laboratory' investigation and *clinical* teaching should be carried out side-by-side and ... one without the other... could never [lead to] a proper comprehension of what *tropical medicine* means'. He then emphasised the fact that the London School of Tropical Medicine (LSTM) had been in close proximity to *clinical* medicine both at the Albert Dock Hospital and at Endsleigh Gardens.[4] The separation of *clinical* medicine from other departments when the LSHTM was opened in 1929 'always appeared to me to be a retrograde step' he continued, and

This reveals a complete lack of understanding of the intimate association of the laboratory side with the *clinical* side which must exist if tropical diseases are to be understood and dealt with properly from the points of view of diagnosis, treatment and prevention.

Wenyon proceeded to outline a more satisfactory plan:

> While the changes which I have [thus] outlined were taking place, a very significant development in the tropical medical world took place, [ie] the foundation at Hamburg of the *Institut für Schiffs- und Tropenkrankheiten*, now, I understand razed to the ground. This had as its pattern the old [LSTM] at the Albert Dock. There were similar hospital arrangements, teaching laboratories and research departments … on a single site. Everything was on a larger scale than [in] London …, and there can be no doubt that the Institute was well organized, possessed a highly competent staff, and was very successful in every way. I paid several visits to the Institute in Hamburg and it was always with a feeling of envy or jealousy that I came away, after having had to make some excuse for the absence of such a centre in London. To me it seemed inexplicable that it was not found possible for London – the centre of the British Empire, with all its Colonial possessions and Dependencies in tropical lands – to found a Tropical Medical Centre at least as good, if not better, than the one in Hamburg.

On the last theme, Wenyon concluded his Address with the following remarks:

> … The present position in London seems to me deplorable. There is no [HTD] and the School of Tropical Medicine is housed in a building devoted chiefly to the teaching and study of hygiene and kindred subjects as applied to this country [the LSTHM]. There seems to be little prospect of the *tropical medical* section expanding. In fact, I understand that for teaching and research in hygiene and … establishment of new departments in this subject more space is urgently required. It does seem, therefore, that there is now an opportunity, not only for formulating plans but for taking definite steps, to establish a *Tropical Medical Centre* in London, where sick people returning from the tropics could receive proper treatment either in hospital or as out-patients, where the teaching of *tropical medicine* in all its branches could be carried out in close association with a hospital for tropical

diseases, and where research into the many problems still awaiting solution could be carried on.

I visualize such a *Tropical Medical Centre* as consisting of a Hospital of perhaps 300 beds, where sick people from the tropics could be examined to determine in the first place whether they are suffering from some tropical disease or not and, if so, where they could have skilled and adequate treatment; an Out-patient Department which is properly advertised, so that casual and impecunious individuals from the tropics could obtain expert advice and treatment; Laboratories and Lecture theatres for the teaching of *tropical medicine*; and Research Departments for research in the various branches of *tropical medicine* and allied subjects. These various sections should, ideally, be in a number of separated buildings located close together on a single site or, if this is found to be impossible in a central position in London, then in a single building of sufficient size to allow of expansion when … necessary.

In order to carry out such a plan satisfactorily it would probably be necessary to build, which is a great difficulty at the present time, though the provision of proper hospital facilities for the ever-increasing number of people who will be returning to this country suffering from tropical diseases might be a sufficient excuse for breaking a rule at the present time. If such a scheme … should be approved … a suitable site in a central position should be secured *at once* [author's italics], for it is certain that if this is not done, no site will be available later …. Having secured such a site, a large notice should be erected announcing that this is the site for the *new Hospital for Tropical Diseases and School of Tropical Medicine*. If this were done the battle for a *Tropical Medical Centre* would be more than half won.

We have heard a great deal lately of Colonial developments [Wenyon declared] and very large sums of money have been mentioned as ear-marked for improvements in our Colonies, not the least of which have been promises for improvements in the general health and living conditions of the natives. I can think of no single object better calculated to give such results in our tropical possessions than the establishment in London of *Tropical Medical Centre*, where sick people from the tropics could be looked after and where medical men going abroad, and others coming here to study, could be taught something about the modern methods of diagnosing and treating the diseases they would encounter, where research would constantly be going on, either at the Centre itself or in various parts of the world to which special teams of investigators had been sent. A great deal has been done recently to extend these facilities at the *Liverpool School of Tropical Medicine*, which actually came into being a few months before the [LSTM] and it is now in a better position to undertake the treatment of patients and the teaching of *tropical medicine*. This is all to the good, but what is needed is a *Tropical Medical Centre in London* [author's italics]. It would restore the position formerly held by this country, would be a monument to the many pioneers who devoted themselves to the study of tropical diseases and would be a centre of tropical medical activity worthy of the British Empire.[5]

Sir Philip Manson-Bahr CMG DSO MD FRCP (1881–1966)[6] (*see* Figure 12.2) gave his presidential address on 19 October 1947; his title was **The practice of tropical medicine in London.** He drew from his 'practical experiences in consulting practice [in London] during a period of more than a quarter of a century …', and this was based on an analysis of 'some 5,600 hospital records as well as probably almost as many again seen in consultation'. A prominent theme was that although his patients came mostly from *tropical* and *subtropical* countries they did not necessarily suffer from a *tropical* disease.

He first spoke about *malaria,* and dwelt on some of its differential diagnoses.[7] On *blackwater fever* he had this to say:

As a rule when [the disease] occurs in this country it does not give rise to any diagnostic difficulties. … twenty-five cases have been investigated during the period under review, but the numbers have decreased since the introduction of atebrin [maloprim]. … half have been seen in what may be termed 'the pre-blackwater stage'. It must not be imagined that blackwater arising in England is mild in character, for it can be exceptionally severe and rapidly fatal. I frankly admit that this haemolysis may eventuate without [due] warning [and] I am guided by the cachectic appearance of the patient, the enlargement and tenderness of the spleen, the sherry-colour of the urine and … the presence of albumin …:-

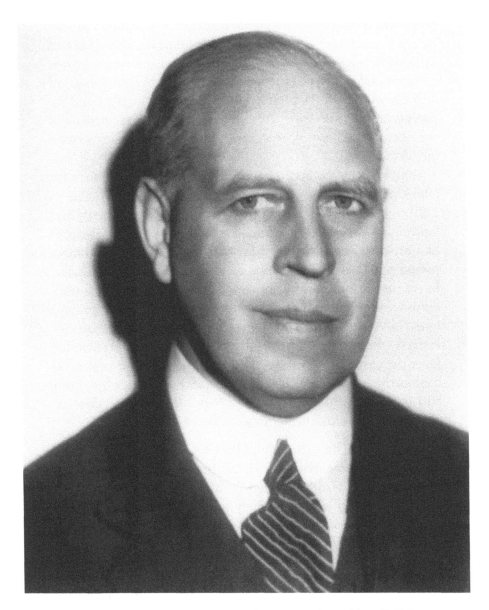

Figure 12.2: Sir Philip Manson-Bahr FRCP – the nineteenth president 1947–9 (reproduced courtesy the Wellcome Library, London).

One morning in March 1933, two Colonial officials recently arrived from the Gold Coast [now Ghana] presented themselves ... Both exhibited the clinical phenomena outlined above and both had scanty [*Plasmodium falciparum*] trophozoites in the peripheral blood. [One] a police officer ... was confident that he could treat himself with a teaspoonful of quinine. [He had a] peculiar greyish-yellow complexion and his [speech was] rather rambling. ... Blackwater supervened at 11pm that night and he was dead 34 hours [later], during which period he passed only 4oz of urine. At autopsy he had acute necrosis of the liver. The other officer ... made an uneventful recovery on atebrin.

That blackwater may ensue after a single infection with [*P falciparum*] under natural conditions was demonstrated in 1927 when I was called to [an] acute case ... [The patient] had landed for one night in Trinidad and returned to England in January of that year. During May and June, ... he suffered from periodic attacks of fever which were not recognized as *malaria*. In August (7 months after his return) he had a rigor and took quinine; immediately blackwater developed and proved fatal. In August 1922, the wife of a Colonial Office official arrived from Nigeria apparently in good health. Blackwater fever developed ... and was so severe that she had universal haemorrhages with melaena. She died 9 hours after the onset and it was [discovered] that she had taken a large dose of quinine the previous night for a severe headache.

Effect of Quinine. These and the following experiences left little doubt [that] quinine constitutes a precipitating factor [in the acute haemolysis]. This was illustrated ... in a lady missionary from the Congo ... who had previously suffered from mild attacks of fever. On admission ... she presented the appearances of an acute [*P falciparum*] infection of the bilious remittent type with [a heavy parasitaemia]. On the one hand she herself realized that she was in danger of dying from *malaria*: on the other she was equally convinced that she would succumb to blackwater if she was dosed with quinine. She was right! After an injection of ... quinine intramuscularly she died within 14 hours of blackwater.

My most sensational experience was in [a man who] at the end of 3 months' leave in England, was found to have [*P falciparum*] *malaria*. Blackwater developed after he had been in bed for 10 days on quinine therapy. He had four separate haemolyses and the haemoglobinuria persisted for 14 days. When the anaemia was very severe … he jumped out of bed, hurled the nurse downstairs, locked himself in and drank twelve bottles of beer. He was found drunk and unconscious on the floor; and after this episode slowly recovered.

Simulating Gastric Ulcer. The epigastric pain and vomiting which precede a blackwater attack may be mistaken for [a] gastric ulcer. … a lady from Nigeria … was sent to England to consult a gastric specialist for persistent vomiting. During a barium meal she had a rigor and developed blackwater fever after taking … quinine. This case was remarkable also because of a pyriform swelling which became visible in the epigastrium and which probably represented a distended gall bladder. During her … illness *amoebic dysentery* and *acute amoebic hepatitis* made their appearance; from all she made a good recovery.

After referring to *Kala-azar*, Manson-Bahr had a good deal to say about *amoebiasis*:

… *amoebic* dysentery is one of the commonest complaints for which patients apply to the tropical consultant. … During the period under review there were over 600 cases [at Endsleigh Gardens] under my care and this figure included only those which had been positively diagnosed by demonstration of *E histolytica* or its cysts. …

- … *Amoebiasis* forms a convenient diagnosis, satisfies the patient and therefore tends to be applied to almost any kind of intestinal disturbance; [however] there are many other affections of the large intestine which are accompanied by much the same phenomena.
- There still exists a [tendency] to ascribe pathogenic properties to any species of amoeba found in the faeces.
- *Acute* abdominal pain, especially in the epigastrium or hypochondrium, and extreme meteorism are *not* [author's italics] features of *intestinal amoebiasis*.
- Acute onset, febrile attacks and vomiting are *not* [author's italics] characteristic of *amoebic* dysentery which is usually apyrexial. On the whole, *amoebic* dysentery tends to be a chronic disease.

- Severe anaemia of the pernicious type is *not* [author's italics] an accompaniment of *amoebic* dysentery.
- As compared with [shigellosis] tenesmus is infrequent, whilst loss of weight is *not* [author's italics] a marked feature.
- The presence of *E histolytica* cysts in the faeces does not *always* completely account for the whole clinical picture ... Nor are they the cause of the anxiety neuroses so commonly met with. Of the amoeba it may well be said:-

We seek him here, We seek him there, We seek him everywhere; We may find him in heaven, We may find him in hell, Where you can find him, you never can tell, That damned elusive pimpernel.

Effects upon Health. Amoebiasis of the [colon] may persist for many years without causing a very noticeably disturbance.

A retired [60 year old] Indian official ... sought advice for a supposed rectal carcinoma. In 1910 he had suffered *amoebic* dysentery and subsequently [a] *liver abscess.* After operation there was no recurrence of intestinal amoebiasis till 1941 ... He was then suffering from diarrhoea and tenesmus. *Amoebic* ulceration of the rectum was revealed by proctoscopy and *E histolytica* cysts were numerous ... In 1939 a clergyman of 70 years was referred also as a possible carcinoma of the rectum on account of rectal pain, diarrhoea and dysenteric stools. It transpired that he had lived (1903–1923) in India and Iraq and suffered from *amoebic* dysentery there more than once. ... The same findings were present as in the previous case and he also made a good recovery. A third example was a Danish journalist ... who contracted *amoebiasis* in North Borneo in 1907 whilst on his honeymoon. This was his sole contact with the tropics. From that time onward for 24 years he had suffered from chronic diarrhoea and haemorrhoids. There was gross thickening of the colon with [faecal] *E histolytica* cysts ... He made an excellent recovery and ... in 1939 ... was suffering from constipation [which was] a great and welcome relief.

[*Amoebiasis*] *mistaken for Ulcerative Colitis.* Two cases had been subjected to appendicostomy as a method of treatment, as the result of a dubious diagnosis of ulcerative colitis, but so far from relieving symptoms, the operation ... tended to aggravate them.

In 1935 [I saw] an elderly man ... invalided from the South African war with dysentery and in 1901 this operation had been performed ... for supposed ulcerative colitis. For 35 years his morning toilette had occupied 2½ hours as he was in the habit of washing himself out daily with 3 pints of water. In some blood-stained mucus which exuded from the appendicostomy active *E histolytica* were demonstrated. ... he made an excellent recovery and the appendicostomy wound healed up. In 1932 [I was consulted by] a man of 32 [who was] invalided from Burma with *amoebic* dysentery which had persisted for the 9 years he had been resident in England. Treatment with emetine and EBI [*see above*] had failed so that this operation had been undertaken. ... active *E histolytica* were found ... This time he responded to combined EBI and quinoxyl treatment and the appendicostomy was closed. ...

Differential Diagnosis:
From Gallstones. The [40 year old] wife of a district officer from Northern Rhodesia [now Zambia] sought advice in December 1945. For 2 years she had recurrent attacks of agonizing [epigastric] pain coming on suddenly ... They were apt to occur in the erect, but abated in the prone position. In 1944 [a] diagnosis of *amoebiasis* had been suggested by the discovery of *E histolytica* cysts in the faeces, but emetine therapy had not brought [any] relief. The diagnosis of gallstones was [later] established ...

From Carcinoma. ... a more serious error is to mistake the incipient symptoms of carcinoma of the colon or rectum for *amoebiasis.* ... a fine [43 year old] naval captain ... from Malta [had] for 2½ years ... been treated as *amoebiasis* with emetine, solely on the grounds that the faeces contained Charcot-Leyden crystals! ... he had lost a great deal of weight. A fungating adenocarcinoma of the rectum was revealed [at] sigmoidoscopy ...

Double pathology. ... rectal carcinoma and *amoebiasis* may coexist. ... in 1922 a [50 year old] patient [had] returned to England from Calcutta with *amoebic* dysentery after 32 years residence. When *E histolytica* in the active stage and its cysts were demonstrated in the faeces *amoebic* ulceration was recognized by sigmoidoscopy. Unfortunately, a digital examination was omitted and a small malignant ulcer of the anal margin thereby missed. It should be emphasised that, in addition to sigmoidoscopy or proctoscopy, a digital examination of the rectum is essential.

From Lymphogranuloma. Lymphogranuloma of the rectum or the ano-genital syndrome has [also] to be considered. In 1941 … a woman in Sussex [was] said to be suffering from *amoebic* dysentery with rectal stricture, reputed to be the result of previous residence in South Africa and Malta. This was found to be an advanced case of lymphogranuloma with multiple fistula of [the] buttocks and perineum [sic] and enlarged fibrous inguinal glands. The Frei reaction was positive. She died later of intestinal obstruction. This was undoubtedly an indigenous infection contracted in England.

Hepatic Amoebiasis (Liver Abscess) and Amoebic Hepatitis. Amoebic hepatic abscess may be very easy to diagnose or [it may be] the reverse, for there is a type of case [in which] every ancillary aid fails and the result has to be assessed by the unsatisfactory method of trial and error.

Differentiation [of Liver Abscess] *from Carcinoma and Cholecystitis.* Carcinoma may simulate hepatic abscess, as the deposition of secondary growths is often accompanied by pyrexia, rigors and nights sweats. Sometimes … the demonstration of *E histolytica* cysts in the faeces may divert the diagnostician. … in both [*amoebic* hepatitis and acute cholecystitis] hepatic tenderness may be localized over the gall bladder area. In acute cholecystitis tenderness is confined to the outer margin of the right rectus muscle. Murphy's sign is elicited and, when referred pain is present, it is directed to the angle of the right scapula. The *liver as a whole is not enlarged.* Usually rigors are present and are accompanied by accentuated rises of temperature in place of the clock-like intermittent fever of *hepatic abscess.* The leucocytosis is higher: the direct van den Bergh reaction is raised and there may be deep jaundice.

Jaundice. In *liver abscess … jaundice with bilirubinaemia is rare* unless secondary infection with *B coli, Salmonella enteritidis,* haemolytic staphylococci or streptococci has occurred, or if there is direct pressure on the gall bladder, a most unusual event. Thus a difficult situation arises when the abscess is situated on the inferior surface of the liver in close proximity to the gall bladder.

… a high remittent fever with a temperature about 103°F with severe anaemia, gross enlargement of the liver and rapid wasting should always suggest a [malignancy], ascending pylephlebitis or some other metastatic infection, such as actinomycosis, rather than *liver abscess*. Some of these difficulties may be appreciated [from the following]:

> *Abscess of the quadrate lobe.* A [58-year-old] patient from Southern Rhodesia [now Zimbabwe, underwent an] operation for an acute appendix abscess [in 1925 and] subsequently [suffered] repeated attacks of *amoebic* hepatitis. *E histolytica* cysts [were] found in faeces. In 1934 [he was] treated … for chronic *amoebiasis* with EBI and quinoxyl. The liver was enlarged, but otherwise there was no evidence of *amoebiasis*. In 1935 he was flown … to London with [a] diagnosis of cholecystitis (cholecystogram and localized pain). Operation [revealed] a large abscess in the quadrate lobe. During convalescence, in spite of emetine injection, *amoebic* dysentery intervened [and] responded to treatment …
>
> *Carcinoma may be engrafted on to a liver abscess.* … In 1936 an Indian seaman was admitted for loss of weight and hepatic pain. He [had] *amoebic* dysentery and had recently been operated on for an abscess in the right lobe of the liver. Moreover, *E histolytica* cysts were present in the faeces. [He had a polymorph leucocytosis, and] the fever was high and hectic. At operation numerous carcinomatous deposits were found in the liver apparently arising from the gall bladder bed. … An ex-officer [aged 61] who had suffered from *amoebic* dysentery in Gallipoli in 1915 [and] subsequently had *amoebic* hepatitis, was admitted [in 1931] with a history of recurrence of symptoms of 3 weeks' duration. *E histolytica* cysts had been reported in the faeces. (Probably this was an error, for *Endolimax nana* and *I butschlii* cysts were actually present.) Bile was present in the urine. A large palpable mass in the right lobe of the liver proved at operation to be a carcinoma of the columnar cell type.

Hypernephroma. Grawitz's tumour of the right kidney may produce a somewhat similar clinical picture. In 1934 … a lady missionary from India … was [thought to have] a liver abscess on account of *E histolytica* cysts in the faeces. Symptoms had been present for 2 months. Suspicion was aroused by the presence of [erythrocytes], leucocytes and albumin in the urine. At operation an enormous hypernephroma [which proved fatal] was revealed …

Pseudohaemophilia hepatica. Pseudohaemophilia hepatica[8] a very rare disease (due to lack of blood fibrinogen), occurred in a nurse of 38 from Singapore. [She had] jaundice, clay-coloured stools, and [a right] hydronephrosis, of congenital origin. *E histolytica* cysts were found in the faeces. Her liver was enormously enlarged with a knobbly surface. Biopsy showed marked perihepatitis, foci of round-cell infiltration and early periportal fibrosis.

Calcification of the Abscess Cavity. … calcified hepatic abscesses [may be] revealed by radiography. In one, a pensioner, the calcified abscess was known to have [been present] for 20 years. … abdominal pain [transpired to be] due to a duodenal ulcer. In … a woman of 73, a large calcified abscess was discovered 56 years after [an] original attack of *amoebic* dysentery during which time *E histolytica* cysts had persisted in the faeces. During the whole of this period she had resided in England.

Girdle pain …mistaken for hepatic pain. A woman of 35, … born in Gibraltar [and who] had suffered from chronic dysentery at the age of 4, complained of right girdle pain and spasmodic contraction of the diaphragm with diarrhoea and anaemia. X-rays revealed an oval-shaped calcified abscess … 1 inch from the spine between the 11th and 12th ribs at the level of the 12th dorsal vertebra … [A] surgeon [aspirated] 35 cc of pus. [At a subsequent operation] a cyst removed from the under surface of the liver and adherent to the diaphragm proved to be a calcified suprarenal cyst. …

Posterior root pain … mistaken for hepatic pain. A Colonial official from Mauritius [aged 25 years] was sent home as he had suffered from *amoebic* dysentery and [a] constant right intercostal pain. *E histolytica* cysts [were present] in the faeces.

… he was bent forward [and had] subcostal band-like pain. On examining his back the spines of the 7th and 8th dorsal vertebrae were prominent and tender. X-rays revealed … tuberculosis of the bodies of the 7th and 8th dorsal vertebrae with calcified lesions at the apices of both lungs. … A war pensioner of 25 complained of … right hepatic [pain]. In the Middle East he had contracted *amoebic* dysentery for which he [had been treated] on several occasions. The pain was referred to the angle of the scapula and … aggravated by movement. X-rays of the spine revealed osteochondritis of the 7th and 8th dorsal vertebrae. There were Schmorl's nodes and … narrowing of the intervertebral disc spaces.

Tropical sprue, an entity upon which Sir Philip had done a great deal of research – in Ceylon (now Sri Lanka) in 1912–13 – was the next disease to be tackled. On this topic he made the following comments:

In former years a considerable portion of my practice consisted in the diagnosis and treatment of *sprue*. I have now collected records of 493 cases [in hospitalised patients]. These have been of all degrees of severity and the general impression … is that the disease has become *far less frequent and less virulent in the last 10 years* [author's italics]. At the present moment it appears to be in danger of extinction. With a malady of such obscure aetiology, mysterious in origin, so variable in its course and presenting such a strange combination of symptoms, it is not surprising that when it does arise after prolonged residence in this country the true nature is not recognized or that the syndrome is mistaken for something else. Thus I have had cases referred … as gastric carcinoma, duodenal ulcer, cholecystitis, Addison's disease and pernicious anaemia. Some had even been operated on for gastric ulcer.

Geographical Distribution. [Former] beliefs regarding the limited distribution of this disease may have [to be] revised. … I have diagnosed [it] from Egypt, Malta, Gibraltar and also … Southern Italy. With the exception of one doubtful case from the Sudan and a second from Nyasaland [now Malawi] I have never seen a genuine example … from tropical Africa. … I have [however] treated two men with sprue contracted in India who subsequently were sent ... to Nigeria with active symptoms of the disease. Both made an excellent recovery in that tropical climate ... *Sprue* may also disappear after recovery from some other acute infection. One ... patient contracted cholera in Persia [now Iran] and another recovered entirely after a ... severe attack of pneumonia. One of [my] worst cases was in an Army officer ... in 1930. He recovered [but] returned 7 days later with alcoholic neuritis. Although he was terribly ill then, he had no recurrence of *sprue*! [Another] was ... an ex-soldier [of 23 years] who was found wandering in the streets [of Naples] in an advanced stage of the disease, having lost 70 lb in weight. The ... military diagnosis had been 'anxiety neurosis' and for 5 months in 1945 he had been subjected to psychological treatment. ... he had [previously] been treated for *amoebic* dysentery. ... He was admitted to hospital and within 2 months had made an excellent recovery ...

Other mistaken diagnoses. The main signs [of] the glossitis, [and] loss of taste and smell ... may lead the practitioner astray.

Antral Disease. In 1940 ... a patient of 55 [years] found his way to [an] ENT department with ... antral disease. No improvement followed the customary washing out of the sinuses, but he soon developed a sore tongue and steatorrhoea so that the diagnosis of *sprue* became obvious. Recovery followed routine treatment during which he gained 14 lb [in weight] in as many days. When seen again 2 years later he had recovered. ... after leaving India he had [however] resided 5 years in England before symptoms developed.

Cholecystitis. *Sprue* may be mistaken for cholecystitis ...: In 1941 ... a woman of 59, who had formerly lived in Bombay [now Mumbai], but ... had been in England for 16 years ... had lost 64 lb. The significance of the sore tongue had been missed. A cholecystogram suggested cholecystitis and this, together with dyspepsia and [occurrence of] large pultaceous stools, had suggested [gall-stone disease]; cholecystectomy [was recommended] and she was actually ...being prepared for operation. [She also had] alopecia. She made a wonderful recovery on the generally accepted liver treatment and ... in August 1942 presented a healthy appearance, rubicund and buxom. ... A pleasurable feature was the regrowth of ... hair.

Malignant Disease. The *sprue* syndrome may be simulated by disease of the abdominal lymphatics. [One example] was ... a young woman of 26 from Siam [now Thailand] who had been treated for *sprue* and at autopsy was found to have lymphosarcoma of the mesenteric glands. [Another example was] a man of 49 from Manila who in 1929 ... presented with the classical features of the disease. He made a good recovery and returned to the Philippines. Nine years later he was readmitted ... with a severe relapse which failed to respond to treatment. ... autopsy [showed] an adenocarcinoma of the jejunum with perforation ...

Pellagra and Sprue. Sprue with [a] symmetrical pellagrous rash on [the] face, arms and legs was seen in an ex-schoolmaster from Hongkong in 1938. He had been invalided ... 16 years previously with *sprue*. For the past [18 months there had] been a recurrence of symptoms together with scrotal dermatitis, angular stomatitis and a pellagrous rash. [He immediately responded] to nicotinic acid [and] made an excellent recovery ...

Relapses. The genesis of relapses of *sprue* after a long latent interval is difficult to understand. ... an ex-Service man of the first World War ... contracted sprue in India in 1917. [He] was invalided to England, and treated in the *old* Albert Dock Hospital ... He made a good recovery and served in the [Royal Air Force] from 1939 to 1942. ... Admitted to the *new* Albert Dock Hospital [opened in 1938] in February 1943 [26 years after the initial diagnosis], in a state of advanced *sprue*, he made a good recovery but relapsed again 3 years later. He has now recovered once more with folic acid. An abnormal feature has been the high persisting hyperchlorhydria ... which has persisted throughout ...

Following this account of a disease which has now indeed become rare, Sir Philip gave accounts of: 'fungous infections, ulcerations, leprosy, helminthic infections and eye complications' following tropical exposure. He had a great deal to say about *filariasis* (the most 'classical' of tropical infections):

Any case [of] lymphatic obstruction is ... considered to be due to *Wuchereria bancrofti*. The great majority [however] are not. Thus a lymphatic cyst of the left axilla in a tea-planter from

Nyasaland [now Malawi] was [in 1936] excised and found to be a *cystic hygroma*. ... Agents other than *W bancrofti* may [also] cause lymphatic obstruction. [An] exact replica of ... filarial *elephantiasis scroti* was seen (in 1920) in a market gardener from Berkshire. ... the probable cause was chronic ... psoriasis of both buttocks ... treated daily with chrysarobin for 20 years.

Elephantiasis nostras [which was] resembling ... *filarial* disease was seen in a Norwegian of 23 [years]. This involved the right leg and scrotum and was preceded by attacks of lymphangitis, [an] exact replica of *filarial* fever. He returned to his native land ... after operation.

Epidemic Lymphagitis. An example of 'epidemic lymphangitis' due to a haemolytic streptococcus presented itself in 1936 in an official from Antigua ... This resulted from an injury to the little toe of his right foot. There was elephantiasis of the right leg. Apparently at that time similar cases had been observed on the island ... All *filarial* tests were negative. In the following year [a similar] case was investigated in [a 32-year-old] Army officer ... from Palestine. ... recurrent attacks of erysipelas and lymphangitis were most severe. For the next 8 years he was under observation till the introduction of sulphapyridine which controlled the attacks.

Myelosclerosis. In 1937 a Swedish naval captain [aged 57 years] was admitted [with] possible ... filariasis. He had [sailed] in tropical waters for 22 years and symmetrical solid oedema of both forearms, sternomastoid region and scrotum had developed [together with] a mild hyphochromic anaemia. ... X-ray examination [revealed] dense sclerosis of the bones ... especially in the pelvis and spinal column. The possibility of osteoplastic carcinomatosis was considered, but eventually the [diagnosis was] 'myelosclerosis with leucoerythroblastic anaemia'[9] ...

Calabar Swellings. Infections with *Loa loa* are [usually] distinguished by Calabar swellings, but there are other allergic manifestations ... Urticaria is one of these ... Biopsies of the skin [of patients with an irritating lichenoid eruption on chest and back, accompanied by a high eosinophil leucocystosis] have failed to demonstrate embryos of *O volvulus*. ... allergic swellings with *Dipetalonema* [*Mansonella*] *perstans* [occur] but it is of course impossible to rule out a ... double infection with *L loa*.

The fate of [infection with] *Loa loa* parasite[s] … has always been a matter of interest … … a lady from West Africa (Gabon) … was found [to be] infected with embryos of *L loa* in 1939 and suffered severely from Calabar swellings … for 5 years. In 1945 she presented … with numerous small painful cystic swellings over the body, forearms, palms of the hands and fingers. The Calabar swellings had [then] ceased and [the] microfilariae had vanished. On incision of the swellings cheesy necrotic material was expressed containing calcified remains of adult *L loa*. … death of the adult *L loa* is [therefore] associated in some way with the genesis of Calabar swellings. This [is] another example of 'Parasites lost and Parasites regained'.

Manson-Bahr finished by summing up his immense *clinical* experience:

I have [therefore] recounted a few of the ups and downs of consulting practice in *tropical medicine* in London. The way has led me along the bedrock of medicine and if I have strayed from the seductive path of pure scientific research, it has been because fate led me thither. I am not sorry, because by these means it may have contributed in some measure to the teaching of *clinical* medicine. There have been sad days and [also] joyful ones: there have been failures and some successes. Some of my patients have made light of their ills: 'Give peace in our tum' said one, but 'make and keep me clean within' rejoined another …[10]

Professor H E Shortt CIE MD DSc DTM&H (1887–1987)[11], Colonel IMS (retd) (*see* Figure 12.3), gave his Address in 1949 – on 20 October. His title was '**Tropical medicine as a career**'. This was largely anecdotal, but nevertheless in outstanding literary style. As well as his main topic, he concentrated on some unsolved problems (and research) within the field of *tropical medicine*, and also life in the tropics; he targeted his remarks at the younger generation – who had the unenviable task of clearing up the 'mess' left by the two World-wars:

… Your choice of career [he claimed] is wide open. Are you interested in *clinical* medicine? … Are you interested in *parasitology* or *entomology*? Although the days when you could describe a new species of parasite from every animal caught in nature are past, the amount still to discover knows no end. Are

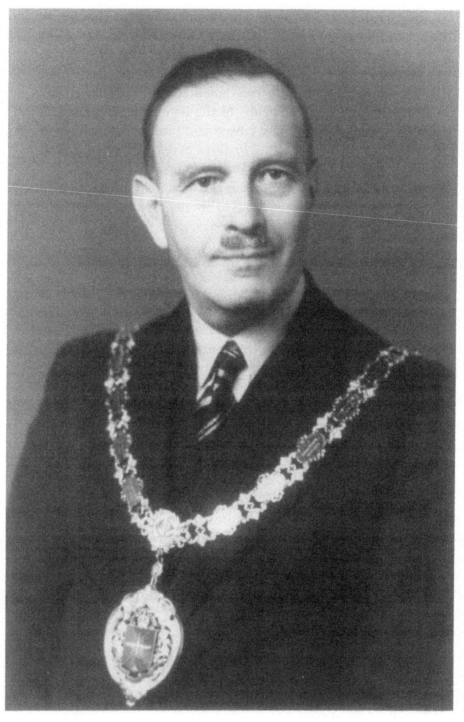

Figure 12.3: Dr H E Shortt FRS – the twentieth president 1949–51 (RSTMH archive).

you interested in *sanitation*? ... Are you interested in *nutrition* and nutritional deficiencies? You have ... one of the widest spaces of all to explore.

... have you some restless fire in your blood which irks you under the restrictions and conventions of modern civilized life in great centres of population like most European countries? Then think of work in the tropics, where open air is cheap and in plentiful supply, where you will often be far enough away from headquarters to feel you are your own master, to take responsibility for your own actions, to make your own mistakes and to rectify them because you have no one else to lay the blame upon. This makes for humbleness while you are building up self-reliance.

He proceeded to emphasise the importance of an enquiring and critical approach to *tropical medicine* and enumerated eight criteria which he felt were *essential* to any scientific enquiry:

... What are the mental and physical disciplines we must undergo to attain our object of a successful career in *tropical medicine*? ... *Tropical medicine* is [merely] an extension of general medicine into new territory and, as such, is almost a new subject. Being practised in new territory much is unknown, and it is, therefore, essential rather than incidental that any approach ... should be made in a scientific spirit of enquiry ... What, then, is this state of mind in which we should approach the problems of *tropical medicine*? It is ... not peculiar to these problems but should become a habit in any scientific enquiry and is called the 'scientific method'. ... As I enumerate and explain these [components], you will notice that some of them are closely related ... and that when taken together as a directive they amount to instructions to observe accurately, to criticize sternly and to allow no personal bias to affect logical conclusions.

- In the *first* place, one must be open-minded, casting aside bias and prejudice of every kind. ... Thousands of times bacteriologists have found moulds growing on their cultures and thrown them away as contaminated. Fleming[12] went farther; he looked at his mould and found it was producing something which destroyed the bacteria around it. It appeared an insignificant effect, but it was the germ of a new idea ... He was open-minded and prepared to accept a possible significance in the phenomenon and the result was *penicillin* and a whole range of ... antibiotics.

- Then one should cultivate [the *second*, or] an 'allergy' to problems. ... Millions of people had seen apples fall from trees but they were not allergic to what, after all, was a very remarkable occurrence, viz the transference of a solid object across space without apparent force applied. Of all the millions who had seen this take place, only Newton[13] was allergic enough to sense a problem and ... carry the matter farther.

- The *third* essential to the scientific method is a passion for facts as opposed to ... impressions. ... A simple example is a ruler, which enables us to say that an object is not merely as long as one's finger but that [if] it is a given number of inches long. Anyone with a ruler can then make comparable observations, and so the statement becomes strictly accurate and verifiable by others. In the same way the microscope extends and makes more accurate the vision of the eye and the stethoscope the accuracy and range of the ear.

- The *fourth* essential ... is a passionless logic and honesty which compels one to give an equal value to all facts ... It must admit the necessity to retrace steps which have been found to lead along the wrong road, and this admission of wrong should be welcomed as keeping one on the right track and in the right faith.

- The *fifth* essential is ... controlled enthusiasm which should make your outlook not static but dynamic. ... It will enable us to sift the likely from the unlikely and so ever edge ... towards the truth until that is finally attained.

- The *sixth* habit to cultivate is the critical mind. ... All unproved hypotheses, even those generally accepted, must be considered at least suspect until finally proved or disproved ...

- The *seventh* attitude to cultivate is to delay your pronouncements on any problem until you have sufficient proof to make no other conclusion possible. A supreme example of this principle was the collection of data by [Charles] Darwin[14] for over 20 years before he enunciated his *theory* of organic evolution.

- The [eighth and last] of your disciplines ... is to work doggedly at your problem along the lines you believe to be correct and not to be discouraged or turned aside when everything seems against you. ...

But there are (Shortt insisted) less serious moments in the practice of *tropical medicine*, and a number of anecdotes followed:

... Do you think from what I have said ... that the pursuit of *tropical medicine* as a career is all serious endeavour without lighter moments of relaxation? ... [Not so, he claimed].

Nowadays, one hardly dares send a worker into the field unless he is provided with living conditions – houses, lights, fan and frigidaires – which we in the past considered to be the luxuries only of large centres of habitation. ... in India we built our own mud and bamboo huts where the work happened to be. These served both for temporary homes and ... laboratories, in fact the latter took precedence. ... in Assam, when working on *kala-azar*, the Governor of Assam visited my field station. ... His Excellency was astonished to see [my family] domiciled in a mud and lath hut in the compound of a good government bungalow while the whole of the latter was used as a laboratory. ... When the monsoon broke my family went up the hills and I was left among the bugs in the mud hut. ... One day, after a week of continuous rain, when I got up in the morning, I saw ... grass growing through the rug! I lifted it up by two corners and shook it vigorously. The damp had rotted it and the rug flew through the air ... while the corners remained in my hands!

I do not mean to infer ... that roughing it is necessary when it can be avoided, but it is certainly a good training in teaching one to 'make do' when all we need is not available.

I often laugh at my initiation into medical research of a young Indian medical man who afterwards became a well known Indian *malariologist*. I was trying to reach a certain tea garden in the monsoon by car along a so-called road across the rice fields. ... Every few yards [my colleagues and I] had to get out and push the car out of the mud or tie ropes round the wheels to act as chains and renew these as they got cut on harder parts of the track. ... It was monsoon, it was raining a tepid flood and steamy hot. On each side of the track stretched flooded rice fields. We were all exhausted and had drunk all the liquid we had. ... As the afternoon wore on, and it looked as if we would be benighted, it became too much for the new recruit who ... began to weep. He was sternly rebuked by [a colleague] who said to him: 'Now, now, ... you needn't weep; this is nothing to what you will endure in the future; this is research work under the Indian Research Fund Association'. ...

If any of you are keen on languages, there is infinite scope for you, and ... no doubt whatever that at least a working knowledge of the language of the people among whom one is working is an immense help ...

[Rickard] Christophers [*see* Chapter 11] and I were swimming in a creek off the river Shatt el Arab, in Iraq. We noticed some Arab children [who were] squatting on the bank opposite to us, and these were continually being reinforced ... We soon realized that we were not being merely admired, either for our swimming or our figures, and that there was an expectant look on some of the faces. At last, partly in exasperation and partly in curiosity, I shouted to them in Arabic, asking them what they were waiting for. One of them with almost an eager look in his eyes, said, 'We're waiting to see the sharks get you!'. ...

[Perhaps] it is surprising what results we sometimes get with what can only be described as Heath Robinson apparatus. ... A great friend of mine, a tea garden doctor in Assam, was lying dangerously ill. He had been diagnosed [with] malaria but he himself thought he had *kala-azar*. I was ... working some 150 miles away, and one day got a telegram from his wife asking me ... to come and see him. On arrival, I found him desperately ill and delirious ... After consultation [with the local medical officer], we decided that the most probable diagnosis was enteric [typhoid fever]. However, we had no culture media, no diagnostic sera and not even a test tube. How could we confirm the diagnosis? I repaired ... to the local Indian butcher and persuaded him to kill a calf. From this ... I extracted bile from the gall bladder into a bottle. On arrival back at the patient's bungalow I found the doctor had unearthed a small tube which would serve as a test tube. Into this we put some of the bile [and] extracted the inner tube from a tyre of the patient's bicycle and, cutting off a piece of rubber, tied it tightly over the mouth of the tube. A hypodermic needle was now thrust through the rubber and left in position. The tube of bile was now boiled for some time in a pan, steam from the boiling tube escaping through the hypodermic needle. When the tube had cooled down, we inoculated the bile with the patient's blood and sent it off to the headquarters laboratory, together with some blood for a Widal test. ... the bile grew a pure culture of *Bacillus typhosus* [*Salmonella typhi*], and the blood gave a positive Widal reaction, ... wonderful nursing by his wife pulled him through.

And there are also, Shortt told his audience, many advantages to be gained from the non-professional viewpoint of life in the tropics:

... We do not work all the time; we also play. Not only do we thus amuse ourselves but we actually have a wider choice of amusements [available] than in the centre of civilization. Many things become possible ... which elsewhere can only be done by the very rich – *now, of course, an extinct class in Great Britain* [author's italics]. I refer to such things as polo, big game shooting, and even ... skiing on the equator. As residents in the country where they exist you can shoot elephants, lions, tigers, leopards, bear, bison, buffalo and what you will at moderate cost or, if you have no desire to kill for tangible trophies, you can photograph these [animals] and still have something to jog your memory in later years ...

And of the *humanitarian and altruistic benefits* which may be achieved by the doctor specialising in research in *tropical medicine*, he had this to say:

In mentioning even a few only of the endless problems awaiting solution, you will realize how widely the net may be cast and that in it are treasures to satisfy every bent. ... many problems require the co-ordination of different lines of attack converging on a given objective. Take, for instance, a syndrome such as *sprue*. It is still a very mysterious condition. ... Think of the joy of directing a successful attack on its hitherto inscrutable obscurity, of lighting up its dark places and so bringing its treatment within the realm of scientifically applied measures based on an adequate knowledge of its aetiology! ... It could be done – therefore why not do it?

And then a few words on the present state of *malariology*: Shortt was clearly alert to disturbances of the fine balance of insect-ecology:

> What of that greatest of all killers of the human race – malaria? Great strides have been made in our knowledge of *malaria* ... We are still a long way from the ideal specific drug or drugs, and ... we are still a long way from ensuring its universal distribution and use. Why is it that so much research is going on in connection with the prevention of *malaria* from many angles? It is because much has still to be learned and only those actively and practically engaged on the work realize how much this is. *We still do not know how much harm, as well as good, we may be doing by the widespread use of DDT* [author's italics]. It must not be forgotten that many forms of insect life destroyed by DDT play their part in the ecology of nature in any given area and that the state of ecological equilibrium has been built up over periods geological in their duration. ... The ... *malaria* parasite which it is the object of *malariologists* to abolish has its place in the ecological picture and ... if they succeed in driving out this devil completely, seven others [will possibly] take its place!
>
> But even if we do not wholly exterminate the *malaria* parasite there are many of the intimacies of its private life we may still pry into to satisfy our morbid curiosity. ... Why does the *malaria* parasite find one kind of mosquito a congenial host and another kind wholly inimical? Why have we not yet discovered the answer to this problem which is common ground to entomologists and protozoologists? Why does the erythrocyte which is host to [*Plasmodium vivax*], develop ... Schüffner's dots? Is there such a thing as malarial toxin ...? If so, why have the biochemists not isolated or even found it? ...
>
> And what of *blackwater fever*? Almost the only established fact [so far] is that the syndrome is connected with malarial infections. Why does the [sufferer] suddenly ... suffer the loss of a large proportion of his erythrocytes and arrive, in a matter of hours, at death's door? ... Could the catastrophe have been prevented? Once it has happened is there any effective means of retrieving the position? ...

And of other human *protozoan* infections:

… do you think [that *African trypanosomiasis is*] no longer a problem? Do you think that … the modern insecticides used to attack the … tsetse flies will supply the complete answer to prevention…? The fact remains that numerous instances could be quoted showing that outbreaks of *Trypanosoma vivax* and *T congolense* have occurred in the apparent absence of tsetse flies. In these cases transmission, normally achieved by the agency of tsetse flies, was probably effected by interrupted feeding of various biting flies such as tabanids and stomoxys, known to be present in very large numbers. But, apart from the disease and its transmission, there is still a great deal to be learned about the *trypanosome* …. … The classification of trypanosomes is still … almost chaotic, especially when we consider the wide phylogenetic range occupied by the genus in the vertebrate kingdom …

[Next, Shortt referred to] the genus *Leishmania*, the cause of kala-azar, oriental sore and espundia. We know the vector in … Indian kala-azar, but … elsewhere in the world the alleged vectors have been incriminated [until now] only on epidemiological grounds and unequivocal scientific delimitation … has still to be achieved. The same remarks would apply to the vectors of the various dermal lesions produced by *Leishmania* …

A good deal of attention has lately been fixed upon *toxoplasmosis*. … we have no idea as to the method of infection, although the parasite is found in mammals, birds and reptiles. The human disease is [usually] manifested in very young children who show encephalitic symptoms shortly after birth and … are already infected *in utero*. In many … cases, the mother does not and never has shown any symptoms of infection yet, … her blood … can be shown to contain antibodies to *Toxoplasma*. …

And next *mycotic* diseases:

[*Tropical mycology* is] an unexplored and labyrinthine jungle [which] is probably one of the least explored branches of *tropical medicine* … The majority of the diseases caused by the mycetozoa do not kill and therefore are less spectacular than the killing diseases such as cholera and plague … but the suffering and disfigurement they cause, their ubiquity in the tropics, their relative refractoriness to treatment and the lack of precise knowledge about them make them one of the major medical problems of the tropics. ...

What about *helminthic* diseases?

> ... *onchocerciasis* ... is caused by a filarial worm of the genus *Onchocerca*. ... It is responsible for nodules in the subcutaneous tissues and eye lesions which may even lead to blindness. Treatment with the newer anti-filarial drugs is now wholly satisfactory. The disease is spread by flies of the genus *Simulium*. In Kenya, where the local vector is *S neavei*, no one has yet [found] the breeding place of this insect.

And now, to *viral* diseases:

> ... *Yellow fever* is a virus disease [of which recent research] has revolutionized our ideas of its distribution, its vectors, its animal reservoirs and its epidemiology and endemiology ... there is still a multitude of lines of enquiry awaiting workers with imagination and application. It offers a wonderful tangle to be unravelled from the intimate association of virus, mosquito, man, monkey and, possibly, other animals.
>
> What of *dengue* fever? This occurs sporadically [and] in severe epidemic form, the latter often in ports ... What happens to the virus in the intervals between epidemics? Are there human carriers or is there [an] animal reservoir? If the latter, why does the virus suddenly concentrate on the human host?
>
> [With] *viral encephalitis,* the series of virus diseases – probably mostly insect-borne – [cause] encephalitis in man and animals in different parts of the world. Among these ... are *St Louis encephalitis, Japanese B encephalitis, Australian X disease, Western equine encephalitis, Eastern equine encephalitis, Venezuelan equine encephalitis* and *Russian far east encephalitis*.
>
> To come to infections in the tropics or subtropics, we have *West Nile virus; Bwamba fever* in Uganda; *Semliki forest virus* and *Bunyamwera virus* both in Uganda [etc] ... The ... pathological findings ... are dependent on the fact that viruses are obligate dwellers in intra-cellular habitats and ... produce their first effects on the cells they inhabit [in the case of the encephalitides] the

cells of the central nervous system. … symptoms will necessarily be related to the parts of the central nervous system involved … A variety of arthropods are [suspected to be] vectors and various animals as reservoirs of these viruses. … The virologist, the entomologist and the epidemiologist, are the workers who should wield the spades to fill in the gaps.

And then a word on invasive *Entamoeba histolytica* infection:

> … *amoebic dysentery* and its complications such as liver abscess [are important tropical diseases]. What are the factors influencing the onset of amoebic hepatitis and its more advanced stage of liver abscess? Why is it that while people in temperate climes [often] harbour … *Entamoeba histolytica*, yet … amoebic dysentery is extremely rare and liver abscess almost unknown? Are nutritional factors involved or are there pathogenic and non-pathogenic strains or even distinct species of amoebae? …

Nutritional problems were also not neglected by Shortt:

> … This subject is assuming an ever-increasing prominence and none can deny its paramount importance in considering any schemes of development … in all countries of the tropical world. It seems paradoxical that in many cases the peoples who live on a soil and in a climate which produces potential sources of food … should suffer from deficiencies of diet … Many of these deficiencies … have been extensively studied, but only those engaged on such work know how small … established knowledge still is in comparison with [what] is essential … before remedial measures can … be formulated on established facts and [then] applied in a manner acceptable to the people concerned … In some cases these deficiencies may be the actual cause of the abnormal conditions they precipitate, while in other[s] cause and effect may be less clear cut and the deficiencies may aggravate diseases due to other causes. In still other[s], the converse may hold and the abnormal states may be the result, not of deficiencies, but of nocuous substances present in the food or water. [In] *endemic fluorosis* in Madras province … a large percentage of the population, and also of the cattle, are affected with bony growths on the long bones and ribs, and complete

rigidity of the spine due to intervertebral ossification leading to great incapacity and, in extreme cases, to death from intercurrent disease, all due to excessive amounts of fluorine in the natural sources of drinking water. …

The physiology involved in *adaptation to a tropical climate* was, Shortt concluded, a further subject which warranted further research:

… As the tropics are opened out for habitation by non-indigenous peoples … a knowledge of physiological variations in hot and humid [or] dry climates will be of great importance in making life not only supportable but pleasant for newcomers. …

Shortt then dealt with the *teaching* of *tropical medicine* (one of Manson's major themes):

… There are openings, both in temperate climes [and] in the tropics … for [teaching *tropical medicine*] and for those with a bent in this direction there could be no better outlet than to pass on [one's] knowledge … to the coming generation of workers. Teaching can be a very humdrum business, both for teacher and student, and the really inspired teacher comes seldom – for the fire must be there – but, when found, is a gift to be cherished, for he can pass on his inspiration, which may be even greater than his knowledge, to generations of students. …

[Such rewards] are intangible and beyond the reach of the levellers, the planners and the income tax collectors. The worker who has succeeded in laying bare some of the secrets of nature and thereby … benefited his fellow men, has his own … reward in the shape of achievement, and who shall say that he has not proved the fallacies of the levellers by the mere fact of rising above mediocrity.

How, then, should the graduate interested in a *career* in *tropical medicine* proceed?:

… On account of the speed of modern transport, the world is [in 1949] a small place, and this alone has enhanced the importance of *tropical medicine*. … How fruitful a method this is could readily be exemplified by names such as Ross, Gorgas, Leishman, James,

Christophers, Sinton, and many others.[15] ... Discipline [in all its forms] is a very valuable thing and indispensable in ... civilized communities. For those ... not fired with martial ardour, love of the sea, or going to strange places by air, there is the *colonial service*. ... There are ample opportunities for work [throughout the Empire] on the clinical, laboratory and public health aspects ...

In the case of those entering the *colonial service*, it used to be customary to take the [DTM&H] before going ... to the tropics. When there arose an acute shortage of recruits [however] this was no longer possible and those entering the service were sent out without preliminary training and had to learn ... in the actual practice of the profession. Such men could later come back and take the Diploma in this country, having already gained ... experience in the tropics. ... perhaps this question could best be left to the *Colonial Office*, with its special knowledge of the conditions of service.

Some [of you] may wish to work completely untrammelled by the rules and regulations of services, whether armed or civil, and ... there are [thus] other openings to consider. Many [of the] major industrial undertakings ... such as the oil industry, the tea and coffee industries, the rubber industry and others less well known, have large interests in tropical countries and maintain large staffs there. Most of [them] now maintain their staff under very favourable conditions as regards pay and general amenities, and among the latter are excellent medical services, the hospitals of which are quite often better equipped than those of official Government organizations. ...

Accordingly life in the topics (Shortt maintained) brings with it lots of excitement and adventure:

... In the life I am advocating you may ... be many things. You may on Monday have to start building a bridge; on Tuesday you may be performing an abdominal operation by candlelight; on Wednesday you may spend half your day burning an anthrax carcass; on Thursday you may be settling a quarrel between two sets of villagers; on Friday you may be taking over, as a temporary measure, the duties of Governor of a province; on Saturday you may actually be doing something connected with *tropical medicine*; and on Sunday you may be taking a church service. ...

He ended his summary of *unsolved* tropical problems with a few remarks about ... exciting times ahead – with more Empire building to be achieved:

> [In 1949] we live in great and stirring times. The days of Elizabethan England, the period of the Napoleonic wars and the time of British Empire building [all] pale into insignificance [and] we live in difficult times, [but] they are great and glorious times, giving the opportunity to do greater things to remedy greater evils, and it is well we should realize our good fortune and be worthy of it.
>
> Now is the time for British youth to be adventurous, to be prepared to welcome and challenge present world problems, and one of the most important of these ... is to fill the unoccupied spaces in the Empire, if possible *with people of our own blood* [author's italics] and with people from our Commonwealth of Nations, the daughter countries which are now vying with the mother country in their influence on world affairs. Even if there were no worthier motives for peopling the waste spaces of the earth, surely the recent world war [1939–45] supplied evidence enough of the danger to their peoples of thinly inhabited countries. The quickest way to achieve this result is to get rid of the causes which make these places waste lands for man, the agents of disease in man and his domestic animals, and [subsequently] create the conditions which will make them suitable and fit to produce food and breed men. ...[16]

Other affairs at Manson House

Financial position after the War

Finances continued to be satisfactory (*see CM*, **17 January 1946**), income coming from subscriptions, rents (tenants and 'occasional lettings' of the hall), advertisements and sale of *Transactions*. However, by 27 March no less than 222 Fellows owed three or more subscriptions; Law 27 had been suspended during the War, but *Council* decided to delete the names of 161 Fellows who owed at least six subscriptions.

At last, the Society had rid itself of the financial burden surrounding the House Fund (*see* Chapter 11). The president (Manson-Bahr) suggested to *Council* on **20 November 1947**, that if future gifts were made to the House Fund (which had now been closed) they should go to the '*Manson Lecture Fund*' (*see* below), a lecture being held every three years.

Tenants

Council considered on both **21 November 1946** and one month later, the 'advisability of continuing to let the three upper floors of Manson House, after expiry of the present lease in 1948'. The alternative was to 'convert the upper part into a Club for Fellows of the Society'; however, it was reluctantly decided that 'the Society could *not* yet afford to forego the rent received from the upper floors'.

On **20 February 1947**, the Treasurer informed *Council* that *The Institute of Petroleum* had agreed to take the three upper floors for five years (from October 1948) at £2,500 per annum, provided the Society reserved the right to use the whole of the first floor in the evenings on eight occasions annually. The lease for this was duly signed on 21 October 1948. The Society's solicitors, Pothecary & Barratt, informed the Secretaries that the British Broadcasting Corporation (BBC) had offered to take out a lease on garage facilities at 4 Cavendish Mews South at a rental of £200 per annum for seven years, inclusive of rates (*see CM*, **21 October 1948**), the previous lease having expired on 11 October. However, the flat and garage had not previously been let separately, and the present tenant of the flat wished to stay there, at £125 per annum. A lease was therefore duly signed by the members of *Council* on 9 December 1948.

Transactions

As has previously been pointed out, this had been a major 'money spinner' since the Society's foundation. In addition to selling copies, it was also a means (via exchanges) of obtaining copies of journals from other societies. *Council* had always exerted very tight control of the contents of this journal, and all published papers had to be approved at *Ordinary* meetings.

Council decided on **11 December 1947** that a *Scientific Editor* for *Transactions* be appointed (this was after Miss Wenyon had stepped down [*see below*]), but in the meantime, Mr H S Pilton be appointed Publishing Consultant, at a fee of £100 per annum; this was unanimously accepted at the following meeting. After renewed discussion, Sir William Macarthur was eventually appointed *Scientific Editor* at an honorarium of £400 per annum. It was not until early 1949 that an *Editorial Panel* was formed, however (*see* 42nd AGM).

The issue of more monographs had been addressed at several *Council* meetings in 1946, 47 and 48; length, print run and whether or not they be sent to *all* Fellows of the Society occupied a great deal of discussion. It was ultimately decided to produce the first to cover Fairley's researches at Cairns, Australia during the war. Also, Clayton-Lane's contributions (based on F W O'Connor's work) on *Filaria* periodicity might, it was aired, be considered. Funding of monographs would also have to be worked out.

Secretarial assistance

Miss Mildred Wenyon had by 1946 completed 25 years as Secretary; her salary was then raised, and a pension of £180 on her retirement was approved. It was reported to *Council* by the Treasurer (Marriott) that the Society's income had increased from £627 in 1921, to £5,366 in 1945, while nearly £30,000 had been raised for Manson House; this had been largely a result of Miss Wenyon's 'energy and foresight'.

On **20 March 1947**, *Council* however accepted her resignation 'with deep regret' after 26 years service, but she agreed to continue with the editorial work of *Transactions* 'for a limited period'; in fact, she continued only until June 1948 (*see CM*, **11 December 1947**). Her retirement was followed by several glowing tributes, before the president (Wenyon) proposed that Miss Norah Hopper be the next Secretary; she was to receive £400 annually.

Office salaries were reviewed (by *Council*) on **20 January 1949**, and the following increases adopted:

Secretary	:	£400 + £25 yearly to £600 per annum
1st Assistant	:	£250 + £25 yearly to £350.
2nd Assistant	:	£150 + £25 yearly to £300.

Present staff members would thus receive:

Miss Hopper	:	£500 per annum
Mrs Langley	:	£300 per annum
Miss Pilton	:	£250 per annum

Meetings

Ordinary meetings continued to be well attended. The *classical* tropical diseases were of course well covered. Also areas of growing significance, many involving chemotherapeutic agents, received attention (*see* Table 12.1). At a meeting on 17 January 1946, the Society was addressed by the American Ambassador to Great Britain, who also presented the Theobald Smith Gold Medal (American Academy of Tropical Medicine) to C M Wenyon FRS.

Fairley told *Council* on **16 May 1946** that *sprue* had 'reached epidemic proportions in certain parts of Burma; but very little … had occurred among prisoners of war: this made it difficult to accept *sprue* as a *deficiency* disease'.

Regarding Wenyon's successor as president, on **20 February 1947** Sir Philip Manson-Bahr had received twelve votes to Dr Norman White's four.

On **26 June 1947** *Council* decided that *Ordinary meetings* would begin at 7.30 rather than 8.00pm.

Honorary Fellows

At a meeting of *Council* on **20 February 1947**, Professor Eugene Pavlovsky (Moscow) was unanimously elected an Honorary Fellow of the Society, and four more Honorary Fellows were proposed on **19 May 1949**:

> Dr N H Swellengrebel (Holland)
> Dr Wilbur Sawyer (USA)
> Maj Gen A J Orenstein (South Africa) and
> Dr Paul Russell (USA)

thus raising the number of living Honorary Fellows to ten.

A Manson Lecture?

Manson-Bahr again raised the question of a *Manson Lecture Fund* on **16 June 1949**; the Society should attempt to raise at least £2,500, and the lecture should be given periodically by a 'distinguished figure (of any nationality) in *tropical medicine*' on some aspect of *tropical medicine*, and it should be well advertised and open to all members of the medical profession.

Table 12.1: Communications at *Ordinary* meetings – 1946–50

Date	Subject	Speaker
1946		
17 January	Medical disorders in East Africa	E R Cullinan
21 February	The war in South-east Asia Command	H L Marriott, I G W Hill, J C Hawksley, R R Bomford
16 May	Tsutsugamushi disease (scrub typhus)	T T Mackie
20 June (39th AGM)	'Paludrine' in malaria	N H Fairley
17 October	Yaws in Lango, Uganda	C J Hackett
12 December	Colonial nutrition	B S Platt
1947		
16 January	Malaria vectors in West Africa	R C M Thomson
20 February	Trypanosomiasis in the Belgian Congo	L M J van Hoof
10 April	Chemotherapy in filariasis	J T Culbertson
15 May	Amoebiasis	C M Wenyon
19 June (40th AGM)	Middle-East Prisoner-of-War camps	S Smith
16 October	Tropical medicine in London (*presidential address*)	Sir Philip Manson-Bahr
11 December	Trypanosomiasis in Nigeria	J L McLetchie
1948		
15 January	Treatment of Leprosy	E Muir
	The eye in Leprosy	E W O'G Kirwan
	Leprosy treated with Diasone	A R D Adams
19 February	Pathology of malaria	B G Maegraith
	The liver in malaria	W H H Andrews
15 April	Tropical disease in captive wild animals	R E Rewell
17 June (41st AGM)	Pulmonary schistosomiasis	M Erfan
21 October	Epidemiology of fungus disease	J T Duncan
	Treatment of fungus disease	I Muende
9 December	Physiology in a hot/humid environment	G P Crowden
1949		
20 January	Kwashiorkor	H C Trowell
17 February	Epidemiology of Yellow Fever in central Africa	A F Mahaffy
19 May	Tropical Disease in Brazil	B Malamos
16 June (42nd AGM)	Chagas' disease in Uruguay	R V Talice

Date	Subject	Speaker
21 July	Malaria in Venezuela	A Gabaldon
20 October	Tropical Medicine as a career (*presidential address*)	H E Shortt
8 December	Vascular disorders in tropical Africa	M Gelfand
1950		
19 January	Malaria in north Holland (1943–6)	N H Swellengrebel
16 February	Chloramphenicol in Tropical Medicine	J E Smadel
18 May	Loaiasis in British West Africa	R M Gordon, W E Kershaw, W Crewe, H Oldroyd
15 June (43rd AGM)	Recent work on Filariasis	F Hawking
6 July	Smallpox in Britain	Sir William MacArthur
19 October	Tropical pulmonary eosinophilia	J D Ball
	Tropical eosinophilia in India	R Treu
14 December	Mite typhus in Burma and Malaya, 1945–50	J R Audy

Warrington Yorke Memorial Fund

On **18 October 1945**, attention was directed to the Warrington Yorke Memorial Fund to establish a Department of Chemotherapeutic Research at the *Liverpool School of Tropical Medicine*; *Council* agreed on a donation of £50.

Controversial matters

DISTINCTION AWARDS

The Registrar of the Royal College of Physicians (RCP) (Dr Harold Boldero [1889–1960]) requested assistance from the RSTMH as to who should receive *distinction awards* in *tropical medicine*. The National Health Service (NHS) had recently come into effect, on 5 July 1948. This, it was said, was a *secret* matter and selection should *not* be confined to degrees and qualifications, but reserved for 'distinctive services to medicine and/or the public'. *Council* on **20 October 1949** was divided on whether this Society should be involved, and requested clarification. The matter was further discussed in December. Sir John Taylor (1895–1974) (a *Council* member) and Fairley (an Honorary Secretary) had apparently met Boldero at Manson House on 16 November 1949. Following that meeting, Boldero had written to Fairley:

I am grateful to you and to Sir John Taylor for meeting me and conveying to me that the *Council* of the [RSTMH] were anxious to assist the College in making recommendations concerning Distinction Awards to Consultants.

At our meeting both you and Sir John Taylor made clear to me that you are a scientific society and that you have among your members many who are not medical practitioners. In fact, the number of members of your Society who may be consultants in the [NHS] is likely to be extremely few, possibly not ten. Therefore your Society is not suitably constituted to take a direct hand in recommendations concerning consultants. We all three agreed that your Society would be well satisfied that this College [the RCP] should consult one or possibly two men, who are members of your Society and who are likely to be consultants in the [NHS], when the College is considering the relevant consultants.

This therefore absolved the RSTMH from any recommendations to this highly questionable, and, to many, a totally obnoxious scheme!

War-time atrocities

Another highly controversial matter was discussed by *Council* on **12 December 1946**. Dr Gerhard Rose had been a Fellow of the Society since before the War; now Dr von Schultz had asked Dr S D Sturton (Professor E Brumpt had previously been approached and would have nothing to do with it) for a certificate of good character; Dr Rose was currently on trial at Nuremberg for alleged experiments on prisoners in concentration camps. Both the president and *Council*, however, agreed on 'no further action'.

Laboratory animals

Council agreed on **18 October 1945** to lend its support to a Committee to consider standardization of experiments on laboratory animals; this decision was apparently approved by the Fellowship.

Involvement with other Societies

Professor T H Davey was appointed as the Society's delegate to the *Royal Sanitary Institute* in Blackpool on 3–7 June 1946. The same society invited delegates to the Congress at Brighton from 23–27 May 1949; Professor

Buxton was nominated. The Health Congress for 1950 was arranged for 24–28 April. The meeting for 1947 took place in June at Torquay, and the name of the delegate was not stated in the minutes, although at the 1948 Congress at Harrogate in May 1948, Professor Buxton was appointed.

The Society was requested by Dr Wilbur A Sawyer of the *American Society of Tropical Medicine* to send at least one representative to the *4th Congress on Tropical Medicine and Malaria* to be held in Washington in May 1948. The names of N H Fairley (since he was ill Sir Philip Manson-Bahr [president] took his place) and J S K Boyd were approved.

Manson-Bahr was nominated as representative on *The Empire Advisory Bureau* for 1948 (*see CM*, 3 **June 1948**).

The *2nd Empire and Commonwealth Health and Tuberculosis Conference* was held in July 1949; it was suggested by Dr [F R] Heaf [1894–1973], Tuberculosis Officer of the LCC, that the RSTMH should sponsor lecture demonstrations and visits to hospitals. *Council* decided that the Society would in fact advertise these.

The Library

A special meeting to decide certain matters relevant to the library took place on **1 September 1949**:

- 237 books which were either 'out of date' or duplicated were disposed of, and offered to Fellows.
- The status of 'exchanges' with other societies was reviewed, and updated.
- The method of using the Florence Frost bequest (*see* below) was discussed.
- Although reference and standard books should be continued, some of the periodicals, it was decided, should *not* be bound and kept.
- This was primarily a *reference* library, and if any Fellow wished to *borrow* a book, he or she must first obtain permission from the Executive Committee.

More gifts to the Society

Donations were now less plentiful than shortly after removal to Manson House.

One from Sir Harold Scott was used to purchase *Stitt's Diagnosis, Prevention & Treatment of Tropical Diseases* for the library (*see CM*, **15 May 1947**).

Dr Florence Frost of California had endowed a gift in memory of Edith Rogers Powers to the library (*see above*); this amounted to $1,000.

Royal matters

At a *Council* meeting on **11 December 1947**, a letter was read from the Home Secretary (Mr Chuter Ede) thanking the president and *Council* for their loyal address on the marriage of Princess Elizabeth (later Queen Elizabeth II) to Philip Mountbatten (later Prince Philip, Duke of Edinburgh – *see* Chapter 13).

Obituaries

The death of Professor Julius Mannaberg (an Honorary Fellow since 1909) in Vienna was announced to *Council* on **27 March 1946**. That of Col S P James (the fifteenth president) on 17 April 1946, was reported to *Council* on **16 May**. The death of Dr Simon Flexner of New York (an Honorary Fellow since 1921) was also reported to *Council* at the same meeting. And on 17 May 1946, that of Professor J W W Stephens (the eleventh president) (*see* CM, **20 June**.) Dr Bernard Nocht's death (an Honorary Fellow since 1937), and also that of Sir Harry Waters (an original Fellow) was announced to *Council* on **16 January 1947**.

Other Society matters

The use of *FRSTM&H* as a *qualification* was *not* approved by the GMC, and was frequently frowned on by *Council* of the Society (*see* for example, *CM,* **9 December 1948**).

At a *Council* meeting on **18 October 1945**, Manson-Bahr had suggested formation of a *Manson Club* – a dining club which would meet after *Council* meetings and 'provide an opportunity of getting to know the younger men'.

At the 42nd AGM, Manson-Bahr drew attention to the gold medals and insignia of Patrick Manson, which were on display in the Fellows' Room, and had been presented by the late Lady Manson-Bahr.

A licence to supply alcohol to Fellows who attended the pre-*Ordinary* meeting dinners was sought (*see CM,* **20 October 1949**). This matter was further discussed by *Council* in December.

At *Council* on **17 March 1949**, the president (Manson-Bahr) suggested restoration of the custom of an *Annual Dinner* for Fellows, when distinguished people should be invited as guests; however, it was decided to leave this for the AGM to decide.

The thirty-eighth to forty-third annual reports

In the year ended 31 March 1945, for the first time for six years, nine *Ordinary* meetings (see Chapter 11) had been held at Manson House, including a laboratory meeting at the RAMC College.

At almost the end of the war (on 31 March 1945), 1,688 Fellows were on the list. However, owing to failure of payment of subscriptions and deaths during the war, this number fell sharply to 1,545. However, the number increased again to 1,646 the following year, and to 1,975 in the year ended 31 March 1950.

The excess of income over expenditure for the year ended 31 March 1945 was £640 2s 0d. At 31 March 1950, the credit balance was £600.

The 41st report recorded the resignation of Marriott from the treasurership.

References and Notes

1   **Lionel Everard Napier** CIE FRCP (1888–1957) qualified at St Bartholomew's Hospital, and served in India and Mesopotamia with the RAMC. In 1919 he joined the School of Tropical Medicine at Calcutta (now Kolkata) where he became the first Professor of Tropical Medicine and ultimately its director. Here, he carried out research into the transmission of kala-azar [R Knowles, L E Napier, B M Das Gupta. The kala-azar transmission problem. *Indian med Gaz* 1932; 58: 321–49; R Knowles, L E Napier, R O A Smith. On a herpetomonas found in the gut of the sandfly. *Phlebotomus argentipes* fed on kala-azar patients. *Ibid* 1924; 59: 593–7]. After several years in the USA, he returned to England in 1946 and became specialist in tropical diseases to the Ministry of Pensions and consultant to Queen Mary's Hospital, Carshalton. His book *The principles and practice of Tropical Medicine* was published in 1946 [*Munk's Roll* 5: 303–4; *Who Was Who, 1951–1960*: 807].

2   **Charles Wenyon** was educated at Kingswood School, Bath; Victoria University, Leeds; University College London; and Guy's Hospital. He became protozoologist to the London School of Tropical Medicine, and was later consultant in tropical medicine to the Wellcome Foundation and Director of the Wellcome Research Institution. His book *Protozoology* was published in 1926. C A Hoare. Charles Morley Wenyon 1878–1948. *Obituary notices of Fellows of the Royal Society.* London: Royal Society 1949; 6: 627–42; Anonymous. Wenyon, Charles Morley. *Who Was Who, 1941–1950*: 1220–1.

3   For further details, and a full biography of N H Fairley *see* Chapter 13.

4   N H Fairley. The Hospital for Tropical Diseases (UCH) London. *Univ Coll Hosp Mag* 1952; 37: 114–18. [*See also*: G C Cook. *From the Greenwich Hulks to Old St Pancras: a history of tropical disease in London*. London: Athlone Press 1992: 338; G C Cook. Evolution: the art of survival. *Trans R Soc trop Med Hyg* 1994; 88: 4–18].

5   C M Wenyon. Presidential address: Tropical medicine in war and peace. *Trans R Soc trop Med Hyg* 1945–6; 39: 177–94.

6   **Philip Manson-Bahr** was educated at Rugby, Trinity College Cambridge and the London Hospital. His distinguished tropical career took him to Fiji, Ceylon (now Sri Lanka) and the Middle-East. Following the 1939–45 war, he was appointed to the Albert Dock Hospital and the Hospital for Tropical Diseases. He was also editor of *Manson's Tropical Diseases* (1921–1960), and received numerous honours, including a knighthood. Anonymous. Manson-Bahr, Sir Philip. *Who Was Who, 1961–1970*: 740.

7   S N Javett, S Sacks. Chronic meningococcal septicaemia simulating malaria. *South African Med J* 1942; 16: 307–8; R Priest. Meningococcal septicaemia resembling malaria. *Br med J* 1942; ii: 129; C H Catlin, E W Bintcliffe, F G Marson. Pyrexia with hypernephroma; report of two cases. *Lancet* 1947; ii: 170–1; J F Loutit, P L Mollison. *Lancet* 1947; i: 401.

8   L E H Whitby, C J C Britton. *Disorders of the Blood* 2nd ed. London: Churchill 1937: 299.

9   *Ibid*: 418.

10 P Manson-Bahr. Presidential address: The practice of tropical medicine in London. *Trans R Soc trop med Hyg* 1947–8; 41: 269–94.

11 **Henry Shortt** was born in the Punjab in 1887, and read medicine at Aberdeen University. He entered the Indian Medical Service and immediately returned to the Punjab. In the Great War, he served in Mesopotamia, at Basra and Baghdad. He returned to India after the war, and carried out research on kala-azar. He later worked on rabies and several other tropical diseases. In the early 1930s he was director of the King Institute of Preventive Medicine at Madras (now Chennai). After World War II, he became Professor of Medical Protozoology at the LSHTM and it was while there that he jointly discovered the exo-erythrocytic cycle of *Plasmodium* vivax. P C C Garnham. Henry Edward Shortt. *Biographical Memoirs of Fellows of the Royal Society*. London: Royal Society 1988; 34: 713–51; Shortt, Col Henry Edward. *Who Was Who, 1981–1990*; T Richards. Doctor, soldier, scientist and shikari. *Br med J* 1987; 294: 1669–70.

12 L Colebrook. Alexander Fleming 1881–1955. *Biog Memoirs Fellows Roy Soc* 1956; 2: 117–27

13 R S Westfall. *The life of Isaac Newton*. Cambridge: Cambridge University Press 1994: 350.

14 A Desmond, J Moore. *Darwin*. London: Michael Joseph 1991: 808.

15 *See* G C Cook. *Tropical Medicine: an illustrated history of the Pioneers.* London: Academic Press 2007: 278.

16 H E Shortt. Presidential address: Tropical Medicine as a career. *Trans R Soc trop Med Hyg* 1949–50; 43: 239–54.

Chapter 13

Completion of the Society's first half-century – in 1957

The fiftieth Annual General Meeting (AGM) took place at Manson House on **20 June 1957**. The Society had successfully ended the year (its Jubilee year) with a balance of £230. However, the highlight of the Jubilee celebrations occurred later that year with a banquet to which numerous distinguished individuals (including the Duke of Edinburgh) were invited. Preparations had begun the previous year, when the president (Gordon) referred to the matter at a *Council* meeting on **10 October 1956**; it was decided that a dinner to which the Patron (HM the Queen) or another member of the Royal Family be invited should be held, some time in the latter half of 1957, and that a sub-committee should be appointed to organise this event. The matter was further discussed at an *ad hoc Council* meeting held at the *Liverpool School of Tropical Medicine* on 15 November. It was reported that although HM the Queen did not attend such functions, the Duke of Edinburgh would probably be pleased to receive an invitation, assuming the date was convenient. The maximum number of attendees should be limited to 400 (in fact on the occasion there were only 231 Fellows and their guests present). The venue should (it was felt) be either the Royal College of Surgeons or the Savoy Hotel. At a meeting on 15 December *Council* was informed by Boyd (an Honorary Secretary) that the dinner would in fact take place at the Royal College of Surgeons in either October or November 1957.

The Duke was somewhat tardy in replying (*see CM*, **20 June 1957**) but it was decided by *Council* that 12 November was the most suitable date; if the Duke could not attend it was suggested that either Princess Margaret or the Duchess of Kent be invited (*see CM*, **20 June 1957**). The Duke however accepted but asked that the speeches be kept short (less than seven minutes); the toasts (it was decided) would be:

- HM the Queen (proposed by the president – Brig J S K Boyd FRS)
- The Guests (proposed by Sir Philip Manson-Bahr)

- Reply on behalf of the guests (Sir Henry Dale FRS)
- The Society (proposed by Prince Philip, Duke of Edinburgh KG)
- Reply on behalf of the Society (president … Boyd)

The event was recorded in detail in *Transactions* and seems to have been an outstanding success (*see CM*, **12 December 1957**). The content of the speeches are preserved verbatim in *Transactions*:

> **Sir Philip Manson-Bahr**: I need hardly express how highly honoured I feel that, on this great occasion, and in this glittering company, I should be invited to propose the Health of our Guests. I need not also stress the great privilege that you, Sir, have conveyed upon our Society and upon all of us here in having agreed to address us. We all know how you have roamed around the world, like some modern Ulysses, to spy out the land and, as a result, we realize that you are no *dilettante* and that you do know what you are talking about! You have most certainly seen for yourself the achievements of British rule and good government in what was once the British Empire, and you have sensed how much better it was to sow the seeds of health, rather than those of hate – all of which serves to create a monument to British genius that will endure; and to counteract to some extent that vulgar slogan of Colonialism bandied about by people who know nothing about the Colonies at all. Perhaps, in this vein, you will permit me to associate the name of Lord Hailey [1872–1969], himself an Honorary Fellow of our Society, and an able assessor of the virtues of Colonial Government. The second edition of his *African Survey* has just made its debut, where he has paid such generous tributes to the victories of *Tropical Medicine*, to the names of the great men who have made them possible, and where he has shown how these benefits have been extended indiscriminately to European and native elements alike. There, too, he has given effect to the words of our motto, 'Zonae Torridae Tutamen – Guardian of the Torrid Zone'. Luckily for us all, it is pretty warm here tonight! It is, Sir, just a century ago since Michael Farraday [1791–1867], the great physicist, was commanded to Windsor to a demonstration before Her Majesty Queen Victoria and the Prince Consort. 'I have in one hand a flask of oxygen, your Majesties', he said, 'and in the other a similar flask of hydrogen. The oxygen

and the hydrogen, your Majesties, will now have the honour to combine to form water'. Possibly in these more modern times, you, Sir, would have felt more inclined to summon some of your atomic experts to have the honour of converting it into wine.

We have tonight a galaxy of stars in the tropical firmament who, to be perfectly up to date, are accompanied, with some exceptions, by their satellites. We are really not good hands at poetry, so I am asking you to put up with just a little doggerel.

> The satellite hath wings of gold,
> The rocket wings of flame,
> Poor Laika had no wings at all
> But she got there just the same!

We are honoured, too, by members of HM Government, by Sir John Macpherson [1898–1971], the Permanent Under Secretary for the Colonies, by Sir Bennett Hance [1887–1958], our good friend of the Commonwealth Relations Office, and by the Earl of Perth, the Minister of State. It is my pleasant task to welcome our foreign guests who have made such a perilous journey to be here with us tonight. These are Professor and Madame Brutsaert from Brussels; Professor and Mrs Wolff from Amsterdam; and we must accord a special tribute to Professor Georges Lavier and his accomplished wife, from Paris. They are very old friends who were with us almost at the beginning and have rejoined us once more. I wish I could make them a suitable address in French, but I can only offer a little Limerick of greeting:

> There was a young man of Boulong,
> Who startled the birds with his song,
> It wasn't the words that frightened the birds
> But the 'orrible Double Entong

I have also to acknowledge the great distinction conveyed upon us by the Presidents of both Royal Colleges – Physicians and Surgeons – Dr [later Lord] Robert Platt [1900–78] and Sir James Paterson Ross [1893–1980], who have come here in unison to see that we behave with due propriety. There are also the Chiefs of the Medical departments of the three fighting services. Sir Alexander Drummond [1901–88], Surgeon Vice-Admiral R C May [1897–1979] and Air Vice-Marshal P B Lee Potter [1904–82], who have always shown themselves to be our firm supporters and good friends.

The Medical Journals are represented by their Editors. Safe in his earth is Dr [T F] Fox [1899–1989], the Reynard of *The Lancet*, more adept, as we well know, with his pen that with his brush, whilst his colleague, Dr [H A] Clegg [1900–83] of the *British Medical Journal* is leaning heavily on his gold-headed cane. Sir Henry Dale [1875–1968], that Nestor of Medical Research, has constantly lent the weight of his great authority to the prosecution of *Tropical Medicine*. Sir Harold Himsworth [1905–93], Secretary of that most useful body, the Medical Research Council, does his best to lead us up the strait and narrow paths of fundamental research with the aid of his team of backroom boys. I feel I must include my sister-in-law, Mrs Hossack, the daughter and only surviving member of the family of Sir Patrick Manson, our founder of half-a-century ago. Let me conclude with a little story of a bewildered boy who shocked his mother by declaring that he could not detect much difference between attending morning service on Sunday or of going to a cricket match. He explained that when he went to church the parson boomed, 'Stand up for God's sake'; but when he went to Lords and peered around to get a glimpse of Dennis Compton, the crowd howled at him with one accord, 'Sit down, for God's sake'. So I will now take the hint and resume my seat, but not before I ask you to drink with me the health of all our distinguished guests, and their ladies.

Sir Henry Dale [Chairman of the Wellcome Trust] …: I am greatly honoured by being called upon to voice the thanks of my very distinguished fellow guests, and my own very hearty thanks, of course, with theirs, to you, our gracious hosts of the [RSTMH], for the privilege, which we are all so much enjoying, of taking part in this commemorative festivity, and for your generous response to the toast which Sir Philip Manson-Bahr has so genially commended to you. Sir Philip's name gives him a family linkage with the very beginnings of *Tropical Medicine*, and of your Royal Society, and his work and his teaching for many years have helped to consolidate its claim to recognition, as a special branch of Medical research and practice.

I know that the others, for whom I am thus called upon to speak, will wish me to say how proud we all are to find ourselves associated, as your guest tonight, with His Royal Highness, Prince Philip, the Duke of Edinburgh, your Guest of Honour on this great occasion. Our programmes tell us that he will presently be speaking on his own behalf; and we are all looking forward to the toast of the Society, which His Royal Highness is to present to us, as the crown and climax of this evening of your Golden Jubilee celebration. May I, then, make only brief mention of one or two points on behalf of your guests?

I am sure that those of us, who are British, will wish me to say how glad and proud we are to be associated, as fellow guests tonight, with the distinguished representatives of *tropical medicine*, and of its institutions, from those European countries which are the nearest neighbours of our own. I think that we may, perhaps, regard the freedom of international co-operation and the sharing of experience, as more natural and more important for medicine as a whole, than for any of man's other scientific, or altruistic, activities; and the presence of these colleagues from other countries should further remind us, if such reminder were needed, that such unrestricted international co-operation has very often been an essential condition for really effective researches dealing with the special problems of *tropical medicine*, many of them extending, without any reference to political frontiers, over all the tropical regions of all the continents.

We, your guests, recognize also what courageous enterprise, what readiness to face primitive and difficult conditions, have often been needed to open the way to a knowledge of tropical diseases and their causes. Many of these pioneers have found their opportunities as officers in the medical services of the armed forces, or of civilian administrations; and these services have a number of distinguished representatives among your guests this evening. We in this country think of Manson in China, Bruce in East Africa, Ross and Leishman in India. These men, and many who followed them, have often done their work under conditions which those of us whose research experience has all been of modern, well-found laboratories, do not find it easy to imagine; on the other hand, I think that such pioneers had a special kind of opportunity – which surely they richly deserved – to open unworked mines of knowledge, and to find nuggets of discovery still plentiful and near the surface. Many of the Fellows of your Society, though their interests were primarily in *tropical medicine*, have also won high distinction in ranges of biological science beyond those strictly related to medicine – in protozoology, botany, helminthology, entomology and the rest. In the study of tropical diseases there has further, and very naturally, been an unusually wide overlap of interest between human and veterinary medicine. We may recall that David Bruce's pioneer work on the African infections due to trypanosomes, and transmitted by the tsetse flies, began with a disease of horses and cattle, though its results were later to provide the clue to the nature of the sleeping-sickness in man. It is on record that your own President, my friend Brigadier John Boyd, now my valued colleague in another connexion, had become so oblivious of the normal limitations imposed by professional etiquette, that he once allowed himself to become responsible for the diagnosis and treatment of an outbreak of amoebic dysentery in a pack of foxhounds at Bangalore. So far as I know, he escaped any such penalty as he might have been expected to incur, for unregistered veterinary practice.

Few of us, your guests, have any direct experience of *tropical medicine*; but I should like to refer, very briefly, to the remarkable influence which its discoveries have had, in promoting, and even initiating, some of the revolutionary advances, during recent years, in medical knowledge and practice in a wider field. Especially impressive, to us who live in temperate climates, has been the introduction of specific and really effective treatment for many of the more familiar bacterial infections, which, for lack of it, had earlier been so tragic in their effects. The sulpha-drugs came first, in 1935, and then the use of penicillin, and all the still expanding range of the antibiotics. We have been watching, indeed, a dramatic and beneficient revolution. I think, however, that we ought to remember that its real beginning was much earlier, some fifty-five years ago, when Laveran and Mesnil had propagated in small laboratory animals the trypanosomes discovered by Bruce and Evans and others, as the causes of tropical diseases; and when that man of rare genius, the late Paul Ehrlich, seized the opportunity thus presented for the really effective launching of his campaign of specific chemotherapy.

There, I think, was the real starting point for the whole of this great pageant of progress in the direct and specific treatment of infections which we are now witnessing.

To mention only one other and quite different example, I think that we should remember that the recognition of the essential dietary factor, which we now call the vitamin B_1, really began with observations made by Eykman and, later, Gryns in the Dutch East Indies, and by your own Fraser and Stanton in Malaya. There, again, was one of the starting points of the revolutionary advance in our scientific knowledge of nutrition, which has already banished, from our community, diseases such as rickets, the once tragic prevalence of which is still remembered. And now this new range of knowledge is being applied to yet other problems of defective nutrition, especially in the tropics.

I must return, however, Mr President, to my primary and very pleasant duty, of expressing the very hearty thanks of us, your guests, for the great pleasure and privilege of taking part in this festival occasion, and for the generous welcome which we have received.

HRH The Prince Philip: Perhaps the Toastmaster ought to have added, 'Fellow of the Royal College of Surgeons, Fellow of the Royal Society and several other organizations', but I would like to warn you that this does not mean I necessarily know what I am talking about this evening!

First of all, I would like to thank you very much for your welcome, and may I also thank you for your invitation to come and have dinner here this evening: I would like, too, to thank you for a very good dinner. I think it is just as well to get that in now, before I warm to my subject, so to speak. The two do not necessarily go together.

May I say at once that I am glad to be here at this, your Golden Jubilee dinner, because it gives me a chance to pay a tribute to the Society and to the members of the Society whose contribution to the relief of suffering in a great many parts of the world is incalculable. In addition, I would like to offer my congratulations on your fiftieth birthday. In doing so I speak for countless thousands of people who have benefited by the work of members of the Society. In fact, the same story of determination and sacrifice and devotion far above the demands of duty is repeated in every case; the causes of these tropical diseases have been searched for and discovered, and the same story is repeated in the perseverance and setbacks and despondence and finally, the triumph as the cure and prevention of each of these diseases was discovered and applied.

I think the Society enshrines a very great tradition. There is obviously a great deal still to do but I think that tonight we can remember the great pioneers and we can look back on their achievements. I am not going to discourse about the pioneers and their achievements – most of you know about them better that I do, and those of you who do not, ought to by now.

In recent years I have been to a good many places, during or since the [1939–45] war, which one might describe as subjected to tropical diseases, and I think I can say it is largely due to the members of this Society that I escaped without anything really serious happening. I thought perhaps you might like to know that as I escaped the consequences, you had at least one satisfied customer. I do not know of the dangers or the names of the diseases I might have contracted, but I have in recent years visited a good many laboratories where they have been tinkering about with these things, and having seen the sort of things they are working at, I am even more grateful that I did not get them.

I can only imagine you go into *tropical medicine* because everything is so much bigger than in European disease. Practically everything you have to cope with in science is very small, but in *tropical medicine* everything seems more huge, with enormous wiggling worms and a tank of mosquitoes and large and fearless flies and big and angry – what do you call them? – snails and lice. Every time I see another example of these horrible things that cause these diseases, my admiration for explorers and the early medical officers in tropical countries grows. The success of *tropical medicine* and the tropical medical specialists of the world has undoubtedly been tremendous and it has benefited both sufferers and potential sufferers, but equally, I do not think there is any denying that the control of these diseases has in many cases created other problems, and these problems are not necessarily medical ones. It is no use closing one's eyes to the fact that these problems do exist. It is no good saying you work with the best intentions and that you left someone else to clear up the mess. I know you are very well aware of this problem, but I do not think there is any harm in repeating the statement, and I do not think there is any harm in repeating it until there is evidence that the same brilliant research which goes into ordinary practical medical problems is also going into the problems of the effect which medical advances may have on the community as a whole. In fact, I really believe that the time has come, and for *tropical medicine* in particular, to extend its scope so that it is not concerned simply with the complete healthy state of the individual but with the complete healthy state of whole communities.

May I once again offer my congratulations and best wishes to the Society on this fiftieth birthday, and I am quite certain that in the next fifty years members of the Society will achieve even more fame than they have so far. So, on behalf of all the people in the world who have been helped by practitioners in *tropical medicine*, I would like to propose the Toast of the [RSTMH], and its President.

The President [Boyd] …: It is my privilege, Sir, as President of this Society, to thank you for the great honour you have conferred on us by proposing this toast, and for the generous things you have said about the Society. I know that I speak for everyone here this evening when I say that this is an occasion which we shall always treasure in our memories.

After listening to three brilliant speeches which, among them, seem to have covered the more important aspects of *Tropical Medicine* from A to Z, I feel that there is little more I can say on this subject, so I shall confine myself to talking of the Society as a whole, which in any case is probably what I am meant to do.

We are proud of our Society and of the way in which its scope and influence have developed in the fifty years of its existence. We are proud of its almost international character, for there are no restrictions of caste or race or nationality. All those whose scientific qualifications are deemed by the Council to be adequate are eligible for election to Fellowship. Thanks to the willing co-operation of some fifty-seven local secretaries, we have now well over 2,000 Fellows on our roll, and the number is steadily increasing. Our meetings are a veritable gathering of the clans of those who share a common interest in *Tropical Medicine*.

The main function of the Society, as laid down by our Founders, is to encourage research into the causes, treatment and prevention of the diseases of man and animals which occur in warm climates, by providing facilities for the exchange of information and ideas. We can say with confidence that our meetings achieve this aim exactly according to the pattern they had in mind.

In staging these meetings we are greatly helped by having our own *permanent* [author's italics] headquarters. Manson House was bought for the Society some twenty-five years ago by the very sagacious and far-sighted officers who guided our affairs at that time, and has proved a most valuable acquisition. It provides a pleasant setting for our scientific meetings and social gatherings, and has come to be pervaded by a spirit of comradeship and good will which is noticeable as soon as the threshold is crossed. In fact the social aspect of our activities is so much enjoyed that I sometimes wonder whether Fellows come to the meetings to hear the scientific papers, or to enjoy the coffee and buns and arguments which follow.

I am sure that the President of the Royal College of Surgeons – whom we welcome here tonight and whom at the same time we thank for his courtesy in allowing us to use these beautiful rooms – I am sure that Sir James will not misunderstand me when I say that I am sorry it has been impossible to hold this dinner in our own home, but it is of course far too small.

I would like to pay a tribute to a Fellow, unfortunately unable to be with us this evening, who did much to make Manson House what it is. I refer, of course, to Miss Mildred Wenyon, sister of one of our most distinguished Past Presidents, who for twenty-six years devoted herself to our interests and reigned at Manson House as Secretary and later as Assistant Editor of the *Transactions*. Our *Transactions* also have played their part in achieving the aim of our Founders. They carry the news of our doings at home to Fellows who are overseas, and conversely afford them special facilities to publish accounts of the work they are doing. Under the guidance of our present gifted Editor, the *Transactions* have reached a standard of which we may well be proud.

I said that I would not speak of our Fellows, but I must make one exception. I find that we have on our roll four original Fellows, Fellows who joined the Society at the time of its formation fifty years ago. They are, Dr E C Girling, Dr J Preston Maxwell, Dr A R Wellington, and last – but by no means least – our Past President, Sir Leonard Rogers FRS, who is still one of the bright stars in our firmament.

I have just looked up Sir Leonard in *Who's Who*. He celebrates his 90th birthday next January. I encountered him a few weeks ago in the Underground Station at Euston Square. He emerged from a compartment about twenty yards nearer the exit than I was, and immediately set off at great speed – so fast that I had to run up the stairs two steps at a time in order to overtake him. I am not at all sure that he did not go two steps at a time also. He was in good shape, full of energy, and was engaged in collecting material for a paper on the prevention of cholera by inoculation. I propose, with your concurrence, to send our congratulations and good wishes to all four Original Fellows.

I would fail in my duty if I did not remind all those who work on *Tropical Medicine* of the debt they owe to their devoted wives. Some help their husbands in their work, others maintain morale by making a home in outlandish corners of the world, and others have perhaps the hardest lot of all, the patient endurance of long and lonely periods of separation. We salute them all.

I have two examples in mind that fall into the first of these categories – one modern, one ancient. We have all, I am sure, been charmed by the appropriate illustrations on our menu card tonight. I am much intrigued by the louse falling off the snail band-waggon. I am sure there is a moral somewhere, but I will leave you to draw your own conclusions. Then the macabre dance of tsetse flies and flying bugs with their appropriate trypanosomes. We read in the Book of Isaiah of the wolf dwelling with the lamb, and I presume this is the modern version. These are all the work of Mrs Gordon, wife of our immediate Past President [*see* below]. It is true that this work was done for the good of the Society as a whole and not for Professor Gordon in particular – but the principle is the same.

The second example goes back to the early days of the century, and I assure you that it is a true story, for it was told to me by someone who was present at the time. The scene is a tent somewhere in the wilds of Zululand. Sir David Bruce, another ex-President, had just been listening to the claim of one of his juniors that he has discovered a new species of trypanosome. Turning to his wife, who accompanied him on all his expeditions – 'Mary', he said, 'let me have *camera lucida* drawings of 10,000 of these trypanosomes, so that we can measure them up and decide if this is really something new'. The drawings were duly made, and indeed were only one of many series of 10,000 which the patient Lady Bruce produced.

Finally, a few words about the future of this Society. It has been said that the Society was founded at a very fortunate time – Manson, Ross, Bruce, in *tropical medicine*, Ehrlich in chemotherapy, Wright and Leishman in the preparation of typhoid vaccines, had opened up new fields. These leads were quickly explored by others and in these last fifty years one problem after another has been solved; so much so that some might say the end is in sight and there are no more worlds left to conquer. Nothing could be farther from the truth. There are innumerable problems, both in the diseases peculiar to hot countries and in the everyday diseases of world-wide incidence, which require special study. There are also, as you have said, Sir, problems related to the application of new methods of prevention and treatment in impoverished and undeveloped countries, and these are perhaps among the most important. There is no lack of material. I predict that in the years ahead our Society and its Fellows will have as much to do as they have had in the past; and if there should be a centenary banquet in fifty years' time [which there was not] our successors in those days will have as big a list of triumphs to record as we have here tonight. This rests with the younger generation on whose shoulders the mantle of Elijah will fall. I sincerely hope that these young Fellows will take the trouble to read back numbers of the *Transactions* – and particularly the one which gives an account of this Banquet and all that has been said. If they do, they will find inspiration in your words, Sir, as we who are present tonight have done.

Once again, in the name of every Fellow of the Society and of all who are present here this evening, I thank you, Sir, for the encouragement you have given us by coming here and proposing this Toast. ... [1]

The Society in the 1950s

Cantlie's bust

An important matter a few years previously, in the 'run-up' to the Society's Jubilee, was acquisition of a bust of the Founder* (*see* Chapter 1). It was decided by *Council* on **19 October 1950**, that a bust of Sir James Cantlie 'whose original idea it was to form the Society of Tropical Medicine', should be commissioned; the suggestion came from Sir Neil Cantlie (son of the Founder). The 100th anniversary of Cantlie's birth, it was said, would take place on 17 January 1951, and the bust would be unveiled at the *Ordinary* meeting on 18 January 1951. Although it was hoped that Low would undertake the unveiling, in the event Sir Neil Cantlie performed the ceremony himself.[2] The cost would be about £50 – to be paid from the Society's General Accumulated Fund.

International standing of the Society

In the approach to the half-centenary, the *international* standing of the Society abroad seems to have attained a very high level. The following provides evidence of that:

> [When visiting Brussels in 1956]: The President [Gordon] had had the honour of an audience with Queen Elizabeth of the Belgians, who referred to [the RSTMH] and seemed to know much about its work; she said she was aware that the Queen was Patron and that the Duke of Edinburgh was Patron of the Liverpool School [*see CM*, **21 June 1956**].

The Society had previously been asked by the *Israel Society of the History of Medicine*, Tel-Aviv for replicas of its medals, historical pictures, documents, etc – for its medico-historical museum (*see CM*, **21 July 1955**). The question was asked as to the reason behind this! There is however, no clear answer in the minutes!

Manson House

Repairs to, and insurance of Manson House continued to absorb a great deal of the Society's income.[3] Other expenditure was announced by the

---

* This is no longer at the Society's present headquarters – 50 Bedford Square, London WC1B 3DR; furthermore, it is unclear whether or not it remains extant.

Treasurer (Bloom) on 17 January 1952; this amounted to £5,500 (spread over seven years) and was largely a result of modernisation of the lift, and repair of subsidence damage. Repairs to Manson House (including strengthening the floors – *see* below) also absorbed a significant amount of the budget for 1955.

Rather depressing news was received in early 1952; the Treasurer reported that he had recently received correspondence from the Town Clerk's office indicating that the Society was no longer exempt from rates; although this matter was contested, and again discussed on **18 February 1954**, it was assumed that this was a *fait accompli*!

On a more positive note, Fairley pointed out to *Council* on **15 May 1952** that: 'Manson House had practically doubled in value since it was bought and was now a very valuable asset'. He felt that it was [thus] worthwhile keeping it in a 'good state of repair'. The Society was notified in 1954, by the Ministry of Housing and Local Government that the House 'had been included in one of the lists of buildings of architectural and historic interest, under the Town and Country Planning Act of 1947' (*see CM*, **21 October 1954**).

A new lantern was purchased for Manson House as a gift from the American Fellows of the Society in February 1950. Miss Grieve, Matron of the HTD, wrote to the Society in 1954 in appreciation of free use of the hall for the 'nurses' dance' in December of that year.

TENANTS

The *Institute of Petroleum* (IP), which held a four-year lease (due to expire in October 1952) requested a ten-year extension; they also asked for sixteen *free* meetings instead of twelve, to be held each year in the lecture-hall. However, the ground landlords would only permit this if the *head* lease (which stipulated that the upper floors were to be used for residential accommodation and *not* offices) was surrendered, and a *new* lease taken 'at a ground rate of £500 per annum' (instead of £100 per annum at present). In the event, the Society decided *not* to surrender the lease, but an additional £200 was paid to the ground landlords 'while the upper part was let as offices'.

The District Surveyor refused to allow the front room on the first floor to be used as a library unless the floor was adequately strengthened, and he informed the IP Secretary that he was 'considering serving a dangerous structure notice'. In the event, the IP 'stayed put' but were unwilling to exchange contracts for the new letting until satisfied that the premises were safe for use. At a later meeting of *Council* on **11 December 1952**, a letter was read from the IP Secretary indicating that they were now satisfied that the necessary work for strengthening the floor was in hand and agreed to exchange of the lease.

The IP later broke their lease on 11 October 1956 but asked for a three-month extension. Two alternative tenants had enquired (*see CM*, **21 February 1957**); *Ferranti Ltd* had an interest. However, provided negotiations with Howard de Walden Estates proved satisfactory, *Central Advertising Agency* would take the upper floors at £2,850 per annum for 21 years (*see CM*, **17 October 1957**). This was later approved; however, the RSTMH would have to pay the increased ground rent of £400 per annum instead of £300.

The flat at 4 Cavendish Mews South was de-controlled from October 1958, and the sitting tenant was offered an extension at an increased rent of £250 per annum. Although the lease to the BBC of garages at 4 Cavendish Mews South had expired, they wished to remain for a further three years at £275 instead of £200 per annum.

The Fellowship and other Society matters

The Fellowship remained fairly steady numerically (at 1,500–2,000). It will be recalled that formal *election* took place at an *Ordinary* meeting, but *Council* gave prior approval of names 'going forward'. There had for long been discussion as to whether technicians should be elected to the Fellowship. At a *Council* meeting on **11 December 1952**, it was decided that laboratory technicians 'would *not* normally be eligible for election as Fellows unless they had made some outstanding contribution to *tropical medicine* or parasitology …'.

Honorary Fellows

On **18 October 1951**, Fairley (president) proposed three new Hon Fellows:

- Lord Hailey GCSI
- Sir Charles Martin, and
- Dr L W Hackett

These were unanimously endorsed by *Council*, and on **17 February 1955**, Dr Albert Schweitzer, despite his lack of 'original contributions to the literature of *tropical medicine*' was also made an Honorary Fellow.

OTHER MATTERS INVOLVING FELLOWS

Grassi centenary. A message from the RSHTM, and a note in *Transactions* marked the centenary of the birth of Battista Grassi (1854–1925) in Italy (*see CM*, **18 March 1954**).

Manson memorial. Manson-Bahr informed *Council* that a plaque would be unveiled at Old Meldrum (the birthplace of Manson) on 7 July 1954, the Society being represented by Sir George McRobert.

Memorial to the late General L Van Hoof. Contributions were invited for a bronze plaque to be unveiled at *L'institut de Médicina Tropicale 'Princess Astrid'*, Leopoldville on September 1954; the Society contributed 1,000 Belgian francs.

Award to Rogers. The gold medal of the *Société de Pathologie Exotique* was awarded to Sir Leonard Rogers in 1956. This award was presented by the Cultural Attaché of the French Embassy at the 49th AGM on 21 June of that year.

Swellengrebel portrait. Ten guineas were contributed to a fund for a portrait of Dr N H Swellengrebel (Holland) – an Honorary Fellow – of the Institute of Tropical Hygiene, Amsterdam on his retirement.

Manson House staff

Council on **17 March 1955** once again reviewed staff salaries; they recommended that:

- The Secretary's (Miss Hopper) salary be increased *immediately* by £30 per annum to £690, and by further increments of £30 at intervals of three years to a maximum of £750.
- The Assistant Secretary's (Mrs Langley) salary be increased by £15 per annum to £400, and by further increments of £25 at intervals of three years to a maximum of £450.

It was also recommended that the Executive Committee adopt a 'contributory pension scheme' for the Secretary.

Miss Pilton left the Society in 1954 after nine years' service, in order to get married; the Society gave her £100 as a wedding present (*see CM*, **18 February 1954**).

Meetings – 1951–7

Every two years since its origin, with two exceptions, a new president assumed the major office of the Society. Elected (as is the case today) by *Council*, he began his duties at the AGM, in June. After the first few years, the presidential address took place in the following October; edited versions of the four addresses for the period under review are given below.

Details of presentations at *Ordinary* meetings for the 1950s are of course, to be found in the Society's *Transactions* (*see* Table 13.1). On **16 February 1950**, Dr Joseph Smadel of the Department of Virus and Rickettsial Diseases, Army Medical Center, Washington had spoken on 'Chloramphenical (Chloromycetin) and *Tropical Medicine*' (*see* Chapter 12). Amongst the discussants at that meeting were: Sir Alexander Fleming FRS (1881–1955) and Sir Howard (later Baron) Florey FRS (1898–1968). There had since foundation of the Society in 1907, been a great interest in anti-malarial agents, and an *Ordinary* meeting on 17 July 1952 was entirely devoted to pyrimethamine ('*Daraprim*') – a *new* folic-acid antagonist.

It was intended to hold a special meeting in July 1951 when overseas visitors to the *Festival of Britain* who possessed an interest in *tropical medicine* would be invited (*see* below). With Fairley (president) in the chair, Sir Harold Scott spoke on '*Some British contributions to Tropical Medicine*' and Dr C J Hackett showed two films: '*Chemotherapy of experimental amoebiasis*' and '*Medical aspects of venomous snakes*'.

Dr Albert Schweitzer (1875–1965) (now an Honorary Fellow – *see above*) was present at an *Ordinary* meeting on **20 October 1955**.

CLINICAL MEETINGS

The first *clinical* meeting at the Hospital for Tropical Diseases (HTD), St Pancras Way (which had been opened in May 1951) was held on 15 July 1954:

> Sir Neil Hamilton Fairley, in welcoming the Fellows and visitors [who numbered about 120], gave a brief outline of the functions of the Hospital. He pointed out that before 1939 it had been customary for the Society to hold annual *clinical* meetings at the *old* Hospital for Tropical Diseases … Endsleigh Gardens. After the war the temporary hospital in Devonshire Street was quite inadequate for such a purpose, nor did the *new* hospital at St Pancras provide the necessary facilities until the Rowland Ward Hall was opened [that] year [1954]. He said he hoped that [that] meeting would be the first of a series of [annual ones] which would be as popular as they were in the past.

Table 13.1: Communications at *Ordinary* Meetings – 1951–57

Date	Subject	Speaker
1951		
18 January	FOREAMI organisation in Belgian Congo	R Mouchet
15 February	Miracil D in schistosomiasis in Egypt	J Newsome
17 May	Pathology of malaria	B G Maegraith, E S Jones, W H H Andrews
21 June (44th AGM)	*Mycobacterium leprae* in *Macacus rhesus* and Man	H C de Souza-Araujo
19 July	Tissue phases of malaria parasites	H E Shortt
18 October	Schistosomiasis (*presidential address*)	N H Fairley
13 December	The African Child	D B Jelliffe
1952		
17 January	DDS treatment of Leprosy	E Muir
	Sulphones in Leprosy	R G Cochrane
21 February	Residual insecticide campaigns	G Macdonald
	Efficiency of insecticides	A B Hadaway, F Barlow
	Newer insecticides	J R Busvine
	Resistance to insecticides	C M Harrison
	Synthetic insecticides	J H Barnes
	Standardisation of insecticides	R C M Thomson, R M Gordon, T H Davey
15 May	Animal-man relationship in tropical disease in Africa	J Carmichael
19 June (45th AGM)	Malaria eradication in British Guiana	G Giglioli
17 July	Daraprim	G H Hitchings
	Experimental use of Daraprim	I M Rollo
	Clinical trials with Daraprim	L G Goodwin
	Compound 50–63 studies	G R Coatney
	Daraprim in monkeys	C L Oakleyn, D J Trevan
16 October	Absorption in sprue, coeliac disease, etc	A C Frazer
11 December	Ugandan viruses	G W A Dick
1953		
15 January	Filariasis in the cotton-rat	D S Bertram
19 February	Malaria eradication in Mauritius	M A C Dowling
21 May	Leptospirosis in the tropics	J C Broom
18 June (46th AGM)	*Schistosoma mansoni* film	Anonymous
15 October	'Retrospect' (*presidential address*)	F N White

Date	Subject	Speaker
10 December	Haematinic action of penicillin in megaloblastic anaemia	H Foy, A Kondi
1954		
21 January	Epidemic haemorrhagic fever	K P Brown, A Knudson
18 February	Q fever	M G P Stoker
20 May	Endomyocardial fibrosis in Africa	J D Ball
17 June (47th AGM)	African Auxiliary Medical personnel	C C Chesterman
21 October	Kala azar in Kenya	R B Heisch
9 December	The Volta River project	G Macdonald
1955		
20 January	Recent knowledge of loiasis	R M Gordon
	Tabinid fauna in British Cameroons	W Crewe
	Chrysops in British Cameroons	H Oldroyd
	Loa development	B O L Duke
	Larval stages of *Chrysops*	J J C Buckley
	Pacific filariasis	P Manson-Bahr
	Loa loa periodicity	F Hawking
	Loa loa epidemiology	W E Kershaw
17 February	Typanosomiasis in British West Africa	H W Mulligan
19 May	Immunology of *Plasmodium* spp	A Corradetti
15 June (48th AGM)	Sir David Bruce's research	Sir William MacArthur
18 August	Animals and birds of East Africa (film)	P Manson-Bahr
20 October	Host-parasite relationship in filariasis (*presidential address*)	R M Gordon
8 December	Mycetoma in the Sudan	P H Abbott
1956		
19 January	Treatment of amoebiasis	A R D Adams, A W Woodruff
16 February	Studies on abnormal haemoglobins	A C Allison
17 May	Gold Coast Medical Field Units	B B Waddy
21 June (49th AGM)	Parasites in Brazil	P C C Garnham
10 October	Sea-snake bite research	H A Reid
13 December	Insecticide-resistant insects	J R Busvine
1957		
17 January	Toxoplasmosis (clinical and epidemiological)	C P Beattie
	Serology of toxoplasmosis	I A B Cathie

Date	Subject	Speaker
	Toxoplasma sp in animals	R Lainson
21 February	Heat disorders	W S S Ladell
16 May	Diagnosis of amoebiasis	W P Stamm
	Virulence of *Entamoeba histolytica*	R A Neal
	New amoebicidal drugs	G Woolfe
20 June (50th AGM)	Research in Uganda	A J Haddow
17 October	Dysentery (*presidential address*)	J S K Boyd
12 December	*Wuchereria malayi* in Malaya	J F B Edeson

A similar event was held under Fairley's direction for the years 1955 and 1956.

The Manson Oration

Sir Philip Manson-Bahr suggested (and it was accepted by *Council*) on **18 February 1954**, that since the London School of Hygiene and Tropical Medicine (LSHTM) had a Manson lecture, this should be titled the Manson *Oration* (to be 'in line' with the Harveian and Hunterian orations). It was hoped that the *BMJ* or *Lancet* would publish it. It could be given by the Manson medallist, but this should *not* be compulsory. The lecturer should receive an Honorarium, and there should be no definite interval between the orations. The Liverpool School gave £100 to this fund. The Society also received £50 for the fund from the LSHTM (*see CM*, **25 July**). The oration was the subject of a good deal of discussion at the *Council* meeting on 17 October 1959. It was decided that the oration should be delivered by 'an eminent man on any aspect of *tropical medicine* or *tropical hygiene*' – at intervals of not less than three and not more than five years. The first oration took place in 1958. The fund then stood at £412.

Chadwick Lecture

This was delivered in 1950 and was supposed to be given every 3–4 years, but discussion arose on **18 March 1954**, when Fairley suggested that Professor Edward Ford (Sydney) should be requested to give a Chadwick lecture that year.

Heat effect(s)

Council debated on several occasions in 1955 the classification of the effect of *heat* on the human body. It was agreed that the three armed services should be involved, and that the RSTMH should be represented by Woodruff (*see CM*, **8 December 1955**).

Transactions

The Society's journal continued to occupy a great deal of time and energy, and was frequently discussed at *Council* meetings and AGMs.[4] Proceedings of the *Ordinary* meetings (*see above*) continued to be reported in detail.

The question of 'unsuitable' advertisements submitted to *Transactions* was once again discussed on 18 January 1951. It was agreed that the Editorial Panel should seek alterations to unsuitable advertisements (*see* below). As an example, *Council* suggested that 'quinine is still *the* most effective drug in severe malaria' should be altered to '... *a* most effective drug'. Furthermore, the name of the sponsoring body should, they considered, be included.

In October 1951 disquiet was expressed at the standard of printing of *Transactions*; John Wright of Bristol, and F J Parsons of Hastings and London had submitted estimates; this change resulted in a higher charge for the journal. It was at last agreed to begin subsequent volumes from January, rather than July of each year (which had been the case since 1907).

Dinners and other entertainment

The major and best attended dinner during this period was undoubtedly the Jubilee banquet (*see above*). However, a licence to sell alcoholic drinks at *Ordinary* meetings had by then been obtained (*see CM*, **19 January 1950**), and led to the origin of the *Dining Club*. A dinner was, for example, held before the *Ordinary* meeting on 18 July 1951. Previously, dinner had been provided at J Lyons & Co of Oxford Street Corner House; for that *before* the laboratory meeting on 16 November 1950 a charge of 4s a head was made (*see CM*, **19 October 1950**).

On 11 December 1952, Col Robert Drew was elected to serve on the 'Wine Club' Committee; he took the place of Professor Frederick Murgatroyd (1902–51) who had recently suddenly died of a presumed myocardial infarct. Dr H J O'D Burke-Gaffney was later appointed to serve (with Bloom and Drew) on the 'Wine Committee'. Further reference to the 'Wine Club' is to be found in the minutes of the 46th and 50th AGMs; Group Captain W P Stamm was elected to the Wine

Committee at the latter meeting. The Treasurer (Bloom) reported in 1955 a favourable balance for the Dining Club of £31 17s 8d (*see CM*, **15 June 1955**).

The current president (Fairley) donated £200 'to establish a fund permitting the occasional entertainment' of distinguished visitors from abroad by the president and *Council* at Manson House (*see CM*, **18 June 1953**).

Gifts to the Society in the 1950s

Further gifts to the library were recorded at *Council* meetings on 15 March 1951, 13 December 1951 and 17 January 1952. A book – '*Microscopium*' – a history of the microscope – was received from the Anglo-Netherland Society. Sir Leonard Rogers donated £200 to the Society in stock in the *Dundee and London Investment Fund* (*see CM*, **15 October 1953**).

'Several articles of silver' which had belonged to Manson were presented by Mr David Manson to the Society in 1955 (*see CM*, **20 January 1955**). A further gift of a rose bowl and cigarette box – which had also belonged to Sir Patrick – was made by Manson-Bahr on **10 October 1956**.

Involvement with other societies and conferences

A proposal for joint meetings with the *Tropical Medicine Societies of Western Europe* was explored in October 1950; this would be restricted to England, France, Belgium and Holland, and it was envisaged that the first meeting would be held in London in 1951. However, owing to the *Festival of Britain*, accommodation in London would, it was felt, be difficult and the Dutch Society was therefore asked to host the first meeting. The following year, 1952, would also be unsuitable as the *5th International Congress of Tropical Medicine & Malaria* was to be held there that year (*see CM*, **14 December 1950**). It was thus agreed that 1953 would be more suitable to all western European societies and further, that meetings should be held every three years. However, the *5th International Congress of Tropical Medicine & Malaria* was later postponed to 2–8 September 1953, and later changed to 18 August – 4 September of that year (in Istanbul); therefore the Secretary (Boyd) asked *Council* on 21 February 1952 whether the Joint European meeting could, after all, be held in London in 1952? Owing to financial constraints and the 'altered economic circumstances', *Council*, however, rejected this proposal also. The meeting was thus 'indefinitely postponed'.

A special RSM programme for the *Festival of Britain* would be held in June–July 1951; the Council of the Royal Society was, it was reported, working closely with the RSM; *Council* agreed that the emphasis from the RSTMH's angle should be on Britain's contribution to *tropical medicine* and that various senior members (Scott and Shortt) would give lectures on 18 and 19 July 1951 (*see* above).

At a *Council* meeting on **16 October 1952**, Boyd announced that he was attending the meeting of the *American Society of Tropical Medicine and Hygiene* [ASTM&H) in November at Texas – the president elect of which was Dr Sodeman. The idea of an *International Society of Tropical Medicine* was discussed at a later meeting (*see CM*, **19 February 1953**); the intention also was to discuss the *Congress of Tropical Medicine and Malaria* at Istanbul (*see* above) later that year. The RSTMH had, incidentally, been invited to send a representative to that Congress. The president (Fairley) suggested however, that before reaching a conclusion, they should get the opinion of the American Society *via* Dr F L Soper, its president.

At a meeting of *Council* on **19 March**, Napier referred to a *Conference on Medical Education* which would be held in London in August 1953. He desired to know whether the RSTMH was to be represented, because he felt that *tropical medicine* should be taught to undergraduates. It was agreed that a Sub-Committee – Maegraith, Napier and Woodruff – should be appointed 'with authority to co-opt other Fellows …'. This Sub-Committee produced guidelines for stressing the importance of *tropical medicine* in the undergraduate curriculum (*see CM*, **21 May**, **18 June**, **16 July 1953**). *Council* decided however, that since this was an *international* conference, recommendations should be focused on teaching in *temperate* countries only. It was later agreed that Napier should represent the Society at that meeting.

Dr Henry de Boer (T H Davey had originally been invited) represented the Society at the *Royal Sanitary Institute*'s Health Congress at Margate on 22–25 April 1952. That for 1954 was held at Scarborough from 27–30 April, and Professor Davey this time represented the RSTMH. Dr Burk-Gaffney represented the RSTMH at the Congress at Bournemouth (26–29 April 1955) and also that at Blackpool (24–27 April 1956).

Council was requested to send a representative to attend the Dinner to be held to mark the 50th anniversary of the ASTM&H at Louisville, Kentucky on 12 November 1953. The *Congresso General de Medicine* invited delegates for the meeting at Rosario, Argentina from 7–12

November 1955, but this was subsequently declined (*see CM*, **19 May 1955**). Professor Maegraith attended the first meeting of the *Egyptian Society of Parasitology and Tropical Medicine* in 1956 (*see CM*, **10 October 1956**). Sir Gordon Covell represented the Society at the first AGM of the *UK Committee for the WHO of the United Nations* on 7 April 1956; he also represented the Society at its 2nd AGM on 6 April 1957. Professor P C C Garnham and Dr Burke-Gaffney represented the Society at the Health Congress of the *Royal Society of Health* at Folkestone from 30 April – 30 May 1957. The *6th International Congress on Tropical Medicine and Malaria* took place in Lisbon on 5–13 September 1958; Shortt represented the RSTMH.

A joint meeting of the *Canadian* and *British Medical Associations* was held in Edinburgh from 18–24 July 1959; it was decided that the *clinical* meeting at HTD that July should be 'open to [a group of] visiting Canadian doctors', and that there should be a special meeting at Manson House.

A later minute records that representatives were requested to attend: *A conference on the Supply of Experimental Animals* – January 1958 (J D Fulton), and the Health Congress of the *Royal Society of Health* at Eastbourne 28 April–2 May 1958 (Burke-Gaffney) (*see CM*, **12 December 1957**).

Royal matters

At a *Council* meeting on **21 February 1952**, an Hon Secretary (Boyd) read a letter of condolence addressed to HM the Queen from the Society on the death of its Patron, King George VI, which was signed by the president (Fairley); the Society duly received a letter of thanks from the Home Secretary (Sir David Maxwell Fyfe). *Council* heard on **19 June 1952** from the keeper of the Privy Purse that HM Queen Elizabeth II had accepted patronage of the Society.

Decoration of the exterior of Manson House for the coronation of Elizabeth II in 1953 was discussed at a *Council* meeting on **11 December 1952**; it was decided that the Executive Committee 'should conform with whatever was being arranged in Portland Place'. The Queen's thanks for a loyal address submitted on the occasion of her coronation were received from Sir David Maxwell Fyfe (*see CM*, **16 July 1953**).

The Home Secretary also thanked the president and Council on behalf of HM the Queen for their loyal address on the occasion of the death of Queen Mary.

Obituaries

Council minutes continued to record the deaths of *all* Fellows of the Society. However, former presidents, Honorary Fellows and other distinguished individuals in *tropical medicine* always received special mention. Among these were the following: Professor W A P Schuffner's (Amsterdam) (an Honorary Fellow) death was announced to *Council* on **19 January 1950**; he had died on 24 December 1949; that of Clifford Dobell (*see* below) was also announced at the same meeting. The death of Sir Arthur Bagshawe (1871–1950), an original Fellow of the Society, past-president, Treasurer and Trustee, was announced to *Council* on **18 May 1950**. Professor Emil Brumpt's death (an Honorary Fellow since 1923) was also announced to *Council* on **18 October 1951**. Dr Wilbur A Sawyer's (an Honorary Fellow since 1949) death was reported to *Council* on **13 December**. The sudden and unexpected death of Professor Frederick Murgatroyd (1902–51) (*see* above) was announced to *Council* on **17 January 1952**. The death of Low (1872–1952), a past-president, Trustee, as well as being a joint founder of the Society, was announced by the president (Fairley) at a *Council* meeting on **16 October**. At the *Council* meeting on **19 January 1956**, the deaths of Professor P A Buxton (1892–1955) (a former vice-president) and Sir Malcolm Watson (1873–1955) (a former member of *Council*) were announced. The death of Brigadier J A Sinton VC FRS (1884–1956), Manson Medallist who had died on 25 March, was announced to *Council* on **17 May**.

The Manson Medal (the highest honour conveyed by the RSTMH) was presented to Mrs Sinton (following Sinton's death), at the 49th AGM. The death of Scott (1874–1956) (a past-president) was reported to *Council* on **10 October 1956** and Professor K Shiga's (an Honorary Fellow since 1907) death was announced on **21 February 1957**.

Presidential Addresses 1951–57

The first Address of the 1950s was delivered on 18 October 1951 by Sir Neil Hamilton Fairley KBE MD FRCP FRS (1891–1956)[5] (*see* Figure 13.1), then Senior Physician at the HTD. Earlier that year the HTD had moved from 23 Devonshire Street to 4 St Pancras Way NW1. Although Fairley had carried out a vast amount of pioneering work on *malaria* (especially chemoprophylaxis and chemotherapy) as well as other diseases, he chose to speak on: **Schistosomiasis and some of its problems**. He had, he told his audience, been associated with this field of research for thirty-five years; investigations to be described were 'mainly ... confined to work undertaken during, and subsequent to the first world war'. He began with an historical review of *schistosomiasis* in Egypt during World War I (1914–18):

> Japanese investigators had worked out the life [-cycle] of *Schistosoma japonicum* ... by 1913, and their work was confirmed by Leiper and Atkinson[6] in China and Japan the following year. In January 1915, Leiper[7] had come to Egypt ... and he and his colleagues [soon] established the existence of two distinct species of bilharzia worms affecting man there, thus terminating the controversy between Looss and Sambon regarding the duality of the two species. *S haematobium* presented distinctive morphological features, laid terminal-spined eggs and developed in a fresh-water snail, *Bulinus contortus*, while *S mansoni* produced lateral-spined eggs and developed in *Planorbis boissyi*. Leiper[8] also outlined efficient measures for the prevention of [infection] in troops stationed there. Early in 1916 a febrile illness affecting Australian troops was found to be due to intestinal schistosomiasis.
>
> It was from the Tel-el-Kebir group that Lawton[9] first described the early toxic features associated with *S mansoni* infection in Egypt. Symptoms included fever, urticaria, abdominal pain, enlargement of the liver and spleen, emaciation, bronchitis and diarrhoea. Clinically, some resembled typhoid fever [and] others bronchopneumonia. Eosinophilia was common and this suggested the possibility of helminthic infection [leading] to the finding of lateral-spined ova in the stools. These early clinical features resembled the urticarial fever known as 'Yangtse River fever' in China and 'Katayama disease' in Japan ... associated with early *S japonicum* infection.
>
> Later [in 1916] I found [continued Fairley] that an early clinical syndrome characterized by urticaria, oedema, toxic pains and eosinophilia with or without fever was occurring in troops infected with *S haematobium* alone; they had been bathing some 6 weeks previously in a sweet water canal at Serapium, where only infected *bulinus* snails could be found.[10] [However, a reinvestigation of Lawton's cases showed many to have terminal-

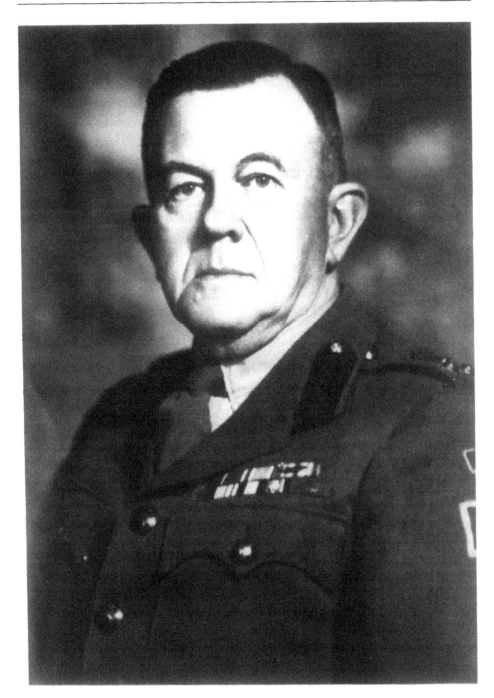

Figure 13.1: Sir Neil Hamilton Fairley FRCP FRS – the twenty-first president (reproduced courtesy the Wellcome Library, London).

spined ova in their urine as well as lateral-spined ova in the stools.[11]] The Rifle Range Canal at Tel-el-Kebir was re-examined and infected *bulinus* and *planorbis* snails were found by Manson-Bahr (*see* Chapter 12] and myself; also stools collected in adjacent fields showed lateral – and terminal-spined ova. Monkeys were experimentally infected from snails ... and our field observations constituted ... complete confirmation of Leiper's work.[12]

Of *experimental pathology* in monkeys, Fairley had this to say:

As the pathological basis of this early clinical syndrome was ... unknown 35 years ago, monkeys (*Cerophithicus aethiops*) were experimentally infected with cercariae of either *S mansoni* derived from naturally infected *P boissyi*, or with those of *S haematobium* derived from *B contortus*; snails of both species were collected from the village of El Marg, near Cairo.

The distribution of the two species ... in the vascular system was accurately determined in the early stages of infection and ... deposition of ova in the various organs was demonstrated by digesting the tissues with caustic soda. The characteristic lesion ... in the liver, intestine, bladder and lungs resembled miliary tubercle; it was named the bilharzia pseudotubercle [consisting] of one or more ova surrounded by giant cells, epithelioid, mononuclear and plasma cells and numerous eosinophil leucocytes. When ova were more numerous central degeneration or caseation sometimes resulted; fibroblasts appeared later and finally fibrosis occurred. Three types of lesion were produced experimentally: (1) [the] pseudo-tubercle; (2) [the] papilloma; and (3) verminous arteritis and phlebitis resulting from worms impacted in the distended thrombosed vessels. The fourth type of lesion – the [schistosoma] granuloma – was *not* encountered. Bilharzia pigment was identified as haematin for the first time.[13]

And as to *diagnosis*, Fairley then described in detail efforts to develop a suitable serological test for both *S mansoni* and *S haematobium* infections. Regarding *treatment*:

... McDonagh[14] in England and Christopherson[15] in Khartoum [established] the curative action of tartar emetic in ... vesical schistosomiasis. [The latter] advocated [an intravenous course lasting] 4 to 5 weeks. Its value as a specific in *schistosomiasis* was confirmed in 1919 and … was soon shown to be an effective therapeutic agent for all three varieties of human *schistosomiasis*.

The period 1915–1918 was remarkable for [outstanding] contributions made by British workers on Egyptian *schistosomiasis* … As a result of this work, the lives of many hundreds of thousands of Egyptians have been saved. It is one of the many beneficial contributions conferred on Egypt during the British occupation which has been too readily forgotten [he maintained], not only by the Egyptians but by leading politicians in this country …

Fairley then turned to *distribution* of the disease:

The two African species, *S haematobium* and *S mansoni*, probably originated in the Nile Valley, where Rüffer[16] found … ova in a mummy of the 19th Dynasty. The spread [of the disease] from the Nile Valley through Africa and the Middle East [was] along caravan and trade routes, by immigration or following in the wake of invading armies, or the slave trade. Intestinal *schistosomiasis* (*S mansoni*) was brought to the West Indies and South America by slaves from West Africa. Asiatic *schistosomiasis* … probably originated in the Yangtse Valley … whence it spread to Japan, Formosa, the Philippines and the Celebes.

During the present century perennial irrigation has been a major factor in its spread. Infected immigrants and returned soldiers from Africa, Egypt and the Far East have failed to establish *schistosomiasis* in England, USA, Australia and elsewhere. One endemic case only has been reported in [the] USA … Though cattle *schistosomiasis* is common in certain Oriental countries … human [disease] has never become established … This must be attributed to an absence of the appropriate snail vectors rather than to the standard of sanitation existing among the agricultural population.

… *schistosomiasis* is on the increase in Africa, North-Eastern South America and elsewhere. [WHO] medical experts … regard [it] as Public Enemy No 1 in the Middle East, for wherever perennial irrigation is introduced … a corresponding increase in [its] incidence … soon follows. …

And to the crucially important aspects of *prevention*:

> Only 2 years ago Khalil[17] reported that *schistosomiasis* remained the greatest obstacle to ... progress and ... prosperity of Egypt, that 14 million out of 20 million Egyptians (*ie* 70 per cent) suffered from the disease and that it was responsible directly or indirectly for 25 per cent of ... deaths there.
>
> ... Methods at present favoured include the use of molluscicide, copper sulphate and periodically clearing the canals of vegetation, silt and snails [but these measures] cannot be regarded as having ... materially reduced the incidence of the disease ... until human excretal contamination of canals and irrigation channels is prevented and some suitable system of village and rural sanitation established ... eradication [of the disease] appears unlikely.
>
> Similar conditions prevail where *S japonicum* is endemic, only here the problem of prevention is even more difficult as, in addition to man, a variety of animal vectors may lead to water pollution.

Fairley continued with a note on 'Compliment fixation reactions' [CF] in cattle *schistosomiasis*:

> My interest in cattle *schistosomiasis* dates back to 1922 when the Director of Medical Research in India asked if I would undertake a serological investigation of Indian soldiers who had acquired vesical *schistosomiasis* in Iraq. As the [CF] was known to be of group nature and as there was a potential source of antigen supply in molluscs [infected] with *S spindale* [of which the definitve host is the water buffalo] in Bombay [now Mumbai] Province, an investigation was undertaken ...
>
> Spindale antigen proved even more potent for the serological diagnosis ... in animals and man than that originally prepared from snails in Egypt infected with cercariae of *S mansoni*. ... Later, the reaction was found to be group specific for ... cattle schistosomes and it was shown that sera from animals infected with *S bovis* in India and *S indicum* and *S matthei* in London, also reacted positively with *S spindale* antigen.[18]
>
> *S spindale* antigen also proved highly satisfactory for the diagnosis of vesical *schistosomiasis* in Indian troops and was later found to be equally effective in human [disease] caused by *S mansoni* and *S japonicum*. ...

He then spoke on the degree of susceptibility to man of the cattle disease:

> Relatively little detailed information [exists] on the susceptibility of man to infection with the various species of cattle schistosomes. This has [largely] been due to the difficulty of differentiating on morphological grounds ova of certain species of cattle schistosomes from *S haematobium* in the excreta.
>
> ... There is no evidence [he concluded] that cercariae of *S spindale* ever develop into adult schistosomes in man. ... Instances of human infection with *S bovis* [another species] have been reported in Natal, Southern Rhodesia [now Zimbabwe], and the Belgian Congo. ...
>
> Blackie claimed that in Rhodesia *S matthei* affected man and baboons; terminal-spined ova were reported in the intestine but not the bladder. ...
>
> The whole question of ... susceptibility of man to infection with cattle *schistosomiasis* ... could be readily determined experimentally by exposing human volunteers to infection with different species of cercariae, following the course of the infection by serial [CF] tests, eosinophil counts and daily examinations of the excreta ...

Then a note followed on 'The status of *S intercalatum*':

> *S intercalatum*[19] is a form of intestinal schistosomiasis with terminal-spined eggs in the faeces but not the urine affecting man in the Stanleyville area of the Belgian Congo. ... The adult worms closely resembled *S haematobium*, but there are differences in the ova. ... As there are no recognizable morphological differences between the eggs or schistosomes of *S matthei* and *S intercalatum*, it still remains possible though improbable, that *S intercalatum* may be *S matthei* adapted to man.

Fairley then described the clinico-pathological consequences of infection in man, and referred to an outbreak of Japanese *schistosomiasis* in US and Australian troops during World War II [1939–45]:

> ... more than 1,500 American officers and men contracted this disease and at least 174 army personnel of the Royal Australian Air Force. The early toxic stage with anaphylactic features (Yangtse

River fever) was recognized early and [those] presenting such features were treated … with fouadin. Swimmer's dermatitis was not common and later localizing features were not much in evidence, diarrhoea and dysentery being … infrequent. A number of patients developed neurological features due to ectopic lesions involving the brain.

[In a series reported by Billings *et al*]: Fever of remittent or intermittent type was constant and lasted 1 to 8 weeks. Headache, loss of weight, malaise, anorexia and upper abdominal or epigastric pain were common. Soreness and stiff neck of myalgic type … was present in 84 per cent … while abdominal colic and generalized toxic pains were common. A harsh unproductive cough was frequent. Urticaria and angioneurotic oedema were observed in 52 per cent. Neurological features, including coma, hemiplegia and paralysis, developed in 9.3 per cent.

This was followed by a detailed account of physical signs and faecal analysis:

It has taken a second world war [he maintained] to make evident the difficulty of finding ova in the faeces in mild and atypical … infections, while several writers emphasize that the extent of subclinical army cases is still unknown.

In this comprehensive account of *schistosomiasis* in man, which in most part could not be bettered today, he then dealt with 'ectopic lesions' in man under the following headings: '*central nervous system*', '*conjunctival*' and '*cutaneous*'.

And on to the *complications* of infection:

I … confine my remarks [he continued] to three complications of … doubtful aetiology which Gelfand[20] has failed to find in South Central Africa.

- *Bladder malignancy.* Ferguson[21] first drew attention to the association of bilharzia in the male fellaheen of Egypt and malignant diseases of the bladder, the increased incidence of which he attributed to prolonged irritation caused by eggs of *S haematobium*. In his opinion, 'cancer of the urinary bladder was the irritation cancer of Egypt'.

... though caustic soda digests revealed the presence of calcified ... eggs in a large proportion of females, he pointed out that primary malignant disease of the female bladder was [exceptional].

- ... *Splenomegaly with Cirrhosis* [caused by *schistosomiasis*] resembles Banti's disease clinically and is characterized by hepatomegaly, splenomegaly and anaemia. In the first stage there is slight enlargement of the liver, in the second hepatomegaly and splenomegaly, [and] in the last stage the liver is generally small but there is marked enlargement of the spleen, ascites and perhaps terminal cholaemia.

The classical bilharzial peri-portal pipe-stem cirrhosis was described by Symmers[22] in Egypt and its early stages were studied by Fairley[23] in monkeys experimentally infected with *S mansoni* and *S haematobium*.

In experimentally infected animals, Fairley and Mackie[24] found the pipe-stem peri-portal cirrhosis ... in goats experimentally infected with *S spindale* during the 2nd year of the disease. No generalized fibrosis [or splenomegaly] was present ... In 26 of these heavily infected animals splenic tissue was digested in caustic soda and only three were found to contain ova. ... In the early stages in experimentally infected monkeys (*S mansoni* and *S haematobium*) there is evidence of generalized toxic damage to the liver, but this does not appear to lead to a generalized fibrosis ...

In my opinion [Fairley continued], the hepatic cirrhosis associated with splenomegaly in Egypt and elsewhere is not due primarily to *schistosomiasis*; it is probably of nutritional origin, and apart from malnutrition the condition would probably never be encountered. The localized peri-portal cirrhosis of Symmers could at most only be a minor contributory factor, while intestinal *schistosomiasis* by inducing dysentery, diarrhoea and intestinal hurry, might contribute in a minor degree also by making complete absorption of a diet already deficient in lipotrophic factors such as choline, or sulphur-containing amino-acids such as cystine, more difficult.

Perhaps Newsome's work on baboons repeatedly infected with *S mansoni* while on normal and deficient diets, will throw light on this ... problem.

- *Pulmonary disease (Egyptian Ayerza's disease).* Turner[25] first directed attention to the frequency with which terminal-spined ova were present in the lungs of South African natives. Fairley[26] next described [the] pseudo-tubercles associated with ova in the lungs of monkeys experimentally infected with *S haematobium* and *S mansoni,* and the larger nodular areas of consolidation (bilharzia pneumonia) associated with impacted worms in the pulmonary arterioles. Both [of these] lesions were specially evident in *S haematobium* infections. In these earlier stages *clinical* features may be latent or associated with cough and crepitations over one or both bases; radiography is suggestive of miliary tuberculosis [but] lesions are not so uniform in size. ...

  Both types of ova are found in the lung in Egypt, but *S haematobium* predominates. According to Day[27], if hepatic cirrhosis and portal obstruction develop, the portal collateral circulation may admit the entry of worms and ova of *S mansoni* to the pulmonary arteries. ... Gelfand[28] has found no case of Ayerza's disease (chronic or pulmonale) ... in South Central Africa, though both species are common there, nor does he find pulmonary *schistosomiasis* more prone to occur in the presence of hepatic cirrhosis.

The next area for consideration was *diagnosis* of human infection:

Severe and average infections are readily diagnosed by finding ova in the stools, especially if they contain mucus; milder cases, atypical infections and instances of ectopic *schistosomiasis* may present difficulty owing to the scantiness or absence of ova in the excreta. ... infections may remain subclinical though ova are ... passed in limited numbers in the excreta. In other cases, *schistosomiasis* may be suspected on *clinical* grounds and a positive intradermal skin test ... may support this diagnosis, but *it is essential to get parasitological or serological confirmation if possible* [author's italics]. In selected cases special investigations may have to be undertaken, including sigmoidoscopy, cystosocopy, pylography or radiology of the chest.

Laboratory investigations
These include examination of the urine and faeces for ova and miracidia, rectal snippings or scrapings, snippings from the bladder, and biopsy of pathological material removed at operation. Haematological investigation for eosinophilia and the [CF] test should be performed as a routine. [Fairley then proceeded to describe each of these investigations in detail].

Although the date of the lecture was 1951, Fairley had a great deal to say about serological diagnosis. He proceeded to describe: the intradermal reaction, the complement fixation test, and the anti-cercarial reaction (membrane formation, precipitate formation and agglutination). Although he was convinced of the value of the first two, he felt that:

... anti-cercarial immunity reactions ... are of great biological interest, [but] much more work will be necessary before we can assess either their immunological significance or their practical value in the serological diagnosis of *schistosomiasis*. Apparently no effort has been yet made to correlate the capacity of immune sera to produce precipitate formation around cercariae and their content in complement-fixating antibodies as measured by the standard [CF] test. ...

A short section on 'Acquired Immunity in Man and Monkeys' followed:

Vogel[29] has published some ... results in monkeys (*Macacus rhesus*) indicating that after repeated exposure to cercariae of *S japonicum* over many months, a progressive decrease in ova occurs and immunity to superinfection is finally established so that a dose of cercariae which would have been fatal previously proved quite innocuous. Standen[30] [also] noted ... development of a similar degree of immunity in *M rhesus* in two monkeys repeatedly exposed to cercariae of *S mansoni*, [a final stage being reached] in which both these monkeys were resistant to superinfection and that, in one, ova are no longer demonstrable.

Acquired immunity of this order is not developed against *S mansoni* by all species of monkeys for Newsome ... has found that repeated infections of the baboon (*Papio homadryas*) with cercariae of *S mansoni* do not result in immunity to superinfection.

Acquired immunity does not occur in man after single infections and ... immunity of this type [probably does not result] from repeated exposure to schistosome cercariae over many years. ... the problem is likely to be settled satisfactorily only by experimental superinfection in volunteer patients who for many years have been exposed to repeated infection in highly endemic areas ... such as Egypt. The problem is of importance where therapy is concerned, for if an immunity to superinfection can develop in man, a drug which produces *clinical* rather than *radical* cure may be desirable in heavily infected areas – especially if it can be given [orally]. The ideal drug would reduce the schistosome load to a subclinical level in all three human species, leaving a reduced number of worms to maintain a state of immunity to superinfection.

The remainder of the Address was devoted to 'Reflections on *Treatment*'. He began with a brief reference to emetine, which had been used in this disease by Hutchinson [in 1913][31]; however, sudden death, probably resulting from ventricular fibrillation had been recorded and it had therefore been discontinued. Much was said about trivalent antimony compounds, widely used at that time; the question of *cure* was also addressed:

> ... *Clinical* cure, as judged by the disappearance of symptoms and of ova from the excreta, is readily attained ...
>
> Schistosomes do not [replicate] in ... the definitive host, and [therefore] every course of treatment ... should decrease the number of living worms. Absence of viable ova from the excreta for 3 months has been suggested as a reasonable period to estimate cure ... Even [after one year, however], though demonstrable ova are absent from the excreta, positive [CF] reactions may persist in the absence of *clinical* symptoms for several years.[32] Pifano and Mayer[33] have found that after a course of tartar emetic, 5 per cent of ... positive [CF] reactions became negative and after a second course 32 per cent were negative. They concluded that a

persisting positive test does not signify [presence of] living worms ... therapeutic studies in experimentally infected animals have shown that persisting positive reactions may be associated with (1) residual unisexual male infection; (2) a reduction in parasites associated with a lowered male: female sex ratio in which only [a] few females survive; and (3) so marked a reduction of male and female parasites that the infection remains subclinical and ova no longer appear in demonstrable numbers in the excreta. Whether patients with residual infection of this nature need further treatment is problematical.

He *concluded* with a short review of miracil D ('Nilodin'), used by Germans during the war, in both mice and monkeys. Clinical usage had shown that (although a gastro-intestinal irritant) it possessed anti-schistosomal activity when given orally – unique at that time. However, a large question mark hung over its efficacy in producing *cure*; it was probably most effective (he claimed) in S *haematobium* infections.[34]

On 15 October 1953, Dr Frederick Norman White CIE MD DPH (1877–1964)[35] (*see* Figure 13.2) gave his Address **Restrospect** on some reflections from the past in India, Russia, Poland, and South-east Asia. He was to dwell at length on the Influenza pandemic of 1918 in India. 'It is inevitable,' he began, 'that one as old as I should be chiefly concerned with events of a bygone era [which are] to a regrettable extent autobiographical':

It is just fifty years since I first arrived in India, when *tropical medicine* first became an absorbing interest [of mine]. I should like [to refer to the closing chapter of my seventeen years in the Indian Medical Service (IMS)].

During the latter half of the first World War [1914–18] I was entrusted with the work of the Sanitary Commissioner of the Government of India ... The ... meagre health and medical services had been depleted ... and were only just sufficient for routine work ... Things went persistently badly. In the autumn of 1917 *malaria* was epidemic in parts of Northern India: the *plague* epidemic of 1917–18 was the most severe that India had suffered for eleven years: failure of the monsoon in 1918 resulted in *food scarcity* and high prices: there was considerable anxiety regarding ... importation of various infections, and fresh strains

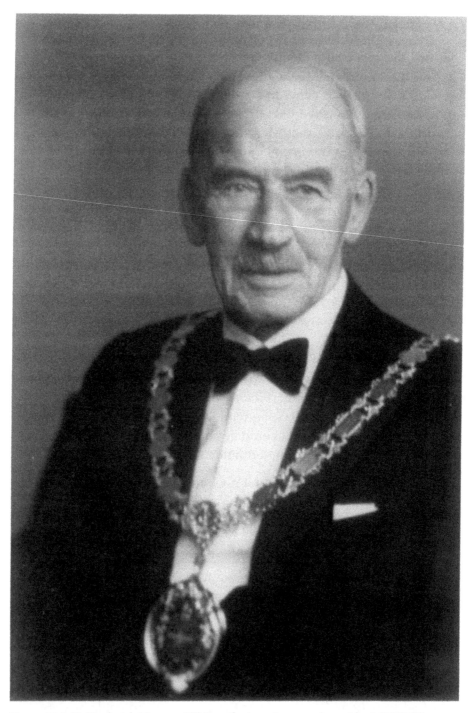

Figure 13.2: Dr Frederick Norman White – the twenty-second president (RSTMH archive).

of infection, with troops returning from overseas: and then came *influenza*.

[The influenza pandemic]

The … wave of *influenza* in the autumn of 1918 in the central, northern and western parts of India and in territories across India's north-west frontier was a catastrophe almost without parallel in the history of epidemics. Within the space of two months it caused the deaths of some six million people in India alone … The so-called Spanish *influenza* had been unduly prevalent in Europe during the spring and early summer of 1918, spreading along lines of communication from western Europe to most parts of the world. It had caused much sickness but little mortality. The pandemic appeared to have died down, when suddenly it flared up again with terrible intensity and almost simultaneously in all parts of the world, except Australasia, but nowhere with the severity that it did in India and adjacent territory. Everywhere adolescents, young adults and people in the prime of life suffered most: the very young and old displayed a surprising immunity. No one who took an active part in … efforts to control the disease in the worst affected parts of India is likely to have forgotten his experiences.

The first reports of alarming mortality were from Bombay [now Mumbai]. My brief visit there was long enough to ascertain the nature of the disease and to satisfy myself that it was not *yellow fever* [YF]. The possibility of … introduction of [YF] into India was, for a time, something of a nightmare … I was very soon recalled to Delhi where conditions were almost as bad as in Bombay, and I stayed [there] for the remainder of those tragic weeks. …

In a report that I wrote for the Government of India on the conclusion of the epidemic I quoted from a report sent me from the Punjab …:

> The hospitals were choked so that it was impossible to remove the dead quickly enough to make room for the dying; the streets and lanes of the cities were littered with dead and dying people; the postal and telegraph services were completely disorganized; the train service continued, but at all the principal stations dead and dying people were being removed from the trains; the burning ghats and burial grounds were literally swamped with

corpses, while an even greater number awaited removal; the depleted medical service ... was incapable of dealing with more than a minute fraction of the sickness requiring attention; nearly every household was lamenting a death, and everywhere terror and confusion reigned.

That gruesome description in no way exaggerates conditions during a few terrible weeks ... Rural areas suffered even more than towns. Some villages in the Central Provinces were literally de-populated. By the end of November mortality rates had returned to normal almost everywhere – and the long war was over.

One reason which prompted this reference to that terrible epidemic is that it was the indirect cause of my leaving India. *Influenza* had spared neither Europe nor America and the Allied countries convened a medical conference in Paris in March 1919, to take stock of the situation and to frame measures, if possible, to prevent the recurrence of a like catastrophe. I was delegated at very short notice to represent the Government of India ... In Paris, after nine years unbroken absence from Europe, I made my first contact with many distinguished European medical colleagues whom I was later to know so well. ...

Life in London.
White then recalled his resignation from the IMS shortly after returning to England. From 1 January 1920, he became a Medical Officer in the *Ministry of Health*. The nascent *League of Nations* (*LN*) (White was seconded to the *Epidemic Commission*) which had just come into being, was asked its advice on epidemics of *typhus* and *relapsing fever* in Poland and Russia in war-devastated Europe. This took him (as a member of an *International Epidemic Commission*) to both of those countries.

The League of Nations (LN).
In addition to *typhus* and *relapsing fever*, White also encountered *cholera* in eastern Europe:

During the twelve years that followed [this] period [he continued] I was privileged to work intimately with medical men and research workers of very many nationalities and in many countries. It was always to obtain whole-hearted friendly collaboration in any work designed to promote the welfare of humanity, or to enlarge our knowledge of the causation, prevention or cure of disease. The contribution to world peace and international understanding which such co-operative work can make is not negligible. That is one reason why the work of the *World Health Organization* [WHO], which has carried on and greatly extended work begun by the [LN's] Health Organization, merits every support.

We received [only] a quarter of the sums we had originally hoped for but ... were able to give ... material assistance to the Health Administrations of Eastern Europe, chiefly Poland, in coping with a difficult and dangerous epidemic situation.

In January 1922, the head office of the *Epidemic Commission* was moved from London to Geneva and ... our activities were incorporated in the newly created Health Organization of the [LN]. I was still styled Chief Epidemic Commissioner but ... acted, in addition, as Rajchman [first Director of the Health Section of the *LN* Secretariat]'s deputy.

White then turned to his involvement in the 'mission to the Far East' ... in 1922–23:

... The Japanese member of the Health Committee, on behalf of his Government, had proposed the despatch of a Mission to the Far East to study the incidence of diseases of international importance in [those countries]; the part played by shipping in the spread of infection; the measures taken to prevent such spread in the ports of departure and arrival, and to make suggestions for the improvement and standardization of port health procedure. ... It was originally intended that the Mission should consist of three delegates of different nationalities but eventually I sailed alone. In the part of the investigation that concerned Hongkong, Shanghai, and part of Japan and the Philippines I had [a member] of the US Public Health Services as an 'unofficial' colleague.

As a prelude to the work of the Mission I attended, as a delegate of the [LN], the first Far Eastern Conference of the League of Red Cross Societies ... in Bangkok in November 1922. [There] my preoccupations were largely concerned with problems of opium growing, drug addiction [etc]. The relative peace and prosperity of the Far East after nearly three years [of] war shattered Europe were more than welcome.

My mission was the first [one sponsored by the *LN*] to visit the Far East, a fact that [greatly] facilitated the inquiry. In 1922 enthusiasm for the [*LN*] was in the ascendant. Many of us believed that a trail was being blazed that would lead to lasting peace. There was an enthusiasm and a spirit of dedication among League pioneers, both in the Secretariat and outside … My association with them is a memory that I treasure perhaps more than any other. There was some evidence of this enthusiasm in several parts of the Far East. The [*LN*] Union in Japan, for example, was an active and very influential body. Thus it was that the amount of co-operation, hospitality and kindness accorded me throughout my … tour was so vastly in excess of my deserts or my expectations. The tour lasted nine months during which all important ports were visited. …

Japan in 1923 had a liberal administration. There I received cordial co-operation, ungrudging help and much hospitality from officials and innumerable health workers. I made contact with several research workers of international reputation, including Kitasato. Baron Kitasato[36] [was] a senator and was too deeply immersed in politics to do any active research but he continued to take a very lively interest in the important work that was being done in the Kitasato Institute; he was looked upon as the father of Japanese medical research. I received much hospitality, kindness and help from him and his associates. Kitasato was one of the original Honorary Fellows of [the RSTMH].

After a few remarks on short visits to Formosa and Korea, White continued:

… To my delight I found Professor [Kiyoshi] Shiga[37] in charge of the medical and health administration of Korea. I had first met [him] at an international medical congress in Bombay in 1908: the fifteen years that had elapsed had aged him but little. [He] was the last surviving original Honorary Fellow of [the RSTMH]. My few days with him in Seoul are a very happy memory. … Shiga very kindly offered to accompany me on my journey through Manchuria. Our party … included Shiga, Miyajima, Tsurumi

(Chief of the Sanitary Department of the South Manchurian Railway) and Wu Lien Teh whose work on plague [must be] familiar …

In Nhatrang … there is a Pasteur Institute, devoted at that time to veterinary research and the production of veterinary vaccines and sera. Its director was [Alexandre] Yersin [1863–1943][38], the discoverer of the *plague* bacillus. He was about sixty years of age but was still an active and enthusiastic research worker. He had many interests but plague was no longer one of them though, incidentally, Nhatrang had long been a minor but interesting focus of endemic rat-*plague*. For him, I think, *plague* had begun to lose its interest as soon as he had isolated its bacillus. Chief among his preoccupations at the time of my visit were cattle *plague*, astronomy, and … experimental work concerned with quinine and rubber cultivation. He loved the Orient and rarely visited France …

My Far East tour provided an admirable opportunity for a comparative study of colonial public health administrations, British, French, Dutch, Japanese, and of the United States as exemplified in the Philippines. There were interesting … differences of priorities and emphasis rather than of fundamentals. Every administration studied had something worthy of emulation.

White continued with some words about *colonisation* (a topical theme today); being of the 'old school', he was obviously very much more positive about it than were the younger generation and the majority of people today:

In these strange days much writing and much oratory is devoted to the denigration of colonization. Colonization and colonies have become words of almost sinister import. Some quite clever people have taken part in this campaign of vituperation but many more much less well informed. For those who have devoted their working lives to the health problems of people in tropical countries such outbursts may often appear fantastic or singularly ill informed. When I hear or read such utterances my mind turns to the countless members of our profession of many nationalities who have done so much for the welfare of colonial peoples, to the research institutes and workers in tropical lands whose discoveries had led to the control or elimination of many diseases that formerly extorted so heavy a toll in suffering and premature death, and to the many who have sacrificed their lives in these high endeavours. Some of them are famous but the memory of many lives only in the hearts of the people among whom they lived and worked. The record is a proud one. Great Britain's pride in her colonial possessions at the dawn of this century was not altogether unjustified: there is very much on the credit side of the account. Fellows of [the RSTMH] need no reminding of … this but it is well that we should sometimes pay a tribute to the memory of our colleagues who have fallen by the way.

The [final] report that was the outcome of my Far East tour contained recommendations regarding the establishment of an *Epidemiological Intelligence Bureau* in Singapore which would be responsible for … collection and regular and rapid dissemination of up-to-date information regarding health conditions in ports throughout the Far East … Throughout my tour I was impressed by the fact that much more information of epidemiological interest and importance was available locally than could be gleaned from health reports etc. Sometimes such information only became significant by the light of knowledge of the behaviour of the disease in question elsewhere. I hoped that the Singapore Bureau … might act as a clearing station for information of this kind and might also be able to co-ordinate inquiries in the different countries into epidemiological problems of interest to the area as a whole.

The proposal for the creation of the Singapore Bureau was approved by the Health Committee and the Council of the [*LN*] and thanks to a generous grant from the *International Health Division of the Rockefeller Foundation* the Bureau was installed and began work in February 1925. Prior to its opening details concerning its function and methods of work were agreed … at a Conference at Singapore which was attended by delegates from the Health Administrations of all countries of the Far East. … The Bureau fully justified itself and did much to facilitate and render more effective port health procedure. In spite of [many] vicissitudes … it still carries on. To its first director … Gilbert

Brooke [1873–1936], the then distinguished port health officer of Singapore, belongs much of the credit for the success and smooth working of the Bureau in its early years.

And White ended this historical 'travelogue', mostly involving India, eastern Europe, and South-east Asia:

> Now that my story approaches its end I am oppressed with a fear that the stories I have conjured up from bygone days can have but scant interest for the present generation [which was probably largely true!]. Delving into the past has enabled me to introduce to you some well known, some little known, colleagues who meant so much to me. Most have joined the great majority but they have been living companions to me during the preparation of this talk. There are many others in many countries, to whom I am equally indebted; they are not forgotten.[39]

Professor R M Gordon OBE MD DSc FRCP (1893–1961) (*see* Figure 13.3)[40] gave his presidential address on 20 October 1955; his title was: **The host-parasite relationship in filariasis.** Then, as now, there was insufficient knowledge of the *host* component of the host-parasite relationship in parasitic infections. Following an introduction which outlined Manson's views on the life-cycle of *Plasmodium sp* outlined in his 1898 text, as well as Bignami's alternative theory, he continued:

> … during the past six years my colleagues and I have been studying certain species of *loiasis, onchocerciasis* and *acanthocheilonemiasis* in Africa and in the laboratories in this country, and it appears to us that … our knowledge of *filariasis* is in much the same state as was knowledge of *malaria* when Manson's book was published [in 1898]. We have [only] a few facts and many conjectures linking them; …
>
> During the course of our investigations, we have paid particular attention to the relationship between [the] host and parasite [and] have come to the conclusion … that a proper understanding of the symptomatology, diagnosis and treatment of *filariasis* is dependent on previous knowledge of the host-parasite relationship between the worm and its vertebrate host, and that it is difficult to plan or to judge the effect of control measures without previous knowledge of the host-parasite

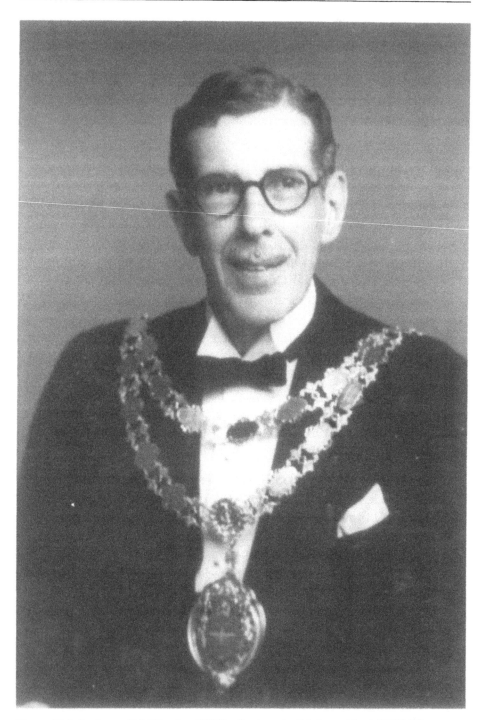

Figure 13.3: Professor R M Gordon FRCP – the twenty-third president (RSTMH archive).

relationship [recognising that] our work has ... concentrated on
Loa loa and its vectors ...

Gordon then embarked on a thoughtful analysis of possible definition(s)
of 'good and bad hosts'; this was followed by a section on the 'host-
parasite relationship between *Loa loa* and its invertebrate hosts'. Before
proceeding, he summarised the major thrust of this discussion:

> ... The facts would appear to be that *C[hrysops] silacea*, when
> observed under laboratory conditions, is an almost ideal host for
> the developmental stage of *L loa*, and that strong presumptive
> evidence exists that it is similarly so in nature. It has been proved
> that a proportion of human beings are naturally ill-adapted
> hosts, and there is good presumptive evidence that [they] can
> acquire some degree of resistance or immunity, which results
> in preventing the appearance of microfilariae in the peripheral
> blood in sufficient numbers for the propagation of the species.
> Finally we have evidence [suggesting] that ... *Chrysops* and
> certain species of monkey are both good hosts for *L loa* and we
> conjecture that this association represents the normal and well-
> established cycle of development, whereas that ... of the human
> strain of *L loa*, although well established in the fly, is badly
> established in man.
>
> I have dealt with one species of filaria, *L loa*, with one species
> of its vectors, *C silacea*, and with its two known vertebrate hosts,
> man and monkey; and ... have tried to indicate the extent of our
> factual knowledge concerning their host-parasite relationship
> and the extent and nature of the gaps in our knowledge. I have
> made no reference to other and more important species of filariae
> which parasitize man, but ... have no doubt that a similar analysis
> would show a similar dearth of factual knowledge, coupled with
> a vast amount of conjecture.

The most fascinating portion of Gordon's address however, concerned
future research requirements on *filariasis*:

> If my summarization of our existing knowledge of the host-
> parasite relationship in *filariasis* is not a gross underestimate
> ... you will agree that it is very scanty in comparison with
> our knowledge of the same subject in other arthropod-borne

infections. Does that really matter however? How much truth is there in our previous contention that a proper understanding of the symptomatology, diagnosis and treatment of *filariasis* is dependent on such knowledge, and that without it great difficulties will arise both when planning control measures and when… judging their effects? …

- As regards *symptomatology*, is it sensible to enter into discussion of the signs and symptoms of *filariasis* when we know so little about the parasite from the time when it disappears beneath the surface of the skin until, some nine months later, it announces its survival by the production of microfilariae? What value could be attached to conjectures regarding the signs and symptoms of *ancylostomiasis* if we had no knowledge of the life-cycle habits and wanderings of the parasitic larvae and adults?
- With regard to *diagnosis*, it appears that the only generally available method of establishing a diagnosis … is by the finding of … microfilariae, many months after the acquirement of infection. This belated method has the added disadvantage that, according to the available evidence, it is the very persons who suffer most severely … who are least likely to show the presence of microfilariae. At one time it was thought that … the disappearance of the micofilariae was indicative of the death of the adult [*Loa*]: but this generalization is misleading, and it appears unlikely that better methods of diagnosis will be evolved until we have a clearer understanding of the host-parasite relationship which is responsible for suppressing the larvae while still allowing the adult[s] to survive.
- As regards *treatment*, it seems reasonable to believe that what has been said about symptomatology and diagnosis applies also to treatment, for how can the efficacy of any form of therapy be estimated when there exists no certain means of deciding (except after a waiting-period of weeks or months) whether the adult[s] have or have not survived? We know that, even when the adult worms have been destroyed, the manifestations of *filariasis* may

persist. How can we prescribe relief for these persistent signs and symptoms when we are ignorant of their cause? My colleagues are now considering whether the ill effects encountered in loiasis can be explained on the hypothesis that they result from a previous sensitization of the patient to the worm or its products, and whether, if this proves to be the case, desensitization can usefully be employed. At present this is a mere speculation, and even if it proves true in loiasis the explanation may not be applicable to other forms of *filariasis*.

- It is when we come to the planning of *control* measures ... and later seek to estimate the success or failure of such plans, that the necessity for further knowledge of [the] host-parasite relationship becomes most evident. How can we confidently plan control measures directed against any particular form of *filariasis* while we lack knowledge of the presence or absence of an animal reservoir? At the present time, plans for the control of *onchocerciasis* and *wuchereriasis* [*Wuchereria bancrofti* infection] are based on the assumption that there is no animal reservoir for either infection. Until very recently a similar view was held regarding loiasis but we now know that that assumption was false. May it not also be false in the case of *wuchereriasis* and *onchoceriasis*?

Quite apart, however, from whether there are, or are not, animal reservoirs for human infections, there remains the problem of whether those species of vectors that are responsible for transmitting *filariasis* to man are in nature also found infected with other species of filariae. It is remarkable that most experienced workers on *filariasis*, while recognizing the fallacy of interpreting the extent of parasitization in the human population by the results of examining the peripheral blood for microfilariae, nevertheless are prepared to deduce the risk of infection from a previous survey of the numbers and infection rate found in the vectors coming to bite man. But what good evidence, morphological or biological, have we that all the forms encountered in these vector surveys are developmental stages of a species capable of infecting man? Already there is evidence that some insect vectors of *wuchereriasis* and *onchocerciasis* are capable of infection in the laboratory with species of filaria which cannot develop in man. It remains to be seen if a similar state of affairs occurs in nature.

Even if satisfactory answers are found to these questions regarding the presence or absence of animal reservoirs of infection, and the identity of the filariae found in the insect vector, there still remains the problem of estimating the extent of control necessary to protect the human population from serious ill effects.

When planning measures for the control of *filariasis* what should be our Plimsoll Line? Should it be similar to that generally accepted for the control of protozoal diseases such as *malaria*? In *malaria* the number of sporozoites inoculated is immaterial, provided that infection results. Nor does it matter whether the person exposed receives an infective bite once a day or once a week; the result is the same, because the individual parasite is capable of reproducing itself, until saturation of the vertebrate host has been reached. In *filariasis*, however, the situation is different: the parasite, although it can produce microfilariae cannot reproduce itself, and each infective form introduced by the vector can result in ... production of only one adult, male or female.

Recent work by one of my colleagues has shown that in *onchocerciasis* the host-parasite relationship is seriously interfered with only after [a] long-continued series of infective bites have been received by the human host. It appears possible, although not proved, that in *onchocerciasis* even a small reduction in the infective density of the vector may lead to a reduction in the incidence of blindness, or even to its complete elimination. If further research confirms this opinion, methods for the control of *onchocerciasis* may have to be planned on a new basis. Until we have settled these questions ... what reliance can we place on deductions drawn from previous surveys, or how can we plan future surveys to be undertaken both before and after the instigation of control measures?

It is to be hoped that no one will interpret these remarks as in any way belittling the value of ... recent advances which have been made in our knowledge of *filariasis*. The very reverse is the case, and I know that, so far as my own colleagues are concerned, they will agree with me ... that the most valuable amongst their many contributions has been their exposure of certain misconceptions, because they have thereby opened up new lines of research.

It would be equally wrong to suppose that anything which I have said ... implies that I believe efforts to control *filariasis* will be of little value until we have acquired more knowledge, or that we should withhold aid from those vast commercial schemes already referred to which are now envisaged in the tropics.

... In war, the statesmen of an ill-prepared country send what aid they can to the point of attack; they do so to avoid immediate disaster, but for final victory they rely on long-sustained study of the enemy's strength and weakness, and on never-failing attention to the improvement of their own weapons of offence and defence. I [firmly] believe that a similar policy is the one most likely to bring [about] success in a campaign directed against *filariasis*.[41]

Brigadier J S K (later Sir John) Boyd OBE LLD MD FRCP FRS (1891–1981)[42] (*see* Figure 13.4), the 24th president, was to open the 51st session of the Society with his presidential address on 17 October 1957: **Dysentery: some personal experiences and observations**. He began by telling his audience that he had spent the previous ten years in administration, and that he proposed beginning by giving a 'somewhat rambling semi-historical narrative' of his experiences is World War I (1914–18). Boyd then compared *amoebic* with *bacillary* dysentery (shigellosis), remarking that no less than four of the Society's evenings since the (1939–45) war had been devoted to *amoebiasis*, but none to *bacillary dysentery*! He continued with these precipient remarks:

... we now have specific treatment for *bacillary* dysentery. But I would remind you that bacteria can become resistant to sulphonamides and [to] antibiotics, and it is by no means impossible that the emergence of resistant strains [of bacteria] may jeopardize the present satisfactory position. ... the Consulting Physician to the Army [is of the opinion] that resistance to sulphonamides has not so far been a problem but that there is evidence suggesting that strains having this property may be developing in some localities. Sonne's bacillus is, of course, resistant to sulphonamides but does not produce [severe] dysentery ...

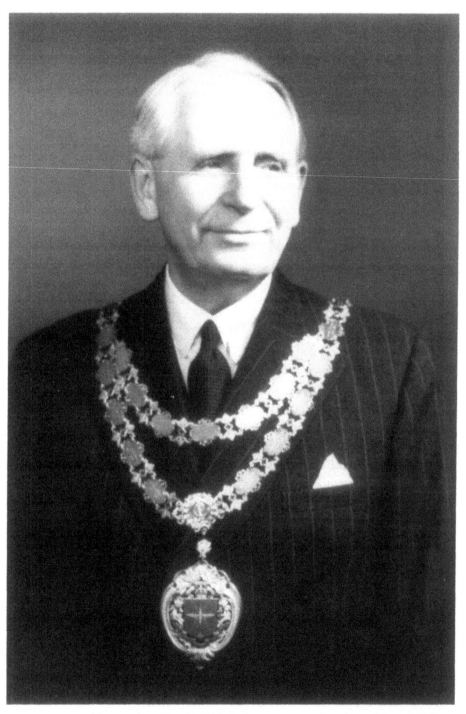

Figure 13.4: Brigadier Sir John Boyd, FRCP, FRS – the twenty-fourth president (RSTMH archive).

Then followed his *personal* reminiscences of the disease in *Macedonia* between 1916 and 18:

> … I began at what I believe our commercial colleagues would call the 'consumer end' during a trek across the Chalcidean peninsula, when I was medical officer to a company of engineers. Fortunately it was not a very virulent organism which attacked me, for I recovered without going into hospital, and was none the worse for it: but it enabled me to learn, from personal experience, the signs and symptoms of *bacillary* dysentery. It is perhaps worth recording that from that day to this – although I have undoubtedly been exposed on many occasions to infection – I have never been re-infected.
>
> My attack occurred early in the first of three waves of epidemic dysentery which swept through the Salonika Army in three succeeding years [*see* Table 13.2]. In 1916 and 1917, there were just under 6,000 reported cases and in 1918 about 9,000. The majority of these were acute, and a number … fatal. Exact death rates are not available, but according to the Official *History of the War*[43] were [somewhere] between 2 … and 3 per cent. Many infections became chronic, and the patients had to be invalided from the Command to Malta and the United Kingdom. … Figures compiled by the Medical Research Council[44] … show that 330 cases from Salonika [were undergoing treatment for an average of] 250.5 days before [they] were fit to return to duty, while 2,319 cases from Gallipoli, of all grades of severity, averaged 75.6 days. In addition to the reported cases [shown in Table 13.2] many others … never reached medical units. In fact [probably] no one who served in the Salonika Army escaped infection.

Table 13.2: Incidence of reported *dysentery* (both *bacillary* and *amoebic*) during World War I (1914–18)*

	1916		1917		1918	
	Total cases	Ratio per 1,000	Total cases	Ratio per 1,000	Total cases	Ratio per 1,000
Salonika	5,987	63.89	5,842	28.89	9,318	58.23
Egypt	5,599	31.19	4,341	23.13	4,906	21.80
Mesopotamia	1,839	50.94	4,960	60.34	5,455	51.12

* Adapted from Vol 1 of the *Official History of the War (1914–18)*[43]

At the time, dysentery took second place to the *malaria* epidemic which decimated the army, but … was nevertheless a serious drain on the efficiency of the fighting forces. The loss of manpower was considerable, and the discomfort and misery suffered [had] a bad effect on … morale. In civilized surroundings, even a mild attack of dysentery is an unpleasant experience: on active service, with no amenities and no proper diet, the term 'unpleasant' is a gross understatement.

The explanation of these epidemic waves was obvious. Those were the days of horse and mule transport. In consequence, manure lay about everywhere, and *Musca domestica* enjoyed an era of uninhibited fertility. [Although] within the lines of established units, a reasonably high state of hygiene prevailed, … elsewhere there were extensive areas which came under the supervision of sanitary squads, too few in number to tackle the problem. The result was a … plague of flies, which swarmed in unbelievable numbers. I recall … one occasion in the summer of 1916 when, after a night march, we came at dawn to a seemingly clean and pleasant transit camp. The first few hours were passed in comfort, but as the sun grew hotter the flies came to life and covered us, the mess table, the food – everything. There was no escape from them, and it was … impossible to eat without getting them into the mouth. Their habits are well known – I believe it was … Balfour [see Chapter 7] who coined the … phrase 'the filthy feet of faecal feeding flies'. Although experiments were carried out which showed that flies did in fact carry dysentery bacilli, both on their feet and in their gut, these did no more than prove the obvious.

One example … illustrate[s] the sort of problem with which we were faced. In the summer of 1918, the General Hospital, to which I was pathologist, was situated on the Kalamaria Peninsula, a few miles south of Salonika. This should have been a salubrious site, but fortunately we had next to us a French veterinary hospital, whose staff had rather primitive ideas about the disposal of manure. As a result, when the warmer weather came, our hospital was invaded by countless flies. Cases of *bacillary* dysentery soon appeared among both staff and patients, and in a week or two the outbreak developed to such an extent that the patients had to be sent elsewhere and the hospital closed. Meantime representations were made at a high level, and the veterinary unit was moved. The skeleton staff left in the hospital was given the task of cleansing the Augean stable. In the compound of the veterinary unit this was a comparatively simple matter, and consisted in raking together the wide-spread collection of manure and burning it on improvised incinerators. But this proved to be only a [minor] part of the problem. The camps were adjacent to the beach, and indeed only separated from it by sandy cliffs some 30 to 50 feet high. We found that enormous quantities of manure had been thrown on to the shore in the hope that it would be borne off by the tide. However, the tide in the Gulf of Salonika rises and falls only a few inches, and so there was a mound of manure several hundred yards long, in which the flies, undeterred by the salinity of their surroundings, were breeding freely. The task of incinerating this sodden mass took several weeks, and it was a long time before the hospital site was declared fit for reoccupation.

By the spring of 1917, I had ceased to be a regimental medical officer and was in charge of a Mobile Laboratory attached to a Casualty Clearing Station through which the casualties of two Divisions passed on their way to base hospitals in Salonika. Here, as elsewhere along the front, *malaria* dominated the picture, but dysentery was also rife. ... The wards were near the laboratory [and] the ... orderlies were very co-operative in bringing fresh specimens in bedpans, and as we were ... permanently on duty, there was never any delay in getting specimens plated. We were ... successful in isolating dysentery bacilli from a high percentage of ... stools, while at the same time microscopic examinations for *amoebae* were consistently negative. Thus it was possible to say with confidence that the dysentery was *bacillary* ... and that *amoebic* dysentery was practically non-existent. While the mucus or muco-pus ... was being searched for *amoebae*, the very characteristic cytological picture which is presented – unexpected cellularity, a preponderance of pus cells, varying numbers of [erythrocytes] scattered among them, and occasional shed epithelial cells and large refractile macrophages – attracted attention. When ... Wenyon [*see* Chapter 12] came from Egypt to Salonika later in the year ... I discussed this with him and was ... interested to find that he agreed [with me] that such a picture was more or less diagnostic of *bacillary* dysentery. Willmore and Shearman[45] recorded a similar observation … this being the first time it [appeared] in print, for it is not mentioned in the 6th, though it appears in the 7th edition of *Manson's Tropical Diseases*.[46] Over the years, my opinion on the significance of this cytological picture has not changed. No other acute diarrhoeal condition of sudden onset produces muco-pus with these characters, and when both this and the clinical signs and symptoms are present, a firm diagnosis of *bacillary* dysentery can be made with confidence. …

Owing to a shortening of our front, my mobile laboratory was closed down in autumn, 1917, and I spent the rest of my time in Salonika as pathologist to a general hospital. Here for some months I worked two mornings a week [next to] the army protozoologist, looking for *amoebae* in the stools of subjects [with] chronic dysentery. Unfortunately I have no record of the total number of cases examined nor of the number of *amoebic* infections … but there were certainly not more than five positives. I mention this in confirmation of our findings during the epidemic season and to emphasize the fact that *E histolytica* played a trivial part in the dysentery [of] the Salonika army. … in the *Official History of the War*[47], … it is stated that *amoebic* dysentery comprised about 3 per cent of … cases of dysentery admitted to hospital during the campaign.

Boyd followed this with his experiences in Gallipoli, Egypt and Mesopotamia:

… in the 3 months from August to October 1915, a high proportion of the 120,000 casualties evacuated from the Peninsula [in the Gallipoli campaign] was caused by dysentery, and it is claimed that 65 per cent … were due to *amoebic* dysentery[48] … but in November and December 1915, and January 1916, *amoebic* dysentery disappeared and the incidence of the *bacillary* type increased. These findings were received at home with considerable scepticism, which was justified by subsequent investigation of the convalescents carried out by Wenyon [*see above*], … and … O'Connor[49] who were sent for this purpose. They found that, of 246 men who had been evacuated from Gallipoli with a history of dysentery, only 6.5 per cent were carriers of *E histolytica* cysts, while among 1,137 men with no history of dysentery, 4.5 per cent were carriers.[50] Various other investigations in the Eastern Mediterranean area produced [similar] results ... while serological tests carried out at home and on the ... serum of convalescents gave evidence that the majority had suffered from *bacillary* dysentery. The ... opinion expressed in the *Official History*[51] is that, while *amoebic* dysentery undoubtedly occurred in Gallipoli, most of the cases, as elsewhere, were *bacillary*.

In *Egypt*, the incidence of dysentery of all types was considerably lower than in Salonika [*see* Table 13.1] while the admissions to hospital of cases of *amoebic* infection varied, in different years, from 2 ... to 7 per cent of all dysentery cases. Thus a careful examination of 659 active cases of dysentery and diarrhoea by the protozoologist to the Mediterranean Expeditionary Force revealed that 7.7 per cent were *amoebic*. However, when this group was [divided] into British ... and Indian troops, only 1.9 per cent of the British cases were *amoebic*, while 15.7 per cent of the Indian cases were due to this infection.[52] Examination of the native population of Egypt revealed that a high percentage – 13.5 per cent of 524 healthy natives – were passing cysts and from this [it] was concluded that *amoebic* dysentery was [significantly] more frequent ... among them than [in] British troops. In the light of recent work which suggests the existence of non-pathogenic strains of *E histolytica* it is by no means certain that this is a valid conclusion. In *Palestine*, figures ran at approximately the same level ...

In *Mesopotamia*, the incidence of *amoebic* dysentery was higher than elsewhere, and in one series of 309 patients suffering from *bacillary* dysentery [some] 26 per cent showed active *amoebae* containing [erythrocytes] in their stools.[53] ...

Thus, the records from the different fronts all tell a similar story. *Amoebic* dysentery had a random distribution, and admissions to hospital ran at a relatively constant level throughout the year. In the chapter on *Amoebic* Dysentery in the *Official History of the War*[54] ... the authors ... state ... that 'epidemics of *amoebic* dysentery do not occur'. In contrast, *bacillary* dysentery occurred in epidemic waves, mainly in late summer and autumn, but to a lesser extent in spring, and was everywhere the predominant type.

Boyd's remarks on the *E histolytica* carrier-state are of interest, especially in view of relatively recent research on invasive and non-invasive strains:

> During and immediately [after] the 1914–1918 war, numerous experienced protozoologists, [including] Clifford Dobell [1886–1949], did a vast amount of work on the problems of amoebiasis, and in particular on the significance of the symptomless carrier ...[55] As the result of this work, it came to be realized ... that *E histolytica* is a common parasite in Britain and in other temperate regions as well as in the topics, it being estimated that several million of the inhabitants ... who had never been overseas, were infected. Nevertheless, disease caused by this parasite is practically unknown except in those who lived, or have lived, in subtropical and tropical countries. ... [Dobell later agreed] that *E histolytica* could live in man as a harmless commensal. However, in 1918 [it was decided that] carriers could be set free in a community without exposing either themselves or the community to any grave risk. The soundness of this decision is borne out by the fact that there was no outbreak of *amoebic* dysentery after either the first or the second World War. According to Hoare[56] the total number of clinical cases recorded in Great Britain in the course of thirty-five years among those who have never been abroad does not exceed three dozen.

Boyd proceeded to deal with dysentery (both *amoebic* and *bacillary*) in *India* between the wars:

> ... While most bacteriologists who worked in the Mediterranean area during the First World War were left in no doubt that *bacillary* [dysentery] was much more common than *amoebic* dysentery, this idea was by no means acceptable [by workers] in India ... Under field conditions in war, the dysentery wards and the laboratories were usually in close proximity, so that stools when received in the laboratory were freshly passed, and in consequence there was a high percentage of isolations of *dysentery* bacilli. In India, however, one laboratory had to serve several hospitals, and fresh specimens were the exception ... The result was that dysentery bacilli were rarely found [and] a significant proportion of such bacilli as were isolated ... were inagglutinable with the available diagnostic antisera [while] on the other hand, the identification

of *E histolytica* lay with the microscopist. No rigid tests had to be passed, and there can be no doubt that the criteria of identification were often laxly applied ... Furthermore, an inconclusive report on the microscopic findings in a specimen from which no dysentery bacilli had been isolated left the clinician to exercise his own judgement ... This was the unsatisfactory state of affairs which existed ... in India in 1924 and [Manifold] launched the attack which was to put an end to it. [He persuaded] the sceptics that *bacillary* dysentery was the prevalent type in India as elsewhere, first, by his own extensive investigations[57] and later, by [his] active part ... in re-organizing and re-equipping military laboratories throughout the Army and in arranging for efficient training of the staff. ...

... figures in the Annual Report of the *Public Health Commissioner with the Government of India*, 1935, [show] the incidence of dysentery, diarrhoea, and colitis* for the years 1920 to 1925 ... compared with that for the years 1930 to 1935 [*see* Table 13.3]. [58] The striking feature in [this table is] the greater precision of diagnosis and the switch from *amoebic* to *bacillary* infection. If the percentage of *clinical* dysentery appears to be high, it must be remembered, first, that ... very selective desoxycholate medium ... had not then been devised, and second, that a considerable proportion of the cases occurred in outstations from which specimens for laboratory tests had to be sent by post.

The relative incidence of *amoebic* dysentery in British [and Indian] troops is of interest. [Between 1930 and 35] *amoebic* dysentery was significantly more common in British than in Indian troops, a complete reversal of [that] in *Mesopotamia* during the [1914–18] war. The figures relating to Indian troops are of particular interest because they show that active *amoebic* dysentery is not a disease of much importance in the indigenous population of a country where pathogenic [strains] of the amoeba are [relatively] common ... The significant fall in the incidence of liver abscess [*see* Table 13.4] affords conclusive evidence that

---

* ... *clinical* dysentery is diarrhoea in which the stools contain mucus of indefinite character, but in which neither [*E histolytica*] nor dysentery bacilli are found. In 'simple' diarrhoea, the stools contain no mucus. Colitis is – or should be – a non-dysenteric inflammatory condition of the mucous membrane of the colon.

Table 13.3: Incidence of *dysentery* in the Army in India (1920–35)[*]

	British Other Ranks				Indian Other Ranks			
	1920–1925		1930–1935		1920–1925		1930–1935	
Average Strength	59,218		55,613		120,771		120,771	
	No. cases	% (exc. Diarrhoea)	No. cases	% (exc. Diarrhoea)	No. cases	% (exc. Diarrhoea)	No. cases	% (exc. Diarrhoea)
Bacillary dysentery	402	7.3	5,470	63.7	241	1.0	7,892	67.8
Amoebic dysentery	3,176	57.8	1,079	12.4	3,272	14.1	814	7.0
Clinical dysentery	497	9.1	1,987	22.8	4,281	18.4	2,767	23.8
Colitis	1,420	25.8	187	2.1	15,485	66.5	167	1.4
Diarrhoea	5,878	–	4,960	–	14,627	–	5,065	–
Total	11,373		13,683		37,906		16,705	

* Adapted from the *Annual Report of the Public Health Commissioner with the Government of India*.[58]

Table 13.4: Incidence of *hepatitis* and *liver 'abscess'* in the Army in India*

	Hepatitis; all causes (including amoebic)		Liver 'abscess' (*amoebic*)	
	1920–1925	1930–1935	1920–1925	1930–1935
British troops	948	417	184	46
Indian troops	681	358	84	37

* Adapted from the *Annual Report of the Public Health Commissioner with the Government of India.*[58]

there has been no increase in missed cases of amoebic infection. In terms of the numbers at risk, *amoebic* abscess is more than twice as common in British ... as it is in Indian troops, a figure which is in general agreement with the incidence of *amoebic* dysentery in the two [ethnic groups].

In general, the dysentery which occurred ... in India ... was endemic in nature. A few small outbreaks occurred, attributable to one particular type of dysentery bacillus, but this was ... exceptional. On no occasion did *amoebic* dysentery arise, other than in the form of sporadic cases [and at] all times, *bacillary* dysentery predominated.

And finally in his geographical tour, to the *Middle East* in 1940–43:

... I reached Cairo [continued Boyd] in mid-August, 1940.

A fortnight later I accompanied the Consulting Surgeon on a visit to the hospitals in Alexandria. On the outward journey he complained that he felt unwell and, when returning in the evening, he had some diarrhoea and abdominal pain, a common complaint in those recently arrived in Egypt. Without being seriously ill, he showed no improvement in the next 24 hours, and was admitted to hospital, where Shiga's bacillus was isolated from his stools. Despite the most careful nursing and the best treatment as we knew it then, including massive doses of Shiga antitoxin, he grew slowly and steadily worse and died in a little over a fortnight. About this ... time, the medical specialist of a newly-arrived hospital was similarly infected and, after a more protracted illness lasting just over 8 weeks, he too died.

This type of illness – slow in onset and progress, but quite unamenable to treatment – was new to me. In *Salonika* in the first war, the fatal cases were mainly fulminating in nature, the patient being violently ill from the first, and usually dying in a few days. In *India*, Shiga infections were by no means uncommon, but although always regarded as more serious than Flexner infections, if taken early they responded to treatment. ... in the Middle East the majority of cases ran this milder course, but from time to time others occurred, such as the two [above], which were ... resistant to treatment, and progressed steadily until the patient died. Most of the more serious cases were caused by Shiga's bacillus, but a few Flexner infections also ran a very protracted course and were extremely difficult to cure.

The remainder of Boyd's address focused on *management* of both *bacillary* and *amoebic* dysentery:

... Long before the first World War [1914–18] the recommended procedure was repeated doses of sodium or magnesium sulphate [which] was still standard in 1940. It resulted in more copious stools and probably lessened the discomfort and tenesmus engendered by attempts to void small quantities of sticky mucus, but there is no doubt that when used indiscriminately ... it prolonged the course of a mild attack. ...

The only specific treatment then available was antiserum for ... Flexner ... and antitoxin for Shiga [infections]. The value of the former was very doubtful, partly because Flexner infections were rarely acute enough to warrant its use, and partly because the antiserum often [produced] ... serum sickness 10 days after administration. ... Shiga antitoxin falls into a different category. It is a definite entity [and] capable of quantitative titration. About the middle of 1940 ... supplies of a highly purified antitoxin ... which could be given intravenously [became available]. This antitoxin was repeatedly administered in the two fatal cases [*see above*]. ... The patients felt better, the temperature fell, and abdominal colic was lessened, but in 24 to 48 hours, absorption of fresh toxin from the bowel lesions had restored the *status quo*. ... this preparation was [therefore] a good antitoxin but, as it had neither [a] bacteriostatic nor bactericidal action, it failed to effect cure in established cases. ... when given in the early stages of the illness it tipped the balance in the patient's favour and gave his defensive mechanism a better chance to overcome the infection.

But, as many cases recovered just as quickly without antitoxin, it is impossible to [be certain] that there was any such action.

Introduction of sulphonamide treatment
[In 1941] the situation was completely [revolutionised] by the introduction of sulphaguanidine. [I was working at this time with Fairley (*see* above)] who was on loan from the Australian Army ... We had access to [many] cases in a large General Hospital which at that time took in most [cases of] dysentery ... in British troops stationed in the Cairo area. ... Marshall [in the USA] used [a new sulphonamide – sulphaguanidine] to treat some mild cases of dysentery and enteritis in children, with so much success that he had a large batch prepared and sent it to [Gladwin] Buttle [1899–1983][59] who was then in Cairo. Buttle in turn handed it over to [Neil] Fairley and me. We were ... pleased to have something new to try in the more serious acute cases, as well as in refractory and long-standing infections ...[60]

The results of treatment with sulphaguanidine in the acute cases were at once obvious. There was early improvement, manifested by relief of abdominal pain, ... a decrease in the number of stools ... and in particular by the disappearance of the feeling of ... misery which is a constant symptom in most cases of dysentery. The stools became normal in a few days, appetite returned, and the patient was fit for discharge from hospital in a much shorter time than with any other form of treatment. Most important of all, the occasional resistant and ultimately fatal case of Shiga infection disappeared. Needless to say, some patients reacted better than others ... but we were left in no doubt that we had a specific remedy of great potency.

> ... The first [to be treated] was a Shiga infection of 80 days' duration, which had proved completely resistant to every form of treatment we had tried ... Stools, of which he passed six to 10 daily, were liquid or liquid and semi-solid, always containing mucus or muco-pus, or even frank pus. His pulse and temperature were almost constantly raised and his general condition was poor. He had no appetite and his weight [was reduced] to 7½ stone. The sigmoidoscope revealed well-marked generalized inflammation of the ... mucosa, with a granular surface which bled readily on instrumentation; the lumen was

contracted and the bowel difficult to distend. [He] was started on … sulphaguanidine on 19 January, 1941 … The response was immediate [and] fever subsided, abdominal colic decreased and disappeared, and in a day or two [he] was demanding food … and he had an uninterrupted convalescence. On 19 February, a month after starting treatment, his weight had risen by [almost] two stones … Sigmoidoscopy [that day] showed a red but relatively normal mucous membrane. A few scattered pitted areas, the site of former ulcers, could be seen, but there was no bleeding and the [colon] distended satisfactorily under pressure. The [colon] had in fact practically healed.

The second patient was infected with one of the Flexner group. His symptoms were only moderately severe when he was admitted to hospital 8 days after onset, but in spite of treatment he continued each day to pass three or four stools containing blood and mucus for 3 months, and thereafter more irregularly for a further 2 months. During this time [he had received the] following forms of treatment …: bismuth subgallate, emetine hydrochloride, quinoxyl enemata, stovarsol, eusol enemata, and sedatives such as luminal and bromides. … anti-amoebic treatment was given as a forlorn hope, for at no time was there microscopic evidence of amoebic infection. The sigmoidoscope revealed … numerous small aphthous ulcers [only]. A course of sulphaguanidine was started on the 149th day of his illness, and 4 days later the stools were normal. … the ulcers had disappeared [after 9 days of treatment] and [a] few small red patches, which did not bleed when swabbed, were the only abnormal features. …

Having established the efficacy of sulphaguanidine, we [had to use] our limited supply to the best purpose, while awaiting the manufacture of bulk quantities, which we could not hope to receive for many months. As the vast majority of severe cases were caused by Shiga's bacillus, [we restricted] its use … to treatment of patients … with this more pathogenic organism …

Meantime, attempts were made to use other sulphonamide drugs. Sulphanilamide – of which we had ample supplies – was not particularly successful, but sulphapyridine proved reasonably [effective], though with very unpleasant side-effects.

At a later date, sulphathiazole was tried but was found to compare badly with sulphaguanidine. Sulphadiazine was good, as was sulphamethazine ... but the latter was never produced in bulk. ... [Sulphaguanidine] had no tendency to crystallize in the urine and cause blockage of the renal tubules, a definite danger in a climate where there is intense sweating and where ... the urine is concentrated. ...

Boyd next turned to his experience with a 'bacteriophage' (captured with German stores at the battle of Alamein) in management of shigellosis in the civilian population of Egypt, and also to immunisation. The first proved useless, and the second possessed extremely unpleasant systemic side-effects. Finally, he added a few 'anecdotal' words on *amoebic* dysentery in the Middle East during World War II (1939–45):

> ... the annual admission rate for all types of dysentery from 1941 to 1943 ran at a ... level of about 33 per 1,000 of the total strength. Details of ... relative proportions of *bacillary* and *amoebic* dysentery can be extracted from [the] *monthly reports* ... From August 1940 until June 1943, specimens from [nearly] 65,000 cases of *clinical* dysentery were examined; ... 5.3 per cent [contained] trophozoites of *E histolytica*. This is [similar to the] 1914–18 war, when the figure varied from 2 ... to 7 per cent in different years.
>
> In contrast ...one or two instances of [an] older school ... were encountered elsewhere. Following the occupation of Lebanon and Syria in 1941, an Australian unit took over a Military Hospital in Syria. [Graphs showing the incidence of] *amoebic* dysentery [rose] steadily during the summer months to a peak of considerable height. There was no graph for *bacillary* dysentery – presumably because the number of reported cases was too small. In 1942 and 1943, *bacillary* and *amoebic* dysentery occurred in the Allied troops stationed in this area in the same proportions as elsewhere, with [a] preponderance of *bacillary* infections. [I suspected a] confusion in diagnosis. In 1941, after the capture of Ethiopia and Eritrea, considerable numbers of Eritrean prisoners were brought into Sudan, and the sick from the POW camps were treated in an expanded section of an Indian General Hospital, staffed mainly by captured Italian medical officers [and large

quantities of emetine were being used]. I found that the hospital laboratory was [supervised by] a keen young pathologist, who … demonstrated the microscopical picture on which he made his diagnosis of *amoebic* dysentery … A fresh specimen was procured [and] after a brief search he … waved me to the microscope. The picture was typical of *bacillary* infection – large numbers of pus cells, a few [erythrocytes], and in the centre a globular non-motile refractile object with a diameter of roughly three times that of a pus cell … which he said was a cyst. [It was in fact] one of the large macrophages which are so characteristic … of bacillary exudate. Such mistakes are … common and [represent] lack of training and … experience.

On the microscopical diagnosis of dysentery, Boyd recalled:

… Dobell [had written in 1917][61]: 'Stool examinations made by persons who have not served their apprenticeship … possess no scientific value whatsoever – and for the average worker, a practical training of not less than four to six weeks is [necessary], even under the most favourable conditions …'. His remark referred especially to the examination of faeces for cysts, but … the same applies to the examination of muco-pus for *amoebae*. [The] diagnosis of *amoebic* dysentery should not be made unless active *amoebae* containing [erythrocytes] have been demonstrated …

And he concluded:

… The main points [therefore] are that: [i] *bacillary* dysentery far exceeded *amoebic* dysentery in importance until the efficacy of sulphonamide treatment was discovered: [ii] that, with the possibility of strains emerging which are resistant to sulphonamides (and antibiotics), it remains a lurking danger, for it is only controlled, and not banished: [iii] that active *amoebic* dysentery should be diagnosed *only* when the golden rule is satisfied: and [iv] that we should remember that, as far as this country is concerned, the symptomless cyst-passer, no matter where he acquired his infection, has been proved, by the experience of the aftermath of two wars, to be of no epidemiological importance. Nevertheless, this same cyst-passer and the *amoebae* with which he is infected, present so many problems that I am

confident he will provide material for discussion and argument
at future meetings of [the RSTMH].[62]

So ended the 24th presidential address, and the last in a little more than
fifty years.

Forty-fourth to fiftieth annual reports

The number of Fellows at 31 March 1951 stood at 2,023. Corresponding
figures for the following six years were: 2,113, 2,052, 2,007, 2,013, 2,014
and 2,054.

Despite the escalation in the size of the Fellowship, the Treasurer's
report for the year ended 1952 showed a deficit of over £2,000 of
expenditure over income. An increase in subscriptions the following
year resulted in an improved financial situation, which in the 51st annual
report, for the year ended 31 March 1958, showed a balance of £189.

References and Notes

1   Anonymous. Golden jubilee banquet of the Society. *Trans R Soc trop Med Hyg* 1958; 52: 1–8.
2   Anonymous. The unveiling of the bust of Sir James Cantlie. *Trans R Soc trop Med Hyg* 1951; 44: 481–2.
3   *See* for example: *CM* 1950: 14 December; 1951: 17 May; 44th AGM 1951: 21 June.
4   *See* for example: 48th AGM 1955: 15 June.
5   **Neil Hamilton Fairley** was born in Melbourne, Australia and qualified at the University of Melbourne. He joined the Royal Australian Medical Corps and served initially in Egypt where he developed an interest in schistosomiasis. He later served in Bombay, India where he carried out research on (and developed) tropical sprue. His major research was carried out during World War II in Cairns on malaria prophylaxis and treatment. Following the War he was appointed to the Wellcome chair of *clinical* tropical medicine at the Hospital for Tropical Diseases, London. *See:* J Boyd. Fairley, Sir Neil Hamilton (1891–1966). In H C G Matthew, B Harrison (eds). *Oxford Dictionary of National Biography.* Oxford: Oxford University Press 2004; 18: 948–9; G C Cook. Neil Hamilton Fairley KBE FRCP FRS (1891–1966): Britain's last world-class tropical physician? (awaiting publication).
6   R T Leiper, E L Atkinson. Observations on the spread of Asiatic schistosomiasis. *China Med J* 1915; 29: 143–9.
7   R T Leiper. Report on the results of the Bilharzia Mission in Egypt, 1915. *J R Army Med Cps* 1915; 25: 1–55.

8 R T Leiper. *Ibid*. 1915; 25: 147–92.

9 F B Lawton. The early symptoms following infection by *Schistosomum Mansoni. Ibid*. 1918; 31: 472–9.

10 N H Fairley. Observations on the clinical appearance of bilharziasis in Australian troops, and the significance of the symptoms noted. *Quart J med* 1919; 12: 391–403.

11 N H Fairley. A report of three cases of bilharziasis treated with tartar emetic. *Med J Aust* 1919; 2: 529–32.

12 P Manson-Bahr, N H Fairley. Observations on bilharziasis amongst the Egyptian expeditionary force. *Parasitology* 1920; 12: 33–71.

13 N H Fairley. A comparative study of experimental bilharziasis in monkeys contrasted with the hitherto described lesions in men. *J Path Bact* 1920; 23: 289–314.

14 J E R McDonagh. *The Biology and Treatment of Venereal Diseases, and the Biology of inflammation and its relationship to malignant disease*. London: Harrison and Sons 1915: 625.

15 J B Christopherson. *The successful use of antimony in bilharziasis. Lancet* 1918; ii: 325–7.

16 A Rüffer. *Cairo Sci J* 1910; 4: 3 [cited by Fairley].

17 M Khalil Bey. The national campaign for the treatment and control of bilharziasis from the scientific and economic aspects. *J R Egypt med Ass* 1949; 32: 817–56.

18 N H Fairley. The bilharzia complement fixation reaction in goats infected with *Schistosoma mattheei* and *Schistosoma bovis J Helminth* 1933; 11: 181–6.

19 A C Fisher. *Trans R Soc trop Med Hyg*. A study of the schistosomiasis of the Stanleyville district of the Belgian Congo. 1934; 28: 277–306.

20 M Gelfand. *Schistosomiasis in South Central Africa*. Cape Town: Jute & Co Ltd 1950: 239.

21 A R Ferguson. Associated bilharziasis and primary malignant disease of urinary bladder with observations on a series of forty cases. *J Path Bact* 1911; 16: 76–94.

22 W St C Symmers. Note on a new form of liver cirrhosis due to the presence of the ova of bilharzia haematobia. *Ibid*. 1903; 9: 237–9.

23 *Op cit*. See note 13 above.

24 N H Fairley, F P Mackie. Studies in *Schistosoma spindale:* part III. The experimental pathology in the goat with special reference to verminous phlebitis. *Indian med Res Mem* 1930; 17: 16–51.

25 G A Turner. Pulmonary bilharziasis. *J trop Med Hyg* 1909; 12: 35–6.

26 *Op cit*. See note 13 above.

27 H B Day. Pulmonary bilharziasis. *Trans R Soc trop Med Hyg* 1936–7; 30: 575–82.

28 *Op cit*. See note 20 above.

29 H Vogel. *Zbl Bakt* 1949; 154: 118 [cited by Fairley].

30 D Standen. Experimental schistosomiasis. II – Maintenance of *Schistosoma Mansoni* in the laboratory, with some notes on experimental infection with *S Haematobium. Ann trop Med Parasit* 1949; 43: 268–83.

31 A C Hutchinson. Results in thirteen cases of dysentery treated with emetine. *China Med J* 1913; 27: 243–5.

32 N H Fairley. Bilharzia complement fixation reaction – persistence of circulating antibody after treatment. *Trans R Soc trop Med Hyg* 1936; 29: 356–7.

33 C Pifano, M Mayer. *Rev Sanid Assistencia Social Caracas* 1945; 10: 65 [cited by Fairley].

34 N H Fairley. Presidential address. Schistosomiasis and some of its problems. *Trans R Soc trop Med Hyg 1951; 45: 279–303.*

35 **Norman White** qualified from St Bartholomew's Hospital, and served for most of his career with the Health Organisation of the League of Nations, and the Ministry of Health in London. He was a pioneer in international hygiene. In his early days he had served with the Indian Medical Service. *See*: Anonymous. White, Frederick Norman CIE. *Med Directory* 1964: 2496; [G M R] F N White (obituary). *Br med J* 1964; i: 1572–3; Anonymous. Frederick Norman White (obituary). *Trans R Soc trop Med Hyg* 1964; 58: 367–8; White, Major Frederick Norman. *Who Was Who, 1961–1970*: 1193.

36 **Baron Shibusaburo Kitasato** (1852–1931) was a Japanese bacteriologist. He worked with Robert Koch (1843–1910) and isolated the causative organism of bubonic plague in 1894; however priority was given to Alexandre Yersin (1863–1943).

37 **Kiyoshi Shiga** (1870–1957) was another Japanese bacteriologist who discovered the bacillus of dysentery (*Shigella shigae*) in 1897. After working with Paul Ehrlich (1854–1915), he became director of the Kitasato Research Institute.

38 **Alexandre Yersin** (1863–1943) was a Swiss-born French bacteriologist and a pupil of Pasteur. Working in Hong Kong in 1894, he isolated a *pure* culture of the organism now named *Yersina pestis*. Kitasato probably also discovered the causative agent of bubonic plague in the same year, but his culture was heavily contaminated.

39 F N White. Presidential address. Retrospect. *Trans R Soc trop Med Hyg* 1953; 47: 441–50.

40 **Rupert Gordon** qualified at Trinity College, Dublin and served with the RAMC at Salonica. He spent most of his subsequent career at the Liverpool School of Tropical Medicine, ultimately becoming Walter Myers Professor of Entomology and Parasitology. He received many awards for his researches into tropical diseases. *See*: Gordon, Rupert Montgomery. *Who Was Who, 1961–1970*: 440–1.

41 R M Gordon. Presidential address. The host-parasite relationship in filariasis. *Trans R Soc trop Med Hyg* 1955; 49: 496–507.

42 **John Boyd** qualified at Glasgow University in 1913. He served in the RAMC at Ypres and Salonica. He then trained in bacteriology, and was appointed to the Royal Army Medical College. He later served in India. He was promoted to the rank of brigadier in 1945 and became director of pathology at the War Office. He then became director of the Wellcome Laboratories of Tropical Medicine, retiring in 1955. However, he continued contributing to the Wellcome Trust. He was an authority on shigellosis. See: P O Williams. Boyd, Sir

John Smith Knox (1891–1981). In: H C G Matthew, B Harrison (eds). *Oxford Dictionary of National Biography*. Oxford: Oxford University Press 2004; 7: 39.

43   W G Macpherson, W P Herringham, T R Elliott, A Balfour (eds). *History of the Great War based on official documents. Medical Services: Diseases of the war.* London: H M Stationery Office 1922: 1: 550.

44   *Ibid.*

45   J G Willmore,C H Shearman. On the differential diagnosis of the dysenteries. *Lancet* 1918; ii: 200–6.

46   P Manson-Bahr (ed). *Manson's Tropical Diseases* 6th ed. 1917 [cited by Boyd].

47   *Op cit.* See note 43 above.

48   R G Archibald, G Hadfield, W Logan, W Campbell. Reports of the M and H laboratories dealing with the diseases affecting the troops in the Dardanelles. *J R Army Med Cps* 1916; 26: 695–724.

49   C M Wenyon, F W O'Connor. An inquiry into some problems affecting the spread and incidence of intestinal protozoal infections of British troops and natives in Egypt, with special reference to the carrier question, diagnosis and treatment of amoebic dysentery, and an account of three new human intestinal protozoa. *Ibid.* 1917; 28: 1–34, 346–70, 461–92.

50   *Ibid.*

51   *Op cit.* See note 43 above.

52   H M Woodcock. Protozoological experiences during the summer and autumn of 1916. *J R Army med Cps* 1917; 29: 290–300.

53   T K Boney, L G Crossman, C L Boulenger. Report of a Base laboratory in Mesopotamia for 1916, with special reference to water-borne diseases. *Ibid.* 1918; 30: 409–23.

54   C Dobell, D Harvey. In: W G Macpherson, W B Leishman, S L Cummins (eds). *History of the Great War based on official documents. Medical Services: pathology.* London: H M Stationery Office 1923: 277–318.

55   C Dobell. *The Amoebae living in Man: a zoological monograph.* London: John Bale, Son & Danielsson 1919: 155.

56   C A Hoare. Amoebiasis in Great Britain with special reference to carriers. *Br med J* 1950; ii: 238–41.

57   J A Manifold, A J Demonte. Report on an investigation of dysentery and diarrhoea in Poona. *Indian J Med Res* 1928; 15: 601–41.

58   *Annual Report of the Public Health Commissioner with the Government of India for 1935.* New Delhi: Government of India Press [cited by Boyd].

59   Buttle, Gladwin Albert Hurst. See: *Who Was Who, 1981–1990:*

60   N H Fairley, J S K Boyd. Dysentery in the Middle East with special reference to sulphaguanidine treatment. *Trans R Soc trop Med Hyg* 1943; 36: 253–78.

61   C Dobell. Reports upon investigations in the United Kingdom of dysentery cases from the Eastern Mediterranean I – Amoebic dysentery and the protozoological investigation of cases and carriers. *Spec Rep Ser med Res Council Lond* 1917: 4.

62   J S K Boyd. Presidential address. Dysentery: Some personal experiences and observations. *Trans R Soc trop Med Hyg* 1957; 51: 471–87.

Chapter 14

Epilogue to the Society's first half-century (1907–57)

In 1957, *ie* after fifty years, the Society was still flourishing, and its original pattern of events was to remain (more or less) until the unfortunate disposal of its focal point – *Manson House* – in 2004. This was a *clinically-based* Society and its *raison d'être* was to learn about and discuss problems of diseases prevalent in the tropics, in London – the heart of Empire – at various location(s) situated in the 'medical quarter' of London.

There can be no doubt that this Society, probably more than any other organisation, did more to bridge the newly emerging specialty with the well established pursuit of 'medicine in the tropics'.

Although in the early days – until 1920 – the London School of Tropical Medicine (LSTM) was situated some ten miles from the centre of the Metropolis, most founding Fellows and presidents had their residences in the 'medical quarter' and many practised medicine from this location. Removal of the LSTM from its original setting at the Albert Dock Hospital to Endsleigh Gardens, WC1 (where it became the *Hospital for Tropical Diseases* [HTD]) in 1920 must have been a considerable relief to many early officers and presidents of the Society, as their *clinical* practice was then closer to their place of domicile.

Origins and function

Scientific tropical medicine was born in the late nineteenth century. Prior to that 'medicine in the tropics' had been practised for many centuries, but not on a strictly *scientific* basis. The average practitioner in London – and elsewhere in Britain – knew little or nothing about the 'exotic' infections which existed in warm climates. Therefore there was a crying need for a centre in London to discuss and debate this group of diseases. Also, medical practitioners serving in the Empire and Raj came to London on leave (furlough) largely in order to learn more about the diseases they were encountering daily (they had learned little, if anything, about these diseases in their undergraduate days!). Therefore a centre for learning and promulgation of ideas was at that time urgently required.

Presidents

There had been 23 presidents (all essentially clinicians) up to the half century, although in 1957 Sir John Boyd (the twenty-fourth) was just beginning his two-year term. Presidents until the half-century had all served a single term of two years with two exceptions: Dr G C Low (1872–1952) from 1929 until 1933, and Sir Rickard Christophers (1873–1978) during the Second World War from 1939 until 1943. Without exception, all had been medically qualified: twelve (including Boyd) were Fellows of the Royal Society, thirteen Fellows of the Royal College of Physicians, and four were Fellows of the Royal College of Surgeons. No less than sixteen (including Boyd) were knighted. The *presidential address* – which had usually taken place every two years – was originally held immediately the *new* president took office, but later took place in the October following the president's inauguration, to coincide with the beginning of a new session.

Venue of the Society

In early days, the Society lacked a firm base. Early premises at the Medical & Chirurgical Society (later the Royal Society of Medicine [RSM]) had proved less than satisfactory. Limited accommodation at the Medical Society of London (MSL) was considerably better, but far from ideal. What the Society urgently required was a 'home' of its own. In the 1920s, suggestions were made that the Society should move to 23 Endsleigh Gardens (under the auspices of the Seamen's Hospital Society) – where London's *tropical* activities largely took place – but this idea came to nought. Primarily as a result of G C Low's initiative (he had been a joint founder, with Cantlie, of the Society), 26 Portland Place (Manson House) became, in 1931, the Society's house and hub of activity. This building survived World War II (1939–45) almost intact, and continued to be the focus of a fundamentally *clinical* Society for over seventy years. It housed reception rooms, meeting rooms, a library and, above all, a lecture theatre (auditorium); this *permanent* memorial to Sir

Patrick Manson (1844–1922) – first president of the Society – formed the centre of activities (and was identified as such by the 1,500–2,000-strong Fellowship of the Society for all of those years).

Another source of difficulty in early days were repeated attempts by the RSM to absorb 'tropical medicine' under its 'umbrella' of fifteen specialist societies. It must have taken a considerable degree of persistence on the part of early *Councils* to fend off attempts by Sir John McAlister (1856–1925) (Secretary of the RSM) to 'hijack' this fledgling Society!

Council

From early days, the *Council* has been responsible for organisation of the Society's activities. This was the body that 'religiously' vetted all new applicants for Fellowship (to be formally elected at the subsequent *Ordinary* meeting of Fellows). *Council* also elected the future president, and *Honorary* Fellows. The *Honorary Secretaries*, who are responsible for the day-to-day running of the Society, form a degree of continuity, and are responsible for the *Annual Report*. The *Hon Treasurer* has reported frequently to *Council* and remains responsible for the annual financial report at the AGM.

Appointment of *Local Secretaries* throughout the world (reporting back to the Secretaries) was introduced during early days of the Society, and took a considerable proportion of the Secretaries' and *Council's* time.

Executive Committee

Emergence of the small *Executive* Committee – which existed until recently – really came about during World War II – when *Council* was unable to meet for logistical reasons; London was considered a dangerous city during those years. In former days, *Council* met before every *Ordinary* meeting and also at other times. At present however (in 2010), its meetings have been reduced to a mere four annually.

Meetings

Ordinary meetings of the Society – at which all Fellows have the opportunity of attending, and at which a lecture followed by discussion, or a demonstration originally took place monthly, with the exception of

August and September, and this programme took place from 1907 until the disposal of Manson House. Once in a while the *monthly* meeting was held at the Liverpool School – for it has been considered by most of paramount importance that the Society is not seen as a London-dominated organisation, with the exclusion of other centres of tropical expertise.

Laboratory meetings – which usually took place at the Royal Army Medical College, Millbank or the London School of Hygiene and Tropical Medicine – were in former days held at least once a year, and for several years after the opening of the HTD at St Pancras in 1951, a *clinical* meeting was also held at that hospital. Now, there are virtually no *Ordinary* meetings, and the laboratory meeting is held once annually. There is no *clinical* meeting.

The *Annual General* meetings have always been held in June or July, the first having taken place in June 1908.

Transactions

This publication has always been a dominant item in the Society's agenda, as well as being an important source of revenue, and initially took a great deal of the Hon Secretaries' time; before appointment of an editor, all editorial work was accomplished by the Secretaries. *Transactions* was for many years a precise record of the Society's proceedings, and its content was largely under control of *Ordinary* meetings of Fellows. Until relatively recently, each volume of *Transactions* covered one session; however, it now encompasses activities during a calendar year.

This journal was of course costly to publish, but was highly prestigious in former years and an exchange with other *tropical* journals added greatly to establishing a worthwhile library. In recent years *Transactions* has become a *tropical medicine* and *parasitological* journal which is *not* merely a medium for recording the Society's proceedings.

Relations with kindred societies

An interchange of views and representation at meetings of allied societies has always been prominent in the activities of the RSTMH, and invitations to send a representative to their annual meetings took a great deal of the Secretaries' time in the early days.

The Library

In the MSL days, and particularly after acquisition and removal to Manson House, it was a policy of the Society to maintain a library of *tropical medicine* texts – which was especially useful to overseas Fellows on leave in Britain. The Society appointed for a while, an *Honorary Librarian*. However, this enterprise has now been abandoned and the library dispersed.

Other activities

Attempts to establish a Dining Club as well as Society Dinners, were made prior to World War II. However, enthusiasm for dinners was never great, and this initiative has now also been discontinued.

During and immediately after World War II, the Society became extremely concerned about the *future* of *clinical* tropical medicine in Britain. However, this interest soon declined, and has coincided with a rapid downward trend of this specialty!

Royal Connotations

This became a Royal Society in 1920 and King George V was the first royal patron (a tradition which has continued until now); HM Queen Elizabeth II is presently the Society's patron. The Prince of Wales (later King Edward VIII) officially opened Manson House in 1932.

The 50th anniversary dinner was held in 1957 at the Royal College of Surgeons, and Philip, Duke of Edinburgh, was the guest of honour (*see* Chapter 13). The next royal visitor to the RSTMH was the Princess Royal who unveiled the refurbished George Carmichael Low (who took a prominent rôle in the early days of the RSTMH) auditorium at Manson House in October 1994. Thus the Society has preserved its *royal* connections until this day.

Future of the discipline

The current emphasis is rapidly moving away from the *formal discipline* to the older pursuit of 'medicine in the tropics'. The reasons for that have been summarised elsewhere.[1]

References and notes

1   G C Cook. Future of tropical medicine. *Br med J* 1996; 312: 1160; G C Cook *et al*. Tropical medicine as a formal discipline is dead and should be buried. *Trans R Soc trop Med Hyg* 1997; 91: 372–4.

Appendices (I–III)

Appendix I

LAWS

cf the

SOCIETY OF TROPICAL MEDICINE AND HYGIENE [1907]

NAME

(1)   The Society shall be called the 'Society of Tropical Medicine and Hygiene'.

OBJECTS OF THE SOCIETY

(2)   The objects of the Society shall be to promote and advance the study of the diseases and hygiene of warm climates, to facilitate intercourse and discussion amongst those who are interested in tropical and exotic disorders, and, generally, to deal with cognate matters.

CONSTITUTION

(3)   The Society shall consist of Fellows, Honorary Fellows, and Corresponding Fellows, and its affairs shall be governed by a *Council*.

THE COUNCIL

(4)   The President, Vice-President, one or more Auditors and the first *Council* of the Society, shall be elected at a meeting of those interested in *Tropical Medicine*, of which due notice shall be given in the medical journals. The *Council* shall consist of the President, Vice-President and fifteen or more Councillors. By their election [to] the *Council* [they] shall become Fellows of the Society and they shall thereafter admit as Fellows without ballot such applicants for Fellowship as they may approve, but no such admissions may be made after a period of six months from the date of the election of the first *Council*.

The *Council* shall further appoint either from their own number or from the general body of Fellows, a Treasurer, and two or more Secretaries, who, by such appointment, shall, if not already elected, become Councillors.

(5)   The President, Vice-President and *Council* so constituted, shall continue in office until the *Annual General Meeting* to be held in June, 1909, when they shall retire and their places shall be filled in the manner hereinafter provided. They shall, however, continue their powers and functions until their successors are duly appointed and have accepted office.

(6)   Four months before the *Annual General Meeting* to be held in June, 1909, the *Council* shall prepare voting lists containing the names of Fellows recommended by them for election to the offices of President, Vice-President, and Councillor, for the next term of two years. A copy of the lists so prepared shall be exhibited in the Rooms of the Society, and published in such journals, or communicated to the Fellows in such manner, as may be determined by the *Council*.

On the lists so prepared votes may be recorded by all Fellows, who shall, when voting, mark by crosses the spaces opposite the names of the candidates for whom they wish to record their votes, and shall sign their names. All Fellows shall be eligible for the offices of President, Vice-President and Councillor, and spaces shall be left on the voting lists, and votes may be recorded for other candidates besides those recommended by the *Council*. A list, when duly signed by a Fellow and returned to the Secretaries, shall be accepted as a voting paper, and the candidates who have the greatest number of votes shall be elected. The Secretaries shall, on request being made, furnish a voting list to each Fellow, and voting lists returned by post before the date of the election and otherwise in order, shall be accepted.

(7)   Representatives of the Biological Sciences, and of the following Services and Institutions shall, so far as is possible, be included in the first *Council*: The Naval Medical Service, The Royal Army Medical Corps, The Indian Medical Service, The Colonial Medical Service, The London School of Tropical Medicine, The Liverpool School of Tropical Medicine, Cambridge University, Edinburgh University, London University.

(8)   Subsequent elections to the offices of President, Vice-President

and Councillor shall be made in like manner, and shall take place at alternate Annual Meetings of the Society. Retiring Councillors shall be eligible for re-election. The *Council* shall have power to fill vacancies occurring in their number during their term of office. They shall direct and regulate the general affairs of the Society, and shall have power to make Bye-laws for the conduct of business at meetings of the Society, for the maintenance and administration of the Society's rooms, library and property, and for the organisation and direction of publications. Five members of *Council* shall form a quorum.

FELLOWS

(9)   All registered medical practitioners and others interested in scientific pursuits relating to *tropical medicine* whose qualifications are satisfactory to the *Council* shall be eligible for election as Fellows in the following manner:-

Save in the case of Fellows elected by the first *Council* as provided by Law 4, the names of Candidates for election as Fellows of the Society shall be submitted to the *Council* on a form provided for the purpose, which must be signed by two Fellows who have personal knowledge of the nominee. This form shall contain a declaration signed by the candidate that he is willing, if elected, to observe and obey the Laws and Regulations of the Society and to endeavour to promote its honour and interests.

If approved by a majority of the *Council* the proposal shall be read by one of the Secretaries at an *Ordinary* meeting of the Society and a ballot shall be taken when directed by the *Council* at a subsequent meeting. No election shall take place unless ten Fellows vote, and no Candidate shall be elected who does not obtain four-fifths of the votes recorded.

HONORARY AND CORRESPONDING FELLOWS

(10)   Distinguished members of the medical profession and persons of eminence in other departments of science connected with medicine shall be eligible for election by the *Council* as Honorary Fellows.

(11)   Members of the medical profession residing abroad, and others engaged in scientific pursuits bearing on *tropical medicine*, shall be eligible for election by the *Council* as Corresponding Fellows.

(12)   Honorary and Corresponding Fellows shall have the right to attend meetings, to read papers, and to participate in the scientific work of the Society. They shall not, however, be qualified to hold office, or to vote, nor shall they be entitled of right to receive the publications of the Society.

ELECTION OF TREASURER AND SECRETARIES

(13)   The Treasurer and Secretaries of the Society shall continue to act until each new *Council* has been elected and has accepted office. They shall thereupon vacate their offices, and the *Council* shall appoint a Treasurer and Secretaries for the ensuing term of two years. They shall in all cases be eligible for re-election.

THE PRESIDENT

(14)   The President shall not hold office for a period of more than two years, and shall not be eligible for re-election until at least two years have elapsed since his last term of office. He shall preside at all meetings, regulate the proceedings of the Society and *Council*, interpret the application of Laws, decide doubtful points, put resolutions and motions, and shall, besides his ordinary vote, have a casting vote in case of an equality in numbers. He shall sign the minutes, admit Fellows, and present the thanks of the Society to contributors and donors.

In the absence of the President the chair shall be taken by the Vice-President, by an Honorary Vice-President, or by a Member of the *Council*, and upon such Chairman the powers of the President shall for the time being devolve.

THE VICE-PRESIDENT

(15)   The Vice-President shall not hold office for a period of more than two years, and shall not be eligible for re-election as Vice-President until at least two years have elapsed since his last term of office.

HONORARY VICE-PRESIDENTS

(16)   The Honorary Vice-Presidents shall be elected by the *Council* from among the Fellows, Honorary Fellows and Corresponding Fellows of the Society. Past Presidents of the Society may be Honorary Vice-Presidents.

THE TREASURER

(17)   The Treasurer shall receive all moneys and pay them into a bank appointed by the *Council*, to the credit of a separate account kept in the name of the Society. All payments ordered by the *Council* shall be made by cheque signed by him and by one of the Secretaries. The Treasurer shall keep an account of all receipts and payments and shall report the same to the *Council* at each regular meeting; he shall keep a numbered counterfoil receipt book and shall sign all receipts; and he shall present at a *Council* meeting not later than April 30 of each year a report of the financial position of the Society and a statement of the income and expenditure during the previous year ended March 31. This report and statement when passed by the Auditors shall with their report be submitted to the Society for the approval of the Fellows at the *Annual General Meeting*. The Treasurer shall report to the *Council* the name of any Fellow whose subscription is nine months in arrears.

THE AUDITORS

(18)   One or more Auditors shall be appointed by the votes of the Fellows at each *Annual General Meeting*. They shall audit the accounts of the Society and shall present a report to the *Council* before each *Annual General Meeting*.

THE SECRETARIES

(19)   The Secretaries shall conduct all correspondence except in so far as the Council shall otherwise direct. They shall attend all meetings of the Society and *Council* and shall be *ex-officio* members of all Committees. When the chair has been taken one of them shall read the Minutes of the preceding meeting, shall take Minutes of the business, shall mention any gifts received since the date of the last meeting, and shall give notice of candidates proposed for election. The Secretaries shall have charge of and keep a Register of all papers communicated.

TRUSTEES

(20)   The *Council* shall appoint three Fellows to act as Trustees of the property of the Society, and may on any vacancy occurring by resignation or otherwise appoint other Fellows to fill their places. A Trustee on ceasing to be a Fellow of the Society or on becoming a

bankrupt, or compounding with his creditors, or on discontinuing to reside within the British Isles, shall thereby vacate his Trusteeship. The *Council* shall decide on the mode of investing the funds of the Society, and all investments, agreements, leases, policies of insurance, and other instruments sanctioned by the *Council*, shall be made in the names of the Trustees on behalf of the Society. No Trustee shall be held personally responsible for loss or damage to the property of the Society, or for depreciation of investments, provided that such loss or damage does not arise through his negligence or default in the office of Trustee.

INCOME

(21)   The Income of the Society shall be derived from the Composition or Annual Subscriptions of Fellows, from such donations or bequests as may be received from time to time, and from interest, rent and other such sources as may be authorised by the *Council*.

It shall be the duty of the *Council* to carry out as far as possible the wishes and desires of donors as to the objects to which bequest and donations are to be applied.

EXPENDITURE

(22)   The *Council* shall out of the funds of the Society defray all ordinary expenses, and shall pay rents, salaries, wages, and such other charges as may be necessary for the purchase of furniture, apparatus and diagrams, for the safe and efficient maintenance of the premises and property, and for carrying on the general work of the Society. They shall further provide for the issue of *Transactions* and such other publications as may be authorised, and shall be empowered to expend money on expeditions for scientific investigation, on prizes, and on such other purposes as they consider advisable. No extraordinary or annually recurrent expenditure besides that herein authorised shall, however, be undertaken by them without the sanction of the Fellows obtained by a resolution submitted at an *Ordinary* meeting of the Society.

(23)   Except so far as may have been authorised by Law 22, no dividend, division, bonus, or gift, shall be made out of the funds of the Society unto or between any of the Fellows.

SUBSCRIPTIONS

(24) Fellows shall pay an annual subscription of One Guinea which shall become due in advance in April of each year.

(25) Fellows elected during the course of the financial year shall upon admission pay one year's subscription, but shall not be liable for a second subscription at the beginning of the next financial year if their election has taken place after December 31.

(26) The name of a newly elected Fellow shall not be placed on the register of Fellows, nor shall he be entitled to any of the privileges of Fellowship, until after his first annual subscription or composition fee shall have been paid, and if such payment be not made within six months from the date of the ballot for his admission his election shall be null and void.

(27) If the annual subscription or other moneys owing to the Society by a Fellow be not paid within three months after the due date he shall be notified in writing that he is in arrears, and if within four months from the despatch of such notification payment shall not have been made, a further notice shall be sent to him to the effect that unless the sums due are paid forthwith his name may be removed from the register of Fellows. If thereupon such sums remain unpaid until March 31 following, he shall be considered to have withdrawn from the Society, and his name shall be removed from the register of Fellows, unless a reason satisfactory to the *Council* be given by him.

(28) Corresponding Fellows shall upon election pay an entrance fee of Two Guineas, but no further subscription shall be payable by them.

(29) Honorary Fellows shall pay no entrance fee or subscription.

COMPOSITION FEES

(30) A Fellow may at any time pay a composition fee of Fifteen Guineas and be thereby exempted from paying any further subscription, although enjoying all the rights and privileges, and being subject to the same penalties as if he were paying an annual subscription. In the event of a Fellow who has paid a composition fee withdrawing or being removed from the Society he shall not be entitled to the return of any portion of such composition fee.

PRIVILEGES OF FELLOWSHIP

(31)   Fellows of the Society shall have the right to attend all meetings, lectures, discussions and demonstrations sanctioned by the *Council* for their attendance, to introduce visitors, to vote on all resolutions, and to ballot for the election of Councillors and Fellows.

(32)   Fellows shall be entitled to receive a copy of the Society's *Transactions* of each year for which their subscriptions have been paid, and such other publications issued by the Society during that year as shall have been ordered by the *Council* to be supplied to Fellows free of charge. Subject to any Bye-law that may be made by the *Council* they shall be entitled to the use of the library, laboratories and such other premises as shall be set apart for the use of Fellows.

WITHDRAWAL, READMISSION AND REMOVAL OF FELLOWS

(33)   A Fellow may at any time withdraw from the Society on giving one month's notice in writing of his intention to do so, and on paying all moneys due by him to the Society.

(34)   Fellows who have resigned under Rule 33 may, on application being made for that purpose, be readmitted upon such terms as the *Council* may think proper.

(35)   If the conduct of any Fellow shall be deemed by the *Council* discreditable or prejudicial to the interests of the Society, he may be requested by them to withdraw from the Society. In the event of his refusing to do so, his name may be removed from the register of Fellows at a General Meeting, provided that in the notice calling the meeting intimation of the proposed resolution to remove his name shall have been given, and that not less than three-fourths of the Fellows present and voting at such meeting record their votes for his removal. A Fellow thus removed shall forfeit all privileges of Fellowship and claims upon the Society from the date of his removal.

MEETINGS

Annual General Meeting

(36)   An *Annual General Meeting* of the Society shall be held on the third Wednesday in June of each year at 8.30pm. Ten Fellows shall constitute

a quorum, and the business shall as far as possible be conducted in the following order:-

(a) The President, or in his absence a Vice-President, shall take the chair.

(b) A Report by the *Council* on the work of the Society shall be presented.

(c) The Treasurer's Report and Balance Sheet as passed by the Auditors shall be presented, and the accounts submitted for approval.

(d) Auditors for the ensuing year shall be elected.

(e) Resolutions for the alteration of Laws or for other purposes, of which due notice has been given, shall be submitted to the meeting.

(f) Any other business approved by the *Council* not included in the foregoing shall be considered.

ORDINARY MEETINGS

(37) The *Ordinary* meetings of the Society shall be held on the second Wednesday in every month excepting August and September, at 8.30pm or on such other day and at such hour as the *Council* may direct.

(38) Fellows attending meetings shall enter their names in the Attendance Book, and when visitors are introduced, the names of such visitors, with the names of the Fellows introducing them, shall also be entered in the Attendance Book.

(39) The business of *Ordinary* meetings shall as far as possible be conducted in the following order:-

(a) The President, Vice-President, or one of the Honorary Vice-Presidents, or in their unavoidable absence a member of *Council*, shall take the chair.

(b) The Chairman shall order the minutes of the preceding meeting to be read, and thereafter submit them for confirmation as an accurate record of the proceedings. On their being confirmed he shall sign them as correct. He may announce gifts or donations, or make other special communications.

(c)   On days set apart for election of Fellows, the Chairman shall appoint two Scrutineers to take the ballots, and after such ballots have been taken shall announce the result to the meeting.

(d)   The names of Candidates for election as Fellows, with those of their proposers and seconders, shall be read by one of the Secretaries, who shall at the same time announce the date of the ballot for such Candidates.

(e)   The titles of communications to be discussed at the next meeting shall be announced.

(f)   Notice of resolutions or motions to be proposed or moved at a subsequent meeting shall be given.

(g)   Communications and papers approved by the *Council* shall be read.

(h)   The Chairman may introduce any distinguished visitors present and invite them to take part in the subsequent discussion.

(i)   Meetings shall stand adjourned at 10 o'clock, unless a special resolution to extend the time for discussion be carried.

(j)   Notwithstanding anything to the contrary contained in the preceding rules, the Chairman may in his discretion alter or vary the procedure, or postpone any discussion, or allow any Fellow to propose a motion or resolution, not affecting the constitution or finances of the Society, or incompatible with the privileges of Fellows, or the interests of the Society, without notice. On all points of procedure the ruling of the Chairman shall be final.

SPECIAL MEETINGS

(40)   The President or *Council* may at any time call a *Special General Meeting* of the Society; and when requested so to do by a requisition

signed by twelve Fellows, which must specify in the form of one or more resolutions the object for which a meeting is desired, the President shall call a *Special General Meeting*.

(41)   Notice of *Special General Meetings* shall be sent not less than one week previous to the date fixed for the meeting to all Fellows known to be permanently or temporarily resident in the British Isles. The notice shall contain a copy of the resolutions to be submitted, and no business shall be transacted at *Special General Meetings* except the consideration of such resolutions.

ALTERATION AND REPEAL OF LAWS

(42)   Whenever it may seem expedient to the *Council* that new Laws be enacted, or existing laws repealed or altered, such enactment or alteration shall be made at an Annual or *Special General Meeting*. Notice of proposals to enact, repeal, or amend the Laws shall be posted in the Rooms of the Society not less than two months before the date of the meeting, or otherwise communicated to the Fellows as directed by the *Council*. The alterations which it is proposed to make shall in all cases be specified in such notice.

(43)   Any twelve Fellows may submit to the *Council* recommendations for the enactment of new Laws or the repeal or alteration of existing Laws, and such recommendations, with any modification or amendment proposed by the *Council*, shall be submitted to an Annual General, or *Special General Meeting* of the Fellows, in the same manner as if the enactments or alterations had been proposed by the *Council*, as provided by Rule 42.

Appendix II

Presidents during the first fifty years of the (R)STMH

1	1907–09	Sir Patrick Manson GCMG MD LLD FRCP FRS (1844–1922)
2	1909–11	Sir Ronald Ross KCB KCMG MD FRCS FRS, Lt-Col, IMS (1857–1932)
3	1911–13	Sir William Leishman KCB KCMG FRCP FRS, Lt-Gen, AMS (1865–1926)
4	1913–15	Sir Havelock Charles Bt GCVO KCLI FRCSI MD, Major-Gen, IMS (1858–1934)
5	1915–17*	Fleming M Sandwith CMG MD FRCP (1853–1918)
6	1917–19*	Sir David Bruce KCB DSc LLD FRCP FRS, Major-Gen, AMS (1855–1931)
7	1919–21	Sir William Simpson CMG MD FRCP (1855–1931)
8	1921–23	Sir James Cantlie KBE LLD FRCS (1851–1926)
9	1923–25	Sir Percy Bassett-Smith KCB CMG FRCP FRCS, Surgeon Rear-Admiral, RN (1861–1927)
10	1925–27	(Sir) Andrew Balfour KCMG CB MD LLD FRCP (1873–1931)
11	1927–29	Professor John W W Stephens MD FRS (1865–1946)
12	1929–33	G Carmichael Low MA MD FRCP (1872–1952)
13	1933–35	Sir Leonard Rogers KCSI CIE MD FRCS FRS, Major-Gen, IMS (1868–1962)
14	1935–37	Sir Arthur Bagshawe CMG MB BCh DPH (1871–1950)

15	1937–39	Sydney Price James CMG MD FRS, Lt-Col, IMS (1870–1946)
16	1939–43*	Sir S Rickard Christophers CIE OBE FRS, Col, IMS (1873–1978)
17	1943–45*	Sir Harold Scott KCMG MD FRCP FRSE (1874–1956)
18	1945–47	C Morley Wenyon CMG CBE MB BS BSc FRS (1878–1948)
19	1947–49	Sir Philip Manson-Bahr CMG DSO MD FRCP (1881–1966)
20	1949–51	H E Shortt CIE MD DSc FRS, Col, IMS (1887–1987)
21	1951–53	Sir Neil Hamilton Fairley KBE MD DSc FRCP FRS (1891–1966)
22	1953–55	F Norman White CIE MD DPH, Major, IMS (1877–1964)
23	1955–57	Professor Rupert M Gordon OBE MD DSc FRCP DPH DTM (1893–1961)
[24	1957–59	Sir John Boyd OBE, MD, LLD, DPH, DTM&H, FRCP, FRS, RAMC (1891–1981)]

* Presidencies affected by the two world wars (1914–18 and 1939–45).

Appendix III

(R)STMH Minute Books (1907–1957) – *Council* and *Ordinary meetings*

Book No.	Date	
	From	**To**
1	4 January 1907	4 November 1920
2	19 November 1920	17 December 1925
3	21 January 1926	21 November 1929
4	13 December 1929	18 May 1933
5	15 June 1933	1 July 1937
6	21 October 1937	19 October 1944
7	19 October 1944	19 May 1949
8	19 June 1949	19 June 1952
9	17 July 1952	15 June 1955
10	21 July 1955	19 June 1958

Index